EXPOSING SPIRITUALISTIC
PRACTICES IN HEALING

EXPOSING
SPIRITUALISTIC
PRACTICES IN HEALING

Edwin Noyes M.D., MPH

Unless otherwise noted, all Bible texts are from the King James Version.

Published by Forest Grove Publishing, Forest Grove, OR and Omnibook Co.

First Edition, third printing

For e-book purchase: Kindle on Amazon, Barnes and Noble
Book purchase:, Amazon.com, Barnes and Noble
Author contact: Edwina.noyes@gmail.com,
Phone: 503-357-6571

Cover and Graphic Design by Omnibook Co. Graphics & Arts

Illustration Art by Sharon Zeismer& Jerry Sticka

Editing: Pamela Bolton, MSc, RT (R) (CT) (M)

Photos of Battle Creek Sanitarium and Western Health Reform Institute, courtesy of Willard Library.

Diagram of Occultism and One World Government used by permission of Gary Kah

Appendix E "Biblical Research Committee Report on New Age and Seventh-Day Adventists" used with permission

Article in Appendix I "Colon Cleansing" Part II *How to Detoxify Your Lymphatics, What is Detoxification* by Ray Foster M.D. , used with permission Appendix L "Counterfeit Medicine" by Walter Thompson M.D. , used by permission

DISCLAIMER

This book details the author's personal experiences with and opinions about spiritualistic influence involved in use of many alternative and mystical healing therapies. The author is not a healthcare provider.

The author and publisher are providing this book and its contents on an "as is" basis and make no representations or warranties of any kind with respect to this book or its contents. The author and publisher disclaim all such representations and warranties, including for example warranties of merchantability and healthcare for a particular purpose. In addition, the author and publisher do not represent or warrant that the information accessible via this book is accurate, complete or current.

The statements made about products and services have not been evaluated by the U.S. Food and Drug Administration. They are not intended to diagnose, treat, cure, or prevent any condition or disease. Please consult with your own physician or healthcare specialist regarding the suggestions and recommendations made in this book.

Except as specifically stated in this book, neither the author or publisher, nor any authors, contributors, or other representatives will be liable for damages arising out of or in connection with the use of this book. This is a comprehensive limitation of liability that applies to all damages of any kind, including (without limitation) compensatory; direct, indirect or consequential damages; loss of data, income or profit; loss of or damage to property and claims of third parties.

You understand that this book is not intended as a substitute for consultation with a licensed healthcare practitioner, such as your physician. Before you begin any healthcare program, or change your lifestyle in any way, you will consult your physician or other licensed healthcare practitioner to ensure that you are in good health and that the examples contained in this book will not harm you.

This book provides content related to topics physical and/or mental health issues. As such, use of this book implies your acceptance of this disclaimer.

TABLE OF CONTENTS

INTRODUCTION

In 1980 a book *The Aquarian Conspiracy*, made its debut upon the American scene. It quickly became a hit, especially with a special group of people with similar beliefs and worldview, yet they were little known to each other. Author, Marilyn Ferguson, was the publisher of a bi-monthly journal—*Brain/Mind Bulletin* (circulation 10,000) which encompassed research, theory, innovation relating to learning, health, psychiatry, psychology, states of consciousness, dreams, meditation, and similar related subjects. Her position as editor and publisher brought her into contact with voluminous information that had not previously been collected and brought together to be shared with those interested.

She had contact with people from many various professions and vocations. As she received, filtered, analyzed, and published information in her bi-monthly bulletin a mental picture began to slowly form in her mind as she observed a change, a transformation taking place in the core belief system of many people. This change was occurring in individuals and in society at large. It was slow at first, starting in the 60's but picked up momentum in an accelerating manner with each decade. The movement was without hierarchal leadership, organization, or funding. It seemed to be arising everywhere spontaneously by small net-working individuals and groups. This change was seen in medicine, education, social sciences, hard science, and even the government.

This change appeared to follow the aftermath of the social activism of the 1960's and 1970's, and was moving toward a "historical synthesis," i.e., a social transformation coming from a personal transformation—a "heart change," then forming into a worldwide society change. With the publishing of *The Aquarian Conspiracy* the massed information Marilyn had collected, now organized and placed out into the open for all to see, stimulated with even greater speed widespread acceptance and promulgation of these changes of worldview and transformation.

I am sure the reader by this time is asking "What is changing in individuals and society as a whole?" Answer: a change in a person's *core belief system— one's worldview*! Such as Where did we come from? What are we doing here? What is the future? A change from a Western worldview formed mostly from Judeo-Christian concepts of our origin, purpose, and destiny, toward an Eastern pantheistic perspective of "divinity within"— "the godhood of man."

Ferguson proceeded to bring out into the open the methods by which transformation within an individual is initiated, then more fully developed. *Health and healing* is a dominant avenue, and a vast array of techniques has been developed to "heal body and mind." The Christian believes that choosing to follow the Eastern pantheistic pathway separates him from his Savior, Jesus Christ the Divine Son of God. Pantheistic healing techniques are presented with an exceedingly deceptive philosophy and explanation as to how they are believed to effect healing. To accept Satan's counterfeit healing modalities gives him homage and worship.

The purpose of this book is to present information which facilitates making an intelligent choice as to whether or not the reader would choose to participate in a particular healing therapy. Many different methods of healing are promoted as being of true value, but are founded on pagan doctrines originating from a counterfeit story of creation. This book further explains why these different therapies that carry occult or pagan principles in the explanation as to their power to heal, cannot be separated from their attachment to such religions.

On the back side of the cover of this book, *Exposing Spiritualistic Practices in Healing* are listed some popular quasi-healing methodologies that have come into our culture in the past 35-40 years. Most of them are of ancient origin and are only new to us. The concern I present in this text has more to do with the spiritual danger imposed from accepting and using those techniques than from a strictly medical concern. In short, it is my contention that accepting the concepts promoted in the explanation for the *power* behind their healing capabilities might well separate us from eternal life.

Since publishing the book *Spiritualistic Deceptions in Health and Healing* in August 2007, I have encountered individuals who have asked me why I had not written on certain other practices in health and healing that they considered affiliated with spiritualism. I also recognized from personal contacts with people who read the book, and from contacts in seminars I conducted on the subject of spiritualism in healing, that certain topics mentioned in the book needed more information and explanation.

It has been more than 14 years since I started writing *Spiritualistic Deceptions in Health and Healing,* and nine years since its publication. These years have given me time to contemplate these requests, and the effect of the book in bringing an understanding of spiritualism's encroachment into the healing arts. During this time, use of alternative and complementary medicine has rapidly increased and been accepted, as if it were part and parcel of general medicine. Less and less do people have concern as to whether there may be any reason that one should question the value or spiritual safety in accepting and using a particular healing method, that at one time was considered suspect.

This book *Exposing Spiritualistic Practices in Healing*, includes all the information found in *Spiritualistic Deceptions in Health and Healing,* and much additional information has been added to several chapters. This book has eleven new chapters, eight additional appendixes, which include a copy of the 1987 report of the Biblical Research Institute of the General Conference of Seventh-day Adventists on the New Age Movement and Seventh-day Adventists, also doubling of the glossary and index.

Additional information is given on the subjects of meditation, yoga, yoga exercises, cleansing therapy, acupuncture, Reiki, craniosacral therapy, mystical herbology, essential oils, aromatherapy, visualization, crystal and gem healing, psychology, relaxation response, mindfulness meditation, Satan's ground, a counterfeit definition, questions pertaining to *particular steps* of 12 step recovery programs, and an introduction to a well-known author in health and healing subjects.

Many different methods of healing are being promoted as of true value, but are founded in pagan doctrines originating from a counterfeit story of creation. This book further explains why these different therapies that carry occult or pagan principles in the explanations of their power to heal, cannot be separated from their attachment to those religions, and one's use of, and could present spiritual danger.

Edwin A. Noyes M.D. MPH

PREFACE

In the mid 1970's, I began to notice new subjects and terms appearing in brochures announcing medical educational seminars, such as energy medicine, paranormal, holistic medicine, electromagnetic medicine, and strange and unconventional methods of treatment. I well remember the confusion I experienced on reading these brochures. It did not seem appropriate for me to participate in those seminars, yet I was very curious. I heard different opinions from physicians as to whether these new methods were just fads, or possibly based in spiritism. No one that I met really understood, but there were many opinions.

Thus, I began a long study in order to understand the origin, history, and science that might explain these methods of healing. For a period of more than twenty years, my curiosity and study about complementary and alternative medical treatment disciplines continued. Early in the pursuit of understanding these subjects I chose not to include these questionable methods in my medical care.

I found books written by Christian authors exposing these treatment disciplines as spiritistic, and I developed a much greater understanding of the world views of those using and promoting these approaches to medical care. I realized that the use of these healing methods was simply an extension of the *world view and theology* of the practitioners of alternative and complementary, or "energy medicine," as it was commonly called.

Around 1993 or 1994, I decided to stop all of my research and study concerning these methods of healing, as I was satisfied in my own mind as to their origin and the power involved. I felt no burden to go public with my conclusions and continued my medical practice as usual. However, near that time I wrote several short essays about these therapies for a church letter that was circulated to the members of the Forest Grove, Oregon, Seventh-day Adventist church.

In April of 1998, I received a telephone call from Walter Thompson M.D. , Chairman of the Board of 3-ABN television, inviting me to the 3-ABN studios in Frankfurt, Illinois, to participate in a panel discussion of complementary and alternative medical therapies. The discussion by the panel was to be aired over the 3-ABN television network. I was not acquainted with Dr. Thompson and was puzzled as to how he was aware that I had any knowledge of this subject.

The invitation was accepted. I later learned that Dr. Thompson's invitation resulted from the articles I had previously written for the church letter.

The panel for the 3-ABN television program consisted of Walter Thompson M.D. , Dr. Manuel Vasquez, Vice Pres. of North American Division of Seventh-day Adventists, and me. Dr.Vasquez received his doctoral degree from Andrews University. His doctrinal thesis was written on the New Age Movement and its theosophy. The panel had a three-hour discussion of the subject of alternative therapies, which was subsequently aired on television. Later that year, I was invited by Nadia Ivanova, Director of Health Education for the Euro-Asian Division of Seventh-day Adventists (Old Soviet Union), to visit Russia and conduct a seminar on "Mystical Medicine" for the health educators of the Uro-Asian Division. I invited Dr. Thompson and Dr. Vasquez to join me in this seminar in the summer of 1999. 3-ABN Television Network of Russia aired this panel's seminar on their nation-wide TV program.

For the next six years, I returned to Russia and Ukraine conducting seminars for health educators within the church. Dr. Vasquez joined me in September 2003, in Kiev, Ukraine, for a three-day seminar conducted for the Ukraine Adventist Medical Association. In October of 2003, Dr. Vasquez came to Forest Grove, Oregon, my home town, to conduct a seminar for the Spanish Church, in which I participated. At that time, he asked me to co-author a book on the subject of spiritualism in medicine, or "mystical medicine." I agreed to join him in the endeavor. Dr. Vasquez had previously authored two books on the New Age Movement, and had included limited information on alternative medicine. I did not hear from him again. Sadly, I learned later that shortly after the seminar in Oregon, he became severely ill due to metastatic cancer, and after a difficult illness, died in January 2005.

As more requests came to me to return to Russia and Ukraine for additional seminars, I began to tire a bit of the travel and looked for another way to share the message of deception of spiritualism in medical care. The Health Director of the Western Russian Union, Andrew Prokopyev, joined with me in preparing a Russian CD and narrative DVDs, presenting this seminar on mystical medicine, which are now available in that country.

The response I received from the seminars on m*ystical medicine* in Russia and Ukraine were a lecturer's dream. Such attention I had never before received in thirty years of health education teaching. These seminars were attended by lay people and medical professionals. If a participant in the seminar was present throughout and heard the presentation from beginning to end, I received no argument concerning the information presented. During the days of communism in Russia, not only the Bible and certain spiritual writings were secretly typed and copies distributed among believers, but so too might copies be made of instructions of certain alternative medical therapies.

Gwen Shorter, of Homeward Publishing of Yorba Linda, CA reviewed the English text of the seminar of mystical medicine and suggested it be made into a book. I consented. I did not get to discuss with Dr. Vasquez his ideas for a new book that we had planned to produce together, but I do know that he appreciated the material I had prepared revealing the basic origin and history of New Age healing practices. It was this material that I placed in the book, *Spiritualistic Deceptions in Health and Healing*, published in 2007. We now come to this book, *Exposing spiritualistic practices in Healing,* which includes the content of the first book and much additional information. The reason for writing it is that over the past four years since *Spiritualistic Deceptions in Health and Healing* was published I had encountered many questions pertaining to the subject of spiritism in various healing techniques that were not fully answered in the first book. Several people urged me to write again, exposing additional subjects not covered in *Spiritualistic Deceptions in Health sand Healing.*

I have observed a steady growth of acceptance of many previously questionable techniques in healing since publishing the first book. Less and less practicing Christians question the use of these methods. And the acceptance of these techniques into the orthodox practice of medicine has been astounding. Therapies that once were found only in naturopathy or chiropractic practices can now be found in mainstream medicine. I was asked by serval people to investigate psychology for any sentiments of spiritism, and also to examine closely the 12-step recovery programs for the same. This I have done and my finding are presented.

These writings express what I learned from studies pursued over many years. I share them with you so you may have information to aid you in your decision as to what techniques or method you would or would not choose to utilize. My expressions and conclusions may vary with what you understand at this time. I had to change several personal beliefs as I became more informed. I caution you to be slow in rejecting what you learn from this book. Do not harden your opinions if you come across a subject whose exposure you disagree with. Take some time, and do an in depth investigation yourself, so your decision is from an informed position.

In the twenty or more years that I have discussed spiritualistic deceptions in the healing arts, I receive primarily one objection to what I present or have written. It has always been a response of "well, it works." We have been warned that spurious healings by Satan would take place in front of our eyes, yet when it happens we tend to forget the warning, and make our judgment of its value only by whether a person improves or not. That is not a safe way to evaluate. By utilizing the information contained in this book you will be able to make an intelligent judgment in these matters

Edwin A. Noyes M.D., MPH

Addendum:

In the following chapters there more than 800 footnotes containing references, some are Internet web site addresses. Web sites may be altered or may add information and page change resulting in difficulty or inability of opening to the web site and quote. At times web sites are removed from the Internet and are no longer available. If the reader is unable to access a reference, feel free to contact the author. Edwina.noyes@gmail.com

CHAPTER 1
WINDS OF CHANGE

April 6, 1971, *"The Ping Heard Round the World"* occurred. The American ping pong team, while competing in the World Table Tennis Championship held in Japan, received a surprise invitation from The Republic of China for an all-expense paid visit to their country. When the team stepped across a bridge from Hong Kong to China on April 10, the era of "Ping Pong diplomacy" was initiated.

On April 14, Premier Chou En-lai, at a banquet in the Great Hall, invited American journalists to visit China, closed to foreign visitors since 1949. Ping Pong diplomacy signaled change. July 15 of the same year, the American government announced that President Nixon would be going to China for an official State visit the following year. The winds of change were blowing.

Reporters from America did visit China and their stories were read with great interest. Stories of a different kind of anesthetic for surgery caught the attention of Americans more than most other aspects of the China trip. The stories of a man undergoing an appendectomy, and of another person chest surgery while awake, seemed like science fiction. It was the first time most Americans had heard the word *acupuncture*. Glowing stories of what it could do initiated a great desire for further investigation. How surprising it was to hear that it had been around for millennia, and yet the "art" was not generally known in America.

Other changes had been occurring in America for several years. Students on college campuses appearances were different. Instead of nicely dressed young people, the trend was to wear "Farmer Brown" overalls. Cultural values changed. Music interests changed from melodious to the "beat." The Beatles from England descended on the scene and were followed by many copycat groups. Drug use increased. Smoking marijuana became popular, as did Eastern religions. The Beatles made popular Transcendental Meditation in place of psychedelic drugs, because they could obtain a "high" in this manner. The famous Woodstock festival of 1969 was an open expression of changing cultural values and practices. Across the country we saw missionaries of the Eastern religions such as Hare Krishna, and followers of gurus such as Hindu Rajneesh Bhagwan Shree, Maharishi Mahesh Yogi, and Paramahansa Yogananda.

Early in this changing cultural norm of society, transcendental meditation followers quickly became widespread, followed by yoga, and natural childbirth classes. We soon began to hear of many other methods of health and healing, such as aromatherapy, essential oils, applied kinesiology, iridology, and magnet therapy, etc.

Another societal change was the declining number of people believing in a six-day creation of the world. Evolution, as the answer for origins, had been around for a long time, but it was not universal among average Americans. The answer that the pagan gave for his origin began to be a contender in answering the question, "Where did we come from?" Pagan theology also crept in through a movement that suddenly appeared in the mid 1970's—the New Age Movement. Its theology was that of theosophy teachings derived from Vedanta Hinduism, Buddhism, and Western occultism, including belief in re-incarnation.

Beginning in the mid to late 1970's, new medical therapies started to emerge along with the New Age Movement. Advertisements of seminars and conferences promoting and teaching such methods as yoga, transcendental meditation, acupuncture, therapeutic touch, and many other treatment modalities were sent to doctors' offices. These methods of treatment became very popular with non-professionals, and teaching seminars were conducted for the public. Many people with no real training in medical science obtained certificates of expertise, and became practitioners in these various treatment methods. As time progressed, there was an ever increasing awareness of these alternative methods. Also, there was rapid growth in the variety of healing disciplines offered to the public, often by chiropractors, naturopaths, and sometimes nurses and non-medically trained people.

In the 1980's, medical doctors became aware of a variety of different treatment methods that were becoming increasingly popular, and patients told their doctors of trying these methods. Medical offices received invitations announcing seminars and teaching sessions for the various new non-traditional medical treatments. One such invitation came to my office from a Catholic Hospital in Tucson, Arizona, announcing a three-day seminar where the instructors for the meetings were *traditional medicine men* (shamans) from the Navajo Indian Reservation as well as other reservations. I still have that invitation.

Few doctors accepted these methods at first. Newer graduates were more likely to accept them because of the world view many of them held as to man's origin. The methods were, to a great extent, the result of the New Age Movement and the theosophy (pagan theology) taught.

The winds of change continue to blow and now we see a much greater interest in the new (yet ancient) practice methods of these types of medical treatments. They can now be found to some degree in many hospitals, even in prominent medical schools that have adopted and are experimenting with various healing disciplines. Medical clinics are forming across the nation integrating the conventional with the non-conventional style of medical treatment.

Many insurance companies now include alternative health coverage in their policies. The coverage often covers acupuncture, chiropractors, massage and somatic therapies, etc. Some work places promote and finance attendance at fitness centers, athletic clubs, health spas and other wellness centers that are featuring meditation, yoga, yoga exercises, tai chi, and martial arts of various types.

I read in books written by Christian authors exposing these new medical therapies as being spiritistic. As I developed a much greater understanding of the world views of those using and promoting these methods of medical care I realized that belief in, and use of these healing methods was a result of their *world view—pagan theology—nature worship*.

Satan attempts to thwart any blessing God gives to man. Early in the history of the world, he designed a system of health and healing to counterfeit God's methods. That same counterfeit system exists today just as it has through ages past.

"There is a way that seems right unto a man, but the end there of are the ways of death." (Proverbs 14: 12)

The purpose of this book is to unveil the counterfeit system of health and healing.

"Lest Satan should get an advantage of us: For we are not ignorant of his devices." (11Corinthians: 2:11).

The spiritualistic invasion of present-day medical care must be recognized for what it is—not a marvelous new approach to health and healing but ancient methods repainted in silver and gold.

A *"world view"* refers to our understanding and belief as to our origin, purpose, and future, as well as to the power that gave us life. In the Christian's world view, man was created and sustained by a Creator God who is a personal Being. Life, health and happiness come from being in harmony with His laws of the physical world as well as the spiritual realm. Man disobeyed God's law and lost the gift of eternal life in paradise. Man can regain eternal life in paradise by believing in and following after the Divine Son of God, Jesus Christ.

Modern evolutionary theory was introduced approximately 160 years past. According to this world view, we are here as a result of a long, natural process of random selection and chance; and there is no future after death. The evolutionist has no answer as to how, or from where, the *spark of life* came.

What was the world view of the non-Christian regarding his origin, prior to the theory of evolution? We will look to the explanation of creation in pagan religions to find this answer. Many of the treatment methods in the pagan concept for healing are not dependent upon the physical laws recognized in science. There is a looking to a "vital force" or special "energy" supposedly permeating the universe from which all substance is said to have originated. Life is believed to repeat itself in different bodies and creatures. The goal in life is to escape from this cycle of re-incarnation, and enter into the spirit life of nirvana.

How is it that ancient healing practices find their way into modern scientific medicine? Did this change come after random selection, controlled, double-blind, scientific tests conducted to evaluate these procedures before accepting them? Was there solid evidence of value as shown by statistical evaluation? No! None whatsoever!

Why then have these new methodologies been accepted? They are not explained or understood under the recognized laws of science. They have not been shown to make a difference in disorders such as tuberculosis, cancer, diabetes, heart disease, gallstones, fractures, endocrine malfunctions, or other such organic disorders. Those parts of the world that used these practices for health care for thousands of years have dismal record of health. These methods appear to have their influence mainly on disorders where there are great subjective symptoms such as pain, nausea, stress, and various musculoskeletal discomforts.

The best explanation for the questions I have asked above is that an acceptance of, and changing belief in, one's world view has allowed the acceptance of unproven and non-scientific methods. A world view is formed by answering the questions: Where did I come from? Why am I here? Where am I going? The Christian's world view is:

> Man was formed from the dust of the ground and the Creator God breathed into him the breath of life and man became a living soul. (living being NKJ, Genesis: 2:7). Man was created for God's glory, (Isaiah 43:7), and placed in paradise. Then man, by believing and trusting the serpent in the tree instead of God, lost paradise and eternal life. (Genesis: Ch. 2, 3).

> We are invited to believe in the Divine Son of God, repent, accept the merits of His shed blood, receive eternal life and live in paradise of the earth made new. (John 14:1-3).

The above outline of our creation, redemption, and restoration is to be contrasted with the story of the origin of the universe, earth, and man from the pagan and nature worshiper's world view. First, before we explore the pagan's story of creation, let us explore in the next chapter a little more of the story of man's loss of his place in paradise, and the effort of the Great Adversary to distract us from accepting the invitation from Jesus Christ to regain our lost inheritance.

CHAPTER 2
TWO GREAT SPIRITUALISTIC DECEPTIONS

The subject of the great spiritualistic deception at the beginning of earth's history in the Garden of Eden, and a great world-wide spiritualistic deception that is to occur at the end of time, is the theme of this chapter.

In the story of creation, Genesis chapter 1, we are told that God created light and He "saw that it was *good...*" He created land and seas "and God saw that it was *good.*" He created the plants on the third day "and God saw that it was *good.*" He made two lights "and God saw that it was *good.*" On the fifth day, life in the sea was created "and God saw that it was *good.*" On the sixth day He created animals "and God saw that it was *good.*" Then God created man (Adam) and woman (Eve). He looked over everything that He had made "and, behold, it was *very good.*"[1]

The word *good* was used seven times in the story of creation. What did God mean by this expression, "*good?*" Webster's Collegiate Dictionary lists one of the definitions as:

> ...to be in harmony with the moral order of the universe.[2]

God was saying that he had created planet earth and all its inhabitants, and they were in perfect harmony with His laws for the universe. All of God's creations are under His fixed laws. His created intelligent beings are also under His moral law.

> In the light from Calvary it will be seen that the law of self-renouncing love is the law of life for earth and heaven; that the love which "seeketh not her own" has its source in the heart of God; and that in the meek and lowly One is manifested the character of Him who dwelleth in the light which no man can approach unto.[3]

---

1   *King James Bible,* Genesis 1:31.
2   Merriam Webster G. & C., *Webster's New Collegiate Dictionary,* G. & C. Merriam Co. Springfield, Mass. (1977) p. 495.
3   White, E.G.; *The Desire of Ages,* Pacific Press Publishing Assn., Mountain View, CA, (1898), (Presently in Nampa, ID) p. 20.

Every part of creation is in balance and ministers to some other aspect of the creation.

> ...There is nothing, save the selfish heart of man, that lives unto himself.[4]

> Looking unto Jesus, we see that it is the glory of our God to give. "I do nothing of Myself," said Christ: "the living Father hath sent Me, and I live by the Father." "I seek not Mine own glory, but the glory of Him that sent Me."[5]

> In these words is set forth the great principle which is the law of life for the universe. All things Christ received from God, but He took to give. So in the heavenly courts, in His ministry for all created beings: through the beloved Son, the Father's life flows out to all; through the Son it returns, in praise and joyous service, a tide of love, to the great Source of all. And thus through Christ the circuit of beneficence is complete, representing the character of the great Giver, the law of life.[6]

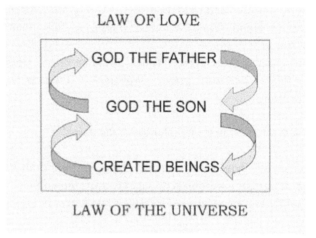

LAW OF LOVE

GOD THE FATHER

GOD THE SON

CREATED BEINGS

LAW OF THE UNIVERSE

Figure 1 Law of Love

Man is placed in a universe that is under the law of God. Government cannot exist without law.

> Immortality was promised them (Adam and Eve) on condition of obedience; by transgression they would forfeit eternal life.[7]

---

4   *Ibid.*
5   *Ibid.,* p. 21; John 8:28; 6:57; 8:50; 7:18.
6   *Ibid.*
7   White, E.G.; *Patriarchs and Prophets,* Pacific Press Pub. Assn., Nampa, ID, (1958), p. 60.

God's law was first broken in heaven by Lucifer. Envious to be *first* was the driving force behind Lucifer's rebellion. He desired that heavenly beings give him the homage due only to God and His Son. He desired to control heaven, and he accused the divine Son of God of having this desire for self-supremacy.

> With his own evil characteristics he sought to invest the loving Creator. Thus he deceived angels. Thus he deceived men. He led them to doubt the word of God, and to distrust His goodness.[8]

The circle of love (law of universe) is broken when we give Satan the honor due God, his deceptions are designed to entice us to do just that.

LAW OF LOVE

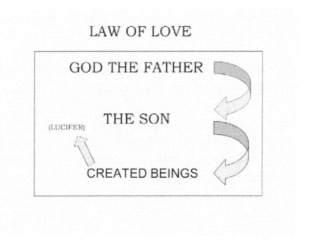

Figure 2. Law of Love broken

To deceive newly created man, Satan appeared to Eve in disguise. He chose the serpent as his *medium*. When Eve wandered from the side of Adam she felt some apprehension, but thought she had sufficient wisdom and strength to discern evil and to withstand it. When she approached the tree of *knowledge of good and evil* the serpent spoke to her. Fascinated, she stayed to listen.

She had no idea that the serpent was being used by Satan, about whom the angels had warned them. Satan, through the serpent, said that if she were to eat of the fruit of the tree, she would gain wisdom and know good and evil. She would become wise as God Himself.

> Satan, the fallen prince, was jealous of God. He determined through subtlety, cunning, and deceit to defeat God's purpose. He approached Eve, not in the

8   White, E.G.; *The Desire of Ages,* op. cit., (1898) p. 22.

form of an angel, but as a serpent, subtle, cunning, and deceitful. With a voice that appeared to proceed from the serpent, he spoke to her. . . .As Eve listened, the warnings God had given *faded from her mind*. She yielded to the temptation, and as she tempted Adam, *he also forgot God's warnings*. He believed the words of the enemy of God[9]. . . .

Eve did not design to rebel against God. However, in believing Satan's lie, she distrusted God, and so came under the penalty of the law, which is death. We, in the judgment, will be held responsible for believing the truth and using opportunities to learn what is truth.

Satan's *great lie* is that disobedience to God does not result in death, but rather will lead to a higher level of existence, and a broader field of knowledge. Had he (the serpent) not received this higher level of existence? Did he not now have the power of speech from eating the fruit?[10] He promised them that they would become wise like God.

Satan tempts men to disobedience by leading them to believe they are entering a wonderful field of knowledge. But this is all a deception.[11]

So, the first use of a *medium,* to gain man's attention and then to draw him into rejecting God's instructions, plunged the human race into sin and under the penalty of death. Satan has used the same pattern of deception since the fall of man. We are warned that the deception of the devil will be world-wide and greatly increased in power at the end of this world's history. Christ foretold this in Mark 13:22.

For false Christs and false prophets shall rise, and shall show signs and wonders, to seduce, if it were possible, even the elect.

In Matthew chapters 24 and 25 we have an enlarged recording of the conversation referenced above in Mark 13. When asked by the disciples about signs of His coming and the end of the age, He not only spoke of certain physical signs, but the real emphasis was on the great deceptions that were to come, so as to lead the saints astray. The parables appearing in these chapters are there to support the message of warning, *to not be deceived*. He said that even the *elect* might be *deceived*. The entire passage of these two chapters is making the point that deception will be almost overwhelming and could cost us eternal life, deception that would cause us to reject salvation through

9   White, E.G., *Signs of the Times,* May 29, (1901).
10   White, E.G., *Patriarchs and Prophets,* op. cit., p. 54.
11   *Ibid.,* p. 55.

Jesus Christ and follow the Prince of this world, Satan, unknowingly. Paul, too, warned of the great deception to come:

> Beware lest any man spoil you through philosophy and vain deceit, after the tradition of men, after the rudiments of the world and not after Christ. (Colosians2:8).

E.G. White, in the book *Spiritual Gifts* Vol. 4, p. 87, refers to this verse as especially referring to the great spiritual deception that is to occur at the end of time.

> Even him, whose coming is after the working of Satan with all power and signs and lying wonders." (II Thessalonians 2:9). And no marvel: for Satan himself is transformed into an angel of light. Therefore it is no great thing if his ministers also be transformed as the ministers of righteousness; whose end shall be according to their works. (II Corinthians 11:14, 15).

Paul also warned Timothy:

> Now the Spirit speaketh expressly, that in the latter times some shall depart from the faith, giving heed to seducing spirits, and doctrines of devils. (I Timothy 4:1).

John, three times in the book of Revelation, wrote about this deception to come:

> And he doeth great wonders, so that he makes fire come down from heaven on the earth in the sight of men, and deceives them that dwell on the earth by the means of those miracles which had power to do in the sight of the beast; saying to them that dwell on the earth, that they should make an image to the beast, which had the wound by a sword, and did live. (Revelation 13:13, 14).

> And I saw three unclean spirits like frogs come out of the mouth of the dragon, and out of the mouth of the beast, and out of the mouth of the false prophet. For they are the spirits of devils, working miracles, which go forth unto the kings of the earth and of the whole world, to gather them to the battle of that great day of God Almighty. (Revelation 16:13, 14).

> And the beast was taken, and with him the false prophet that wrought miracles before him, with which he deceived them that had received the mark of the beast, and them that worshipped his image. These both were cast alive into a lake of fire burning with brimstone. (Revelation 19:20).

Mrs. White adds this warning concerning events of the last days:

> The last great delusion is soon to open before us. Antichrist is to perform his marvelous works in our sight. So closely will the counterfeit resemble the true that it will be impossible to distinguish between them except by the Holy Scriptures. By their testimony every statement and every miracle must be tested.[12]

There will be a false revival. Paul, in his second letter to the Thessalonians, points to the special working of Satan in spiritualism as an event to take place immediately before the second advent of Christ. Speaking of Christ's second coming, he declares that it is

> ...after the working of Satan with all power and signs and lying wonders.[13] II Thessalonians 2:9

Present-day religions teach the imminent coming of a Messiah. Satan has done his best to have the world looking for someone other than the Son of God, a different Messiah.

In the book of Revelation, chapter 11, we learn about the rise of spiritualism and militant atheism —"the beast from the bottomless pit," in the latter part of the 19th century and its dominance in the French revolution. This power did not continue in the position as "head of government" but it did stay alive. It has been an influence in the world ever since and has been growing rapidly. In the last twenty-five years it has actually mushroomed to a place of prominence in the thinking of men. Satan has laid his trap carefully and is preparing to join with the forces of religion in our time.[14] He has been quietly at work to condition people's thinking until total control of their minds, and the rejection of God and His law is accomplished. We have seen in recent years the amalgamation of Eastern religions and their spiritualism with occultism of the West. This neo-occultism and neo-paganism has been planting its seeds of thought through the press, radio, schools, television, and in the churches.

For years the West has been seeing changes in that which is taught in schools, even to an open attack on the Creator God. In the entertainment industry, we see efforts to change the views of people by devaluating Christian concepts and elevating atheistic and paganistic ideas. This same shift is seen

---

12   White, E.G., *The Great Controversy,* Pacific Press Publishing Association, Nampa, Idaho, (1888), p. 593.

13   *King James Bible,* II Thessalonians 2:9.

14   White, op. cit., pp. 588–589.

in music, games, comic books, movies, environmental movements, and in the special focus of this book, that of *health and healing*.

"...TENS OF THOUSANDS OF ENTRY POINTS TO THIS CONSPIRACY."--Marilyn Ferguson

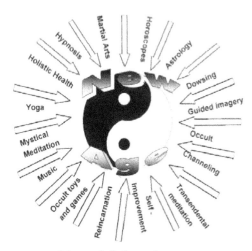

Figure 3 Points of entry.

Satan has developed his plan to deceive man until almost all external influences in our civilization are used as entry points to bring man's acceptance to his world view. In his world view, creation was not a six day event and did not involve a sovereign God. God is nature and nature is god. We are gods and we only need to learn how to bring this "god" within us to its full potential. One of the avenues that Satan uses to deceive man into paying homage to him is in the field of health and healing. He works to get the human race to accept his version of the *origin* of man, and in turn, his false premise of the cause of disease. By accepting Satan's false concepts concerning the causes of disease, and resorting to his unsound methods of treatment, man gives reverence to Satan.

The pivotal book that officially launched the New Age movement was Marilyn Ferguson's *The Aquarian Conspiracy*, published in 1980. This book was "an important New Age manifesto that attempted to announce and popularize what the New Agers chose to publicly display in their Movement." The book set forth futuristic thinking that has become so commonplace in our culture that an entire generation has grown up believing its basic assumptions. One of the key topics in this book was Ferguson's assertion that the radical overhaul of society could be based upon health care **"reform"** -- a **"transformation"** explained in the chapter "Healing Ourselves." Ferguson wrote "The new paradigm of health and medicine enlarges the framework of the old, incorporating brilliant technological advances while restoring and validating intuitions about mind and relationships." (p. 247)[15]

Chapter 4 in *The Aquarian Conspiracy* titled "Crossover: People Changing" lists a number of medical disciplines that Ferguson refers to as *points of entry* and "psychotechnologies," to facilitate change in a person's world view. They include: biofeedback, autogenic training, music in combination with meditation and imagery, psychodrama, self-help programs such as 12 step of AA, all forms of meditation, yoga, EST, Silva mind control, dream journals, Arica, Theosophy, Science of Mind, A Course in Miracles, all body disciplines and therapies, Tai Chi Chuan, karate, Sufi stories, koans, whirling dervishes, etc., etc. In the chapter on *Changeover* further explanation is made as to the steps involved in a change—transformation of an individual. Step one, is experimenting with an *entry point.* Step two, is *exploring* further the entry point and possible additional ones. This going deeper into the healing technique in search of something enticing, actually a beginning of breaking the grip of one's deeply established core values, and allows for a change to a new set of guide lines (pantheistic) for one's life. Step three, *integration*, wherein the individual trusts an inner guru. Contact with an inner guide, an inner child, or as C.J. Jung says "the divine child." This is a stage where contact is made with demons—fallen angels. Step four, *conspiracy,* (def. to breathe together) discovering additional sources of power and the ways to use it, such as self-healing, healing others, and attempting to heal society, a conspiring for renewal. Is it any wonder that the New York Times referred to the book *The Aquarian Conspiracy* as the New Age Bible?

In II Kings l, it is written that Ahaziah, king of Israel, fell and sustained serious injury. He sent a messenger to inquire of Baalzebub, god of Ekron, as to whether he would recover from his injuries. God sent Elijah the prophet to intercept the messenger of the king as he traveled toward Ekron. Elijah sent him back to the king with the question:

> Is it because there is no God in Israel that you go off to consult Baalzebub the god of Ekron? (II Kings 1:3 NIV).

A captain and fifty soldiers were sent to arrest Elijah and to bring him to the king. When they attempted to arrest Elijah, fire from heaven consumed them. The king sent another fifty, who suffered the same fate. The captain of a third group pleaded with Elijah not to allow fire to consume them, and God told Elijah to go with the captain to see the king.

---

15   http.//www.discernment-ministries.org, Feb. 10, 2011

As Elijah faced the king he repeated the question,

Is it because there is no God in Israel that you go off to consult Baalzebub the god of Ekron? (II Kings 1:3 NIV).

Elijah told him that because of this inquiry of Baalzebub he would not recover from his injuries but would die. We must be very careful not to be found "inquiring of the god of Ekron" regarding our physical status. Many sincere Christians are deceived by Satan and are indeed inquiring of the god of Ekron.

In the same manner do men and women dishonor God when they turn from the Source of strength and wisdom to ask help or counsel from the powers of darkness. If God's wrath was kindled by Ahaziah's act, how does God regard those who, having still greater light, choose to follow a similar course? [16]

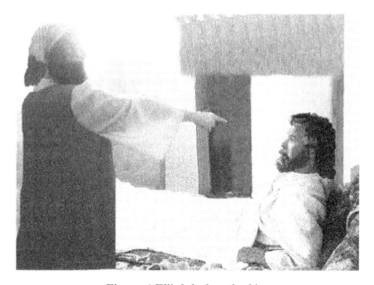

Figure 4 Elijah before the king

Satan has long been preparing for his final effort to deceive the world. The foundation of his work was laid by the assurance given to Eve in Eden:

Ye shall not surely die... in the day ye eat thereof, then your eyes will be opened, and ye shall be as gods, knowing good and evil. (Genesis: 3:4, 5).

---

16 White, E.G., *The Review and Herald*, Jan. 15, (1914); White, E.G., *Prophets and Kings*, The Review and herald Publishing Assn., Hagerstown, MD, (1917),pp. 211,212.

Little by little he has prepared the way for his masterpiece of deception in the development of spiritualism. Spiritualism leads, by word and practice, to the belief in immortality (a spirit life after death), and it often involves communication with the spirit world. Satan has not yet reached the full accomplishment of his designs; but it will be reached in the last remnant of time. Says the prophet John:

> I saw three unclean spirits like frogs...they are the spirits of devils, working miracles, which go forth unto the kings of the earth and of the whole world, to gather them to the battle of that great day of God Almighty. (Revelation. 16:13, 14).

> Except those who are kept by the power of God, through faith in His word, the whole world will be swept into the ranks of this delusion. The people are fast being lulled to a fatal security, to be awakened only by the outpouring of the wrath of God.[17]

As we turn our attention to the advancement of spiritualism into the field of health and healing, let us look again to God's messenger, Ellen White, for guidance in appraising various treatment methods. Those who have been persuaded by apparent achievement of the false sciences will praise them and point out the apparent good they have accomplished, yet without understanding the power that is behind these sciences and the extent of deception.

> ... but it is a power which will yet work with all signs and lying wonders–with all deceivableness of unrighteousness. *Mark the influence of these sciences*, dear reader, for the conflict between Christ and Satan is not yet ended.[18]

Ellen White spoke of three popular therapies of her day, warning of their connection to spiritualism, that of phrenology, psychology, and mesmerism. Let us take a brief glimpse at each of these *mind cure* therapeutic methods.

Phrenology emerged in the 1800's and taught that by feeling the shape of the skull, a person could determine the character and personality of an individual. Phrenology also included *mind therapy*, by pressure placed on certain areas of the skull it was believed that the personality traits and mental makeup could be changed. It was a pseudoscience that taught phrenology as psychological insight and self-knowledge, all originating from within. It contributed to the popular psychology of the nineteenth century and functioned in the same way as psychoanalysis permeated psychology of today. In the mid-

17   White, E.G., *The Great Controversy,* op. cit., p. 561-562.
18   White E.G., *Mind, Character, Personality,* Vol. 2, Southern Pub. Assn., Nashville, TN, (1958), p. 712.

later 1800's phrenology in the USA became part of a counter-culture movement as distinguished by new dress styles, communes, mesmerism (hypnotism), and revival of herbal remedies. It did not make successful inroads into regular medical thought. (See encyclopedia—phrenology)

In the 1800's and early 1900's, the term, "psychology", had a somewhat different meaning than it does today. Noah's 1828 dictionary defines it thus: n. [gr. Soul, and discourse.] A discourse or treatise on the human soul. Or the doctrine of the nature of the soul.

Popular psychologist of the 1800's and early 1900's presented a theory of the "subconscious mind" and focused inward to self-love, self-acceptance, self-improvement, self-worth, self-esteem, self, self, etc., and based their therapeutic methods upon this foundation. Some of the more influential psychologists were believers in the occult and had connection with spirits. Jung had a spirit guide by the name of Philemon. Their "mind cure" theory was to look within our minds to find solutions to life stresses and problems, rather than pointing them to the greatest healer of the mind—Jesus Christ the Divine Son of God. These psychologists, some of who were connected to the spirit world, might use mind altering methods, such as hypnosis, including cocaine, in analysis and therapy for their patients.

Today, psychology is generally considered a science of the mind and human behavior, and has gained some understanding of mental processes, yet it suffers from a solid standard which allows many theories and approaches to mind cure. It is often practiced in a way that presents the same dangers as in the past. (See chapter 19— Psychology)

Mesmerism referred to a therapeutic approach to health that was patterned after the teachings of a Dr. Mesmer who lived in the late 1700's and early 1800's. He was a graduate of the Medical School of Vienna. He was also an astrologer and believed in the association and sympathy of the cosmos, earth, and man. He started his medical practice, after graduation from medical school, by using magnets in an attempt to treat disease. This was an ancient practice that repeatedly, over many centuries came and left the field of medicine. Eventually he found that by just placing his hands over a body, he could get the same response that he did with magnets. This practice evolved into what is now known as hypnotism. In many encyclopedias, Mesmer is called the father of hypnotism, a method of *mind cure*. Mrs. White gave strong warnings against its use.

> This entering in of Satan through the sciences is well devised. Through the channel of phrenology, psychology, and mesmerism, he comes more directly to the people of this generation and ***works with that power which is to characterize***

his efforts near the close of probation. The minds of thousands have thus been poisoned and led into infidelity.[19]

We have reached the perils of the last days, when some, yes, many, 'shall depart from the faith, giving heed to seducing spirits and doctrines of devils.' Be cautious in regard to what you read and how you hear. Take not a particle of interest in spiritualistic theories. Satan is waiting to steal a march upon everyone who allows himself to be deceived by his hypnotism. He begins to exert his power over them just as soon as they begin to investigate his theories.[20]

John, in the Biblical book of Revelation, chapter sixteen, has warned us that spirits of demons will be the method and power by which the world will be brought together to place all men under one system (Satan's), at the end of time. John also points out that there will be another very small group that will not accept the control by this spiritistic power, and they keep the commandments of God and have the faith of Jesus.

This book *Exposing Spiritualistic Practices in Healing* has been written to expose this spiritistic power as it works through health and healing. The scope of this deception is so large and so many different deceiving methods are used that it is impossible to cover them all, so I have focused on revealing the foundation from which the many counterfeit healing methods explain their power and origin. With a reasonable understanding of these principles, it is possible to determine for oneself whether a particular healing modality is real or spiritistic. First it is needful that we look at God's system of health and healing and understand its principles so that we may be able to recognize the counterfeit. The next chapter identifies God's system, and the beneficial effects of following its principles are substantiated by contrasting the results with that of the counterfeit.

---

19   *Ibid.,* p. 711.
20   *Ibid.,* p. 718.

CHAPTER 3

THE STORY OF THE SEVENTH-DAY ADVENTIST HEALTH MESSAGE

The book "The *Story of Our Health Message,*" by D.E. Robinson, is the source of much information used in this chapter concerning the early history of the Seventh-day Adventist (SDA) Church. Robinson was the personal secretary of E. G. White for the last fifteen years of her life. I was a student in a class he taught presenting the history that I am presenting to you. Additional information came from the book, *Historical Perspectives in Health,* by Ruben Hubbard, who was an instructor at the School of Health at Loma Linda, California. Both of these books were based on careful research. Much of the material in the last section of this chapter comes from my own knowledge accumulated through my years in medical work and in the Seventh-day Adventist Church.

For sixty plus years I have been associated in various capacities with medical work, I have seen a complete change in the way the scientific community views the principles involved in the Seventh-day Adventist health teachings. This same viewpoint change has also occurred in the general public. The attitude has moved from disbelief and ridicule to esteem. We have not changed our teachings. Scientific studies have shown the value of these teachings and practices. This presentation will mention several of the SDA scientists whose research has been most responsible for this change in attitude.

BRIEF MEDICAL HISTORY OF PAST AGES

Medical historians have given to the world great insight into the beliefs, practices, and quality of medical knowledge over the past three thousand years. A large body of knowledge of past medical concepts and practices was recorded in Egypt, India, China, and the Mesopotamian valley. These writings have been found, translated, and studied, revealing patterns and changes that occurred over time.

Early in medical history, there was a rational approach to the health of man. By the time of the exodus of the Israelites from Egypt near 1500 B.C., medical writings reveal that concepts and practices in medicine had become irrational and mystical in the Egyptian and Sumerian civilizations.[21] There appears to have been a parallel trend in religious beliefs with medical practices.

The history of Medieval Europe often referred to as the "dark ages," shows this same change from the rational to irrational in religious dogma, health habits, and medical concepts.[22] Advancements in the practice of medicine and the knowledge of physiology occurred within the early Christian church. Several of the early church bishops were physicians, and their writings are available.[23] When the Christian church began to blend with pagan religions, a change took place in European medical practice—a change from rational to irrational and on to mystical.

Medieval Europe experienced the "midnight of the world" in the practice of health and healing, while the knowledge of medicine was preserved by Christian and Jewish physicians within the Arabian Empire.[24] The Christian church at Rome banned the practice of medicine and surgery in the thirteenth century. Sickness was explained as being the result of possession by evil spirits. The practice of "casting out the spirits" became the method of treatment for disease. This ignorance existed for one thousand years.[25] During the renaissance of the sixteenth century, this curtain of darkness began to slowly lift from the land. As knowledge of God revived, a change began in the knowledge of health practices. This change was very slow however, and not until the middle of the nineteenth century did we see the beginning of what is now termed "scientific medicine." The actual practice of medicine throughout America and Europe was similar. In some of the medical centers knowledge slowly increased, but it was a long time before this impacted the average physician's practice.

During the mid-nineteenth century, physicians had no knowledge of physics, chemistry, or physiology. A common treatment was to take one half to one liter of blood from the patient (bleeding), and sometimes more than once per day. If someone had a fever they were put in a hot, dark place without fresh air, fluids, or water. The physician used a variety of toxic substances such as mercury, arsenic, antimony, nicotine, strychnine, opium, digitalis, and others.[26] He also used many herbs. He had no knowledge how

21   Hubbard, Rubin; *Historical Perspectives of Health,* Printed by the Dept. of Health Education, School of Health, Loma Linda University, (1975), pp. 9, 20.
22   Ackernecht, Erwin H.; *A Short History of Medicine,* John Hopkins
23   Hubbard, op. cit., pp. 121, 123, 136.
24   Garrison, Fielding H. , *History of Medicine*, W.B. Saunders and Co., Philadelphia and London, (1929), pp. 126–139.
25   Hubbard op. cit., p. 130–132.
26   Robinson, D.E., *The Story of Our Health Message*, (1965), Southern Pub. Assn., Nashville, TN, (1943,1955, 1965), pp. 22, 28-29.

any of these substances acted on the system; also there existed no guide as to a safe dosage. It seemed that any truly helpful treatment had been discarded.

The most common cause of death was from infectious disease.[27] There was no understanding about microorganisms, or the relationship between dirt, filth, and disease. Personal cleanliness was frequently lacking. The nutritional status was often poor, and the ability of the immune system to respond to disease was depressed.

Medical treatment during this era was, at best, worthless. Most of the time it was harmful, and frequently the cause of death.[28] These conditions paved the way for the emergence of a variety of therapeutic approaches to health and healing. Frequently these methods appeared to be helpful because they did not use the harmful methods employed by the regular medical profession. Doing nothing was much safer than receiving standard medical care. This situation made it easy for alternative methods (which had no true value), to be accepted as being more effective.

The science of nutrition gradually was acknowledged by physicians to have a role in preventing disease by maintaining a strong immune system. Adequate calories, minerals, vitamins, and trace elements are all needed to allow proper functioning of the immune system. It was not known that some methods of food preservation were themselves the cause of various diseases, such as cancer of the stomach and esophagus, or that some minerals and vitamins are lost during certain types of food preparation. Only in the past 50-60 years have we realized the problems caused by the use of too much salt, and the danger of eating pickled and smoked foods.

The large amount of salt used in preserving meats and some vegetables produce "nitrosamines," which are carcinogenic (cancer initiators).

Unhealthful personal habits also contributed to the incidence of illness and early death. Tobacco use started in America and spread throughout the world. Coffee and tea consumption were also widespread and alcohol use was well-nigh universal. Working twelve or more hours per day, seven days a week was not uncommon. The heavy use of some condiments, vinegar, meats, and cheeses laid the foundation for disease.

Occasionally, some reforms were seen in the way people lived and how they dealt with illnesses. However, even if the methods used produced good results and caused no harm, they did not easily gain acceptance. Change for the better was slow. Satan, it seemed, did all in his power to hinder improvement.

---

27   Haggenson, C.D., Wyndham, E.L., *A Hundred Years of Medicine,*(1942), Sheridan House, NY, p. 42. reported in Hubbard, op. cit., p. 154.
28   Hubbard, op. cit., pp. 153-8.

EARLY REFORMS IN MEDICAL CARE

In 1777, many sailors on a long voyage became ill with typhus. It was customary to put sick sailors in the bottom of the ship and deprive them of water or other fluids. They were given drugs that were not helpful and often worsened the disease. The sick sailors were denied fresh air and body cooling measures were avoided. So many sailors became ill on a particular voyage that there was no room for them in the bottom of the ship, the usual location for the sick bay. Therefore, those who were not expected to live were placed on deck. These sick men were so miserable they asked the crew to pour water over them. Since they were not expected to live, the ship's doctor granted their requests. Surprisingly, they recovered. This experience was passed on to other ships' physicians, and when duplicated, the same good result was seen. Due to the prejudice and disbelief of physicians this enlightenment did not prevail and the old methods continued.[29]

In 1812 the benefits of the use of water in treating the sick was accidentally discovered by Vincent Priessnitz, a lad of thirteen, living in Austria. He found that using cold water on a sprained wrist lessened the pain. Sometime later, he was accidentally run over by a wagon and sustained bruises and broken ribs. He was seen by a physician who told him that he would die from his injuries. He again used cold water to treat his injuries. This uneducated lad subsequently began to apply his water treatment to others with good results. He established a "hydrotherapy" clinic in Grafenburg, Austria, and in a short time his fame grew, and people from all over Europe sought treatment. Eventually, doctors who went to his clinic to observe his methods of healing took these treatments back to their countries. As a result water treatment centers were opened in many countries of the world.[30]

Most physicians opposed this method of treatment. They tried to close Priessnitz's institution by appealing to the courts of law, but failed. Remember that in that day the results were outstanding when compared to conventional medical care.

By the mid 1850's, there was public demand, championed by Horace Mann, a famous educator, for teaching physiology and hygiene in schools. Cleanliness was promoted. Sylvester Graham, an American, introduced the use of whole grains and a vegetarian diet. He produced "graham flour," (whole wheat flour) for bread making, and today, in America, "graham crackers" are still made. Also during this time, temperance societies were established to oppose the sale and consumption of alcohol.

---

29   Robinson, op. cit., pp. 28-30.
30   *Ibid.,* p. 31–33.

This revived interest in a wholesome diet and lifestyle. Interest in and application of hydrotherapy therapy peaked in the 1840's and 1850's, and then began to fade. The vast majority of physicians, however, continued with the old ways of practicing medicine. At that same time there also arose a religious revival world-wide, proclaiming the imminent second coming of Jesus. When Jesus did not appear as expected, this church revival faded also.

It was out of this revival that the Seventh-day Adventist Church had its beginnings. For eleven years after the Great Disappointment, a small group of people continued diligently to search their Bibles in an effort to understand why Jesus did not appear on the expected date. As they prayerfully studied the prophecies, they gained a fuller understanding not only of what the prophecies foretold, but also of the requirements of God's laws and commandments. This new knowledge ultimately led to their observance of the Biblical seventh-day Sabbath.

EARLY REFORMS IN SEVENTH-DAY ADVENTISTS' HEALTH

Ellen G. White was part of the small group of Seventh-day Adventists. Around the age of seventeen Ellen started receiving visions from God. In many of her visions she received instructions on how to live in a healthful manner. In 1848, a special message was given to her concerning tobacco, coffee, and tea. It was pointed out that use of these substances was harmful to health, and had a deleterious influence on the mind, and was to be done away with.[31]

In response to a letter, she replied, "I have seen in vision that tobacco was a filthy weed, and that it must be laid aside or given up. Said my accompanying angel, 'If it is an idol it is high time it was given up, and unless it is given up the frown of God will be upon the one that uses it, and he cannot be sealed with the seal of the living God.'... I saw that Christ will have a church without spot or wrinkle or any such thing to present to His Father."[32] Tobacco use was common among the people. Getting the believers to give it up was a slow process which took fifteen years to accomplish.

During this time, through continuing Bible study, the prohibition against the use of swine's flesh was discovered, and there was a movement to abstain from its use. However, in vision, Ellen White was instructed that it was not then the time to promote such change. God would bring about this change at the proper time.[33]

---

31   *Ibid.,* p. 65.
32   White, E.G., *Manuscript Releases,* Vol. 8, no. 592, The Open Door.
33   *Robinson,* op. cit., pp. 62–63.

In 1854, a second message on health was given through Ellen White. This message emphasized three points:

1. Cleanliness of both home and body;
2. Control of appetite, and
3. Use of whole grains in preference to refined flour, and food free from animal fat.[34]

Ellen White commented, after the above message was received: "I saw that God was purifying unto Himself a peculiar people; He will have a clean and holy people, a people in whom He can delight. I saw that God would not acknowledge an untidy, unclean person as a Christian. His frown is upon such. Our souls, bodies, and spirits are to be presented blameless by Jesus to His Father; and unless we are clean in person, and pure we cannot be presented blameless to God. I saw that the houses of the saints should be kept tidy and neat, free from dirt and filth and all uncleanness."[35]

The Seventh-day Adventist Church was first organized at a General Conference meeting in May 1863. In June 1863, God sent another message through E.G. White covering many aspects of health. The central theme was the relationship between health and spirituality, and that care for one's health is a religious duty. The first instructions were to herself and her husband concerning the need to change their habits. The responsibility for leading out in this work of promoting health reform was placed upon Ellen and her husband James White. The message was relevant to eating, working, drinking, and the use of poisonous drugs in medical care. God directed them to use water both inside and outside of the body for the prevention and treatment of disease, and for the promotion of health and cleanliness.

It was made clear to James White that his gloomy and depressed mood was affecting his health. He was to exercise faith in God, and thereby rise above his depressed thoughts. He was to be cheerful, hopeful, and in a peaceful frame of mind because his health depended upon this. *He was to seek improvement in his health by following proper habits of life, rather than by seeking some magic cure, while continuing on with health destroying habits.*[36]

The health information Ellen White received in visions was given one hundred and fifty years ahead of its time, and medical science has substantiated almost everything about which God gave directions.

Ellen White was also instructed in vision to counsel the people to give up the use of flesh foods, as its use would promote disease and have an unfavorable influence upon the mind and the willingness to follow God's leading.

---

34   *Ibid.,* p. 71.
35   White, E.G., *Manuscript Releases* Vol. 6, E.G. White Estate (1854) pp. 221-223.
36   Robinson, op. cit., pp. 78, 79.

Many of the principles of reform given to E.G. White had been promoted by a few people in the years preceding her vision. However, those teachings and most of their good influence had disappeared. I believe God was the source of this prior reform, which had been advocated and supported by a person here, and one there. Now, however, He entrusted it to an organization of believers who were to take it to the world.

The 1863 message emphasized the connection between health reform and giving the message of salvation by faith in Jesus. Habits and diet affect our character and eternal destiny.[37] Even the apparel of the Christian is to glorify God by modesty and appropriateness.

Mrs. White wrote:

> "I was again shown that the health reform is one branch of the great work which is to fit a people for the coming of the Lord. It is as closely connected with the third angel's message as the hand is with the body."[38]

God's message to the church in 1863 was that disease prevention and treatment of illness were to be accomplished by following proper health habits, use of water internally and externally, and following a vegetarian diet, with limited use of eggs and milk. God directed that they were to start an institution for the treatment of the sick. They needed a place where their own members could go for care and be taught proper health habits.[39] There were only thirty-five hundred members in the church at that time. They were to move out in faith as God would lead them. Little did they dream of where He would lead.

---

37 *Ibid.*
38 White, E. G., *Testimonies For the Church,* Vol. 3, Pacific Press Pub. Assn., Mountain View, CA (1948), p. 161.
39 *Robinson,* op. cit., p. 142.

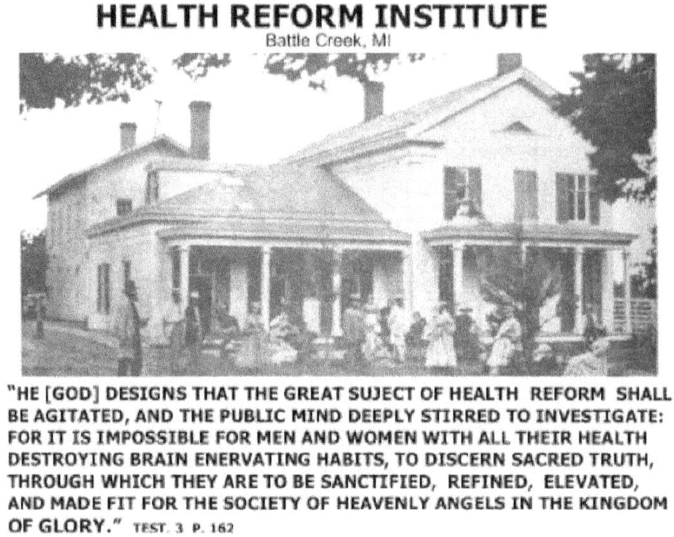

HEALTH REFORM INSTITUTE
Battle Creek, MI

"HE [GOD] DESIGNS THAT THE GREAT SUBJECT OF HEALTH REFORM SHALL
BE AGITATED, AND THE PUBLIC MIND DEEPLY STIRRED TO INVESTIGATE:
FOR IT IS IMPOSSIBLE FOR MEN AND WOMEN WITH ALL THEIR HEALTH
DESTROYING BRAIN ENERVATING HABITS, TO DISCERN SACRED TRUTH,
THROUGH WHICH THEY ARE TO BE SANCTIFIED, REFINED, ELEVATED,
AND MADE FIT FOR THE SOCIETY OF HEAVENLY ANGELS IN THE KINGDOM
OF GLORY." TEST. 3 P. 162

Figure 5. Western Health Reform Institute

"He (God) designs that the great subject of health reform shall be agitated, and the public mind deeply stirred to investigate: for it is impossible for men and women with all their sinful health-destroying, brain enervating habits, to discern sacred truth, through which they are to be sanctified, refined, elevated, and made fit for the society of heavenly angels in the kingdom of glory."[40]

In 1866, the church began to publish a journal on health which soon gained wide circulation. A building was also purchased in Battle Creek, Michigan, to be used as a treatment center. The treatments consisted of physical exercise, hydrotherapy, and a diet free of meat, alcohol, coffee, and tea. Tobacco was not to be used in any of its forms. The institution was called the Western Health Reform Institute.[41]

Basic instructions for a healthy lifestyle were taught at the Reform Institute. A diet of plant foods, whole grains, and an abundance of fruit, vegetables of all types, nuts, and legumes was served. A small amount of eggs and milk was also a part of the menu. Regularity in hours of sleeping, working, eating, and resting was followed. Eating between meals was discouraged. Patients were directed to avoid the use of lard and tallow (grease) in their food. The heavy use of salt and foods preserved in salt or vinegar were to be avoided.

This pattern of lifestyle became the blueprint for many Seventh-day Adventists for the next one hundred and forty years. Pure air, sunlight,

---

40   White, op. cit., *Testimonies* Vol. 3, p. 162.
41   Robison, op. cit., p. 149.

temperance, rest, exercise, proper diet, the use of water, and trust in divine power are the true remedies for health. Trust in God will result in obedience to his physical and spiritual laws. Today, Seventh-day Adventists are recognized by the scientific community as among the longest lived people on earth.

Success of the Western Health Reform institution came by following God's directions.

> ...This institution is designed of God to be one of the greatest aids in preparing a people to be perfect before God...[42] ...They should not depend upon their skill alone. If the blessing, instead of the frown, of God be upon the institution, angels will attend patients, helpers, and physicians, to assist in the work of restoration, so that in the end the glory will be given to God, and not to feeble, short sighted man.[43]

The physicians at the institution were to be highly trained in the sciences, thereby able to command the respect of the patients and the doctors of that day. There were to be no "novices" acting as physicians. They were to be able to explain the treatment methods and to show that they were done on *a rational, scientific basis*; yet, they were to follow the plan God had directed in treatment, not the methods of the world.

The health institution grew rapidly, and subsequently it developed into a medical and surgical hospital as well as being a sanitarium. The medical staff consisted of well-trained physicians, and the institution gained fame through the success of its medical care, and the spiritual atmosphere. Gradually, respect from the medical profession developed,[44] as the institution became so well known that the wealthy and powerful came for care from across America, and also from Europe.

Early in the development of the health institute, a young physician, John Harvey Kellogg, was chosen to be its director. First, he was sent to Bellevue Hospital Medical College in New York City, for a three-year course in medicine to receive the best training possible. This training brought him up to the top level of understanding of the science of medicine that was known in his day. He learned surgery as well. The treatment approach of the hospital remained as God had directed in spite of Dr. Kellogg's exposure to the large hospitals of the day. God directed Dr. Kellogg in his efforts and blessed him in skills and understanding. In his book, *Rational Therapy* (1902), Dr. Kellogg mentions that he had a 3% death rate in surgery and the last 165 cases without a death.

---

42   White, op. cit., *Testimonies* Vol. 3, p. 166.
43   White, op. cit., p. 215
44   Robinson, op. cit., p. 215.

Most hospitals had a death rate of 20-30%. In a letter to Dr. Kellogg, E.G. White wrote:

> My dear brother, as I have before written to you, I know that the Lord had placed you in a very responsible position, standing as you do as the greatest physician in our world, a man to whom the Lord has given understanding and knowledge, that you may do justice and judgment, and reveal the true missionary spirit in the institution which is to represent truth in contrast with error.[45]

Who has been by your side as you have performed these critical operations?

> Who has kept you calm and self-possessed in the crisis, giving you quick, sharp discernment, clear eyesight, steady nerves, and skillful precision? The Lord Jesus has sent His angel to your side to tell you what to do. A hand has been laid upon your hand. Jesus, and not you, has guided the movements of your instrument. At times you have realized this, and a wonderful calmness has come over you. You dared not hurry, and yet you worked rapidly, knowing that there was not a moment to lose. The Lord has greatly blessed you. You have been under divine guidance[46]

> As you looked to God in your critical operations, angels of God were standing by your side, and their hands were seen as your hand performing the work with an accuracy that made the beholder surprised.[47]

HEALTHFUL FOODS PRODUCED

Dr. Kellogg recognized that many people had poor diets and he desired to make available to them more whole grain cereals. Through experimentation he developed breakfast cereals and other wholesome foods. Thus began the great breakfast cereal industry and the beginning of the health food industry. Dr. Kellogg also put a great deal of effort into developing tasty meat substitutes consisting of grains, legumes, and nuts in small proportions.

Ellen White wrote the following to the members of the church:

> I must now give to my brethren the instruction that the Lord has given me in regard to the health food question. By many people the health foods are looked

---

45   White, E.G., *Manuscript Releases,* Vol. 5, No. 260-346, (1990) MR No. 333, Our Health Message.

46   White, E. G., *2 Selected Messages,* Review and Herald Publishing Assn. Washington D.C. (1958), p. 285. White, E.G., 1 *Testimonies*, vol. 8, pp. 187 188.

47   White, E.G., *2 Selected Messages,* Review and Herald, Washington D.C., (1958), p. 285.

upon as of man's devising, but they are of God's origination, as a blessing to His people. The health food work is the property of God, and is not to be made a financial speculation for personal gain. The light hat God has given and will continue to give on the food question is to be to His people today what the manna was to the children of Israel. The manna fell from heaven, and the people were told to gather it, and prepare it to be eaten. So in the different countries of the world, light will be given to the Lord's people, and health foods suited to these countries will be prepared.[48]

Health foods are Gods productions, and He will teach His people in missionary fields to so combine the productions of the earth that simple, inexpensive, wholesome foods will be provided. If they will seek wisdom from God, He will teach them how to plan and devise to utilize these productions. I am instructed to say, forbid them not.[49]

In 1895, Dr. Kellogg patented a machine for grinding nuts and making peanut butter. One of his employees, Joseph Lambert, in 1895, patented a home grinder for making peanut butter.

Peanut butter had been made as far back as the days of the Incas but was not generally used.

As Battle Creek Sanitarium Health Food Company in the mid-1890s forged ahead in making wheat flakes, a coffee substitute, 'caramel cereal', and in developing of vegetable protein meat substitutes–beginning with peanut butter and soon more sophisticated products as "nuttose" and "nut cheese" –a serious interest along these lines began to emerge in Australia."[50]

By 1914, there were many companies in the United States making peanut butter. Many people, not members of the SDA church, also developed special health foods, and now these health foods and stores are found around the globe. However, not every product found in a health food store is really health food.

Adventists also formed companies that produce healthful foods. The SDA Church's breakfast cereal industry in Australia was started in 1898. Today, that company is a major producer of breakfast cereals and soy milk for Australia and New Zealand. The Sanitarium Health Food Co. listed on their web site, has sales of three hundred million dollars a year. It exports to more than thirty countries. The first Health Food store in Australia may well have been the

---

48   White, E.G., *Counsels on Diet and Foods,* Review and Herald Pub. Assn., Washington, D.C., (1938), p. 269.1.
49   *Ibid.*, p. 272.2.
50   White, *Arthur, Biographical Books*/4BIO, Review and Herald Pub. Assn., Hagerstown, MD, Vol. 4 Chapter 30, (1983).

Sanitarium's café and food shop on Pitt Street in Sydney, opening in 1902; and another opened in 1907 on Auckland's Victoria Street, New Zealand. Another large SDA food company, "Granix," is in Argentina, and exports wholesome foods to fifteen nations.

Around the year 1900, Dr. Harry Miller, an Adventist doctor and prior student of Dr. Kellogg's, went to China as a mission doctor. He saw babies dying from starvation because their mother's milk was drying up. He improved on the soymilk which Dr. Kellogg had produced, and started its commercial production in China. He was thus able to provide milk for babies whose mothers were unable to feed them. He also established a health food industry in America and later gave it to the church. The company was known as Loma Linda Foods. When Dr. Miller died at age 95, he was still experimenting in food products.

This work by Dr. Kellogg and Dr. Miller in creating soy products has gained the attention of the medical world and food industries, and soy products are now produced and used around the world.

HEALTH REFORM INSTITUTE INITIATES MEDICAL EDUCATION

The Western Health Reform Institute, later called the Battle Creek Sanitarium and Hospital, started a School of Health in 1878 to train young people in physiology, hygiene, and nutrition. These students then returned to their churches to teach others a healthful lifestyle. This training produced many health educators. In 1883 the hospital was in desperate need of Adventist nurses, so the Sanitarium started a nursing school. The hospital continued to grow in size and fame. There was a need for more physicians who would practice in harmony with the principles of the hospital, and a medical school was therefore opened at the hospital in 1895, called the American Medical College.[51]

---

51   Robinson, op. cit., pp. 249-281.

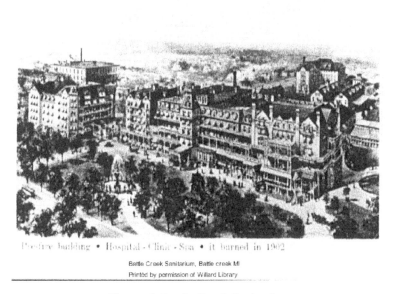

Postive building • Hospital - Clinic - Spa • it burned in 1902

Battle Creek Sanitarium, Battle creek MI
Printed by permission of Willard Library

Figure 6. Battle Creek Sanitarium

Many of the graduates of this medical school spread across America, and others went abroad, often starting similar sanitariums. Most of these institutions also developed nursing schools.

SUBTLE TEACHINGS

We have been learning of the rapid growth and expansion of the health work. However, around 1898, a problem slowly and insidiously developed. It was a subtle belief and teaching of pantheism promoted by Dr. Kellogg, which spread to some workers and ministers. Dr. Kellogg had been influenced by a relative who was a Baptist minister. The idea was that the righteousness of God was in the air we breathe and the water we drink, and when we take of these substances we obtain the righteousness of God.[52]

While Ellen White was in Australia, she was shown in vision this problem of pantheism, and wrote a letter to the General Conference at its 1899 meeting, warning of this hidden subtle teaching. She advised them to strongly deal with it. She wrote letters to Dr. Kellogg many times concerning his belief, warning him of his danger, but to no avail. The teachings continued to spread causing the fall of some leading ministers.[53]

---

52 *Ibid.*, p. 314
53 *Ibid.*, p. 312–317.

The Sanitarium was totally destroyed by fire in 1902. Dr. Kellogg immediately made plans to rebuild on a grand scale. Ellen White was directed in vision to counsel him that they should build small. However, Dr. Kellogg went ahead with plans for a 1000 bed institution.

To raise money to pay for a new sanitarium he wrote a home medical book called the *"The Living Temple."* Pantheism was subtly woven into the content of the book. The church's publishing house refused to publish it, so Dr. Kellogg had it published by another company. The refusal to publish this book was a further step in the separation of Dr. Kellogg and the Sanitarium, from the Seventh-day Adventist Church.

God had not yet withdrawn all of His blessings from the medical institution and after the Sanitarium was rebuilt, it continued for some years to be a center of influence and medical missionary activities.

The spread of pantheistic teachings continued to cause increasing division between the church leadership, and Dr. Kellogg and the hospital. In 1906 it was recognized that there would be no turning back, and the church and the Sanitarium separated. The title of the hospital was not in the name of the church, and the property was lost by the church. The Sanitarium continued to function, but by 1910, no more medical students applied for admission and the school was closed. The hospital continued operating without association with the church but also eventually closed.[54]

> Be not deceived: many will depart from the faith, giving heed to seducing spirits and doctrines of devils. We have before us now the alpha of this danger. *The* omega will be of a most startling nature.[55]

Dr. Kellogg was teaching the *theology* of pantheism. Today, the *practical* aspect of pantheism is in the therapeutic modalities of health and healing taught by Eastern religions and the New Age movement. Pantheistic heresy caused the loss of the Battle Creek Sanitarium and nearly split the church. Today, this same spiritistic influence could again deceive us. E.G. White wrote speaking of the subtle teachings of Dr. Kellogg:

> I am instructed to speak plainly. 'Meet it,' is the word spoken to me. "Meet it firmly and without delay"... "In the book *The Living Temple* there is presented

---

54   *Ibid.*, chap. pp. 312-334.
55   White, E.G., *I Selected Messages,* Review and Herald Pub. Assn., Washington D.C., (1958), p. 197.

the alpha of deadly heresies. The omega will follow, and will be received by those who are not willing to heed the warning God has given."[56]

SANITARIUMS STARTED IN CALIFORNIA

While these changes between the church and the sanitarium were occurring, God was leading in movements occurring in southern California near the city of Los Angeles. The Conference in this area consisted of 1100 people.[57] In 1901, God had shown E.G. White that medical institutions were to be started in this area. In 1904, the Southern California Conference bought two properties, each with buildings and land so as to be able to start a sanitarium; one was called Paradise Valley Sanitarium, and the other Glendale Sanitarium. The Conference was young and poor. These institutions had been bought with a small down payment with the principal to be paid on time. Though this purchase caused the Conference to be heavily indebted, they moved out in faith.

In another vision in 1901, Mrs. White was shown a special property in southern California that was to develop a medical institution which would become a great educational center.

White visited the two sites that the Southern California Conference had purchased, and said that neither of these institutions was the one that was to be a special educational center. In 1905, another property sixty miles east of Los Angeles which consisted of land, orchards, and buildings, which were perfect for a sanitarium, was for sale at a much reduced price. A Pastor Burden who lived near the property carefully inspected it and realized its value, but there was no money available even for a down payment. The Conference officers were burdened with the two medical facilities they already had. Mrs. White told Pastor Burden that he was to borrow the money himself for the down payment. By the time he secured money the price had dropped even further. The purchase was in May 1905, and in June 1905, Mrs. White visited the grounds; she looked about and recognized it as the property shown her in vision.[58]

D.E. Robinson, in his book *The Story of Our Health Message,* chapters 28-31, tells the exciting, marvelous story of God's providence in securing the property and providing money for completing the payment.

---

56   White, E.G., *Selected Messages Book 1,* Review and Herald Publishing Assn., Washington, D.C., (1948), p. 200.
57   Robinson, op. cit., pp. 335-342.
58   *Ibid.,* p. 350.

The location was called Loma Linda, a Spanish term meaning "pretty hill." It was located in a rich agricultural valley with a deep well producing pure water in abundance. There was a single small hill rising up out of the valley with the future sanitarium building on top giving a wide view of the valley and nearby mountains. A train track running directly to Los Angeles went through the property.

In November 1905, the first class of nursing students started, and in September 1909, the first class of medical students began their study. The school took the name "College of Medical Evangelists." Mrs. White was shown that the Medical School at Loma Linda:

> ...is to be of the highest order, because those who are in that school have the privilege of maintaining a living connection with the wisest of all physicians, from whom there is communicated knowledge of a superior order.[59]

Soon the school was graduating physicians and nurses who spread out across the United States and to many countries around the world. As the graduates of the American Medical College in Battle Creek had done, so now these Loma Linda graduates followed in starting sanitariums and hospitals in America and in other nations. Over time, the medical school added schools for medical technologies, dietetics, and developed teaching programs to train physicians in specialties.

In 1953, a dental school was opened, and in 1967 a School of Public Health. The name "College of Medical Evangelists" was changed to Loma Linda University when the school joined with nearby La Sierra College. About this same time, the church established a medical school in Montemorelos, Mexico, and in recent years a dental school was added in the Philippines as well. Another medical school is to be found in River Platte, Argentina, medical schools in Africa, and the church has established an affiliation with the Christian Medical College in India making it possible for Seventh-day Adventist students to attend. Loma Linda School of Public Health has, and is, offering postgraduate courses of Master of Public Health & Doctorate of Health Sciences and others.

WORLD INFLUENCE OF LOMA LINDA AND THE HEALTH MESSAGE

Let us look at what has occurred since 1848, when the first vision on health was given to E. G. White for the people that were preaching the soon

59   White, E.G., *Counsels to Parents, Teachers, Students,* Pacific Press Pub. Assn., Mountain View, CA, (1913), p. 480.

return of Christ, and the importance of keeping the commandments of God. A few hundred people have grown to more than nineteeen million. The lifestyle initiated by God's directions in the early history of the church has brought blessings of improved health. Life span has increased, and Seventh-day Adventists are recognized as a group of people among the longest lived in the world. The health food industry started by Dr. Kellogg has spread around the globe. Great companies are producing foods for breakfast from cereal grains. Most of these companies are not associated with the Church; still great blessings have come from the health food industry. Meat substitutes in many countries are being produced. Soymilk and soy products are presently the object of great study worldwide by nutritional scientists. Vegetarianism has been shown to be a safe way of life.

World influence from the SDA Church and its lifestyle and medical work is also seen through the work of the business professionals who operate our hospitals and medical institutions. This work has developed into a highly specialized occupation. A few years ago, Chinese governmental officials asked the Seventh-day Adventist Hospital Administration to come to China and teach up-to-date methods of hospital administration.[60]

Battle Creek Sanitarium had been a world leader in teaching a healthful lifestyle. Its reputation in medical care had drawn the rich and famous from America and other countries. It was the pattern for many other institutions here in America as well as in foreign countries. The loss of Battle Creek Sanitarium and its schools was a tremendous blow to the Church, but God again directed in establishing His health work through Loma Linda University, a medical institution that has, as well as several of its graduates, earned international respect.

Loma Linda Medical School heart surgery team, under the leadership of Drs. Ellsworth Wareham and Joan Coggin, initiated travels to foreign countries to teach physicians and surgeons of those countries the skills and techniques needed for performing heart surgery. Many children with heart defects were operated on during those visits. Some governments requested the visits of the surgical team so as to bring an elevated standard of medical care and to share knowledge with their surgeons. With Dr. Leonard Bailey's leadership, Loma Linda has become a center for heart replacement in children. Loma Linda is the place to go for proton treatment of various cancers by Dr. Slater and his team.

By far the greatest influence of the Seventh-day Adventists health message, which God directed to be shared with the world, has come from studies of the life style and longevity of church members.

---

60   Personal conversation with Ralph Watts, prior President of South East Division of SDA, July 2003.

Mervyn Hardinge M.D. , Dr. P.H., Ph.D. Professor Emeritus, School of Public Health, Loma Linda University, in the prologue to the book *Vegetarian Nutrition*, edited by Joan Sabate M.D., shares with us some extremely interesting information relative to the early studies of vegetarians. He enrolled in Harvard University in 1948 to pursue a doctoral degree in nutrition. He chose for his thesis a comparison of vegetarians versus non-vegetarians. Nutritional scientists did not believe one could get adequate nutrition without the use of animal flesh. His study showed that nutritionally, vegetarians are equal to non-vegetarians. His paper was published in The Journal of Clinical Nutrition, 1954.

Nutrition studies up to that time focused primarily on protein, minerals, and vitamins and little to no attention was given to fats or carbohydrates. Due to the study's comparison of vegetarian to a non-vegetarian diet, Dr. Hardinge studied fats as well as protein, and he separated animal fat from plant fat. Blood analysis of the participants of the study included a blood cholesterol test (at that time in medicine almost all blood cholesterol tests were performed only to be compared with a basal metabolism test for thyroid function).

The study showed a direct relationship between the amount of animal fat and cholesterol consumed to the blood level of cholesterol. Little attention was given by the scientific community to the adequacy of the vegetarian diet as was reported, but there was great interest in the reports on the association of fat and cholesterol levels. It was the start of the world's scientific investigators' fascination with fats—animal fats, saturated fats, polyunsaturated fats—and cholesterol in relationship to the great epidemic of vascular disease in much of the world.

In 1958, Drs. Frank Lemon and Richard Walden of Loma Linda University initiated a scientific mortality study of 23,000 Seventh-day Adventists extending over twenty-five years, which revealed less heart disease, less cancer and an extended life in comparison to other Californians of equal educational and financial status. These findings led to an additional study initiated in 1974 of 34,000 Adventists (Adventist Health Study # 1). This study was designed to discover what in the life style and diet made the difference between Adventists and the comparable Californian. The lifestyle and diet of the Adventists were identified as the reason for improved health and longevity of Adventists. Similar smaller studies of Adventists living in Australia, Norway, Japan, New Zealand, The Netherlands, and the Caribbean Islands have revealed the same trend. For those Seventh-day Adventists men who followed carefully the Adventists lifestyle and vegetarian diet from near age 35-40 onward could expect to live nearly 12 years longer than their counterparts.

A small study comparing 5000 SDA physicians to 2300 Southern Californian University physicians, showed a nearly 50% reduced risk of dying from heart disease for the Adventists physicians. Analysis of Adventist Health Study # 1 for the effect of nut consumption on heart disease revealed that eating nuts 5x's, or more/wk. reduced the incidence of heart attack deaths by approximately 50%. At the time of this study doctors were advising patients to avoid nuts because of their high fat content. Later on, similar studies done by other university medical schools revealed similar benefits from nut consumption.

Adventist Health Study # 2 of 97,000 (25,000 black) Adventists, led by Gary Frazer M.D. of the School of Public Health of LLU, has been underway for nearly 22 years. The U.S. government has funded the study with one objective being to discover why the black population in America has a higher rate of disease and reduced life span in comparison to the Caucasian. Since Dr. Hardinge's research article appeared in the prestigious *American Journal of Clinical Nutrition* (1954) another 300+ scientific peer reviewed articles have been published in numerous scientific journals about Adventists.

Additional world recognition has been as a result of the Five Day Stop Smoking program initiated by Dr. J. Wayne McFarland and Pastor Elman Folkenberg. These programs have been presented around the world, helping many thousands to stop smoking, and at the same time have introduced the participants to a better lifestyle. The founding principle of the program is, that the power of God can and will change habits and lives.

The late U.D. Register Ph.D., Professor of Nutrition at Loma Linda, by his scientific work, was able to change the attitude of the governing bodies in the American Dietitians Association, and so brought Loma Linda's School of Dietetics into full accreditation. Due to the vegetarian proclivities of the school, they had not received full recognition prior to this.

Dr. McFarland, Dr. Hardinge, and Dr. Register spent much of their lives teaching not only at the medical school, but also in camp meetings, and special conferences around the United States, and in many other places world-wide. They were loved and respected by the medical students for their humility and love of God. This I know personally, as they were my teachers.

A special supplement of the *American Journal of Clinical Nutrition* Sept 1999, (a prestigious journal in nutrition) was dedicated to Dr. Hardinge and Dr. Register. This special issue of the Journal contained the reports given at the Third World Congress of Vegetarianism held at Loma Linda University. To God be the glory.

CHAPTER 4

BABYLONIAN SPIRITUALISTIC MYSTERIES IN HEALTH AND HEALING FROM EDEN TO BABYLON

This chapter reveals how Satan created a counterfeit system of health and healing, which had its beginnings in the Garden of Eden, based on the lies that the serpent told Eve at the Tree of the Knowledge of Good and Evil:

> And the serpent said unto the woman, you shall not surely die: For God doth know that in the day ye eat thereof, then your eyes shall be opened and ye shall be as gods, knowing good and evil. (Genesis 3:4, 5).

In Colossians Paul wrote:

> See to it that no one takes you captive through hollow and deceptive philosophy, which depends on human tradition and the basic principles of this world rather than on Christ. (Colossians 2:8, NIV).

Ellen White tells us this verse points to the danger in man's philosophy and of blindly following the traditions of men. It especially points to the deceptions to come in earth's final events before the second coming of Jesus.[61]

In the book *The Great Controversy*, Ellen White wrote:

> The last great delusion is soon to open before us. Antichrist is to perform his marvelous works in our sight. So closely will the counterfeit resemble the true that it will be impossible to distinguish between them except by the Holy Scriptures. By their testimony every statement and every miracle must be tested.[62]

To be able to identify a counterfeit, we must know the true. The foundation of the true system of health and healing is presented in the book *Ministry of*

---

61   White, E.G., *I Testimonies,* Pacific Press Pub. Assn., Mountain View, CA, (1948), Now in Nampa, ID, pp. 290–302.
62   White, E.G., *The Great Controversy,* Pacific Press Pub. Assn., Mountain View, CA, (1888), p. 593.

Healing by E.G. White. Eight types of influence affecting our spiritual and physical health are presented as true remedies and are often referred to as the

> Eight Laws of Health: These are: pure air, sunlight, abstemiousness (no use of harmful substances and temperate use of wholesome products), rest, exercise, proper diet, the use of water, and trust in divine power...[63]

To trust in God means we not only acknowledge Him, but we also follow all of his laws, both physical and spiritual. When we seek for our wellbeing through God's system, we will realize that God works through His laws to impart health and healing.

When man is out of harmony with God's laws, changes occur that allow sickness and disease to manifest in our bodies. In Eden, following Eve's disobedience, a change began, which over time produced a condition that we call "disease."

> Disease is an effort of nature to free the system from conditions that result from a violation of the laws of health.[64]

God has blessed us with knowledge that when applied, results in restoration of health. As we choose to be in harmony with His ways, He imparts His healing power to us. God has given great knowledge of His laws through the sciences of chemistry and physics, and we are to use that part of science that is in harmony with His laws. Present-day medical science endeavors to learn more of the physical laws that govern us, but it is not perfect and does not recognize the Great Author of life.

However, there has been a movement among some clinical practitioners to accept types of treatment modalities, that I believe, are not in harmony with the laws of God. The objective of this book is to present information that will enable the reader to differentiate between God's system and the system of the great deceiver. Satan's methods of treating disease often referred to as "alternative" or "complementary," have not been shown to be dependent upon these laws. The term "mystical medicine" is also used in reference to these treatment methods.

Those who believe in God are warned that at the end of time God's people will face deception by "miracles." Revelation 13:14 and 16:14 identify the power behind these miracles as: spirits of devils working miracles.

---

63   White, E.G., *The Ministry of Healing*; Pacific Press Pub. Assn., Mountain View, CA, (1905), Now in Nampa, ID, p. 127.

64   *Ibid.*, p. 127.

The devil, too, advocates the use of air, pure water, sunlight, exercise, rest, proper diet, and temperance, but instead of total trust in the Creator, he teaches that the power of healing is to be found within *self*. We are led to believe that by using certain varied treatment modalities, we can activate this power that is inherent in *self*, to bring about not only restoration of health, but the elevation of one's consciousness to the level of godhood.

CREATION–TEMPTATION–FALL–DELUGE

When God called his creation "very good," He was saying it was not only perfect in design and beauty, but also in total harmony with the laws of the universe.

Adam and Eve, as long as they remained in obedience to God's laws, were to enjoy immortality. To break from this harmony, they were told, would result in death. Eve's sin was that she did not believe God, and accepted the lie told by the serpent that she would not die.[65]

Lucifer had accused God of having an imperfect system. He said that *man,* the created being, could not keep God's commandments.[66] He, Satan, had an antidote for the problem. He would introduce a "pinch of *self*" into God's "selfless" society. By the change he proposed, he promised to bring balance to the system that God had called "good." He, the devil, saw that in the creation, there was harmony by the presence of opposites, such as light and dark, day and night, land and water, sun and moon, warm and cool, and in pro-creation, male and female. He charged God with withholding from man the knowledge that would make him wise like God. He said that God had withheld the knowledge of "evil" because it would balance with "*good*" and bring enlightenment and even *godhood* for themselves. There would be no death, as God had used the threat of death to scare them and keep them from this knowledge.[67] He promised a new system which would bring harmony, equality, transformation, oneness, completeness, enlightenment, immortality, and finally *godhood* for man.

This promised utopia was already the experience of man except he was created and never could become God. Lucifer wanted to be God and was jealous of the Son of God. Eve was deceived into disbelieving God and believing Satan's lie to obtain what was already hers.

---

65   White, E.G., *Patriarchs and Prophets,* Pacific Press Pub. Assn., (Nampa, ID, 1958), pp. 53, 55.
66   *Ibid.,* p. 42.
67   *Ibid.,* chapter p. 54.

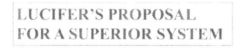

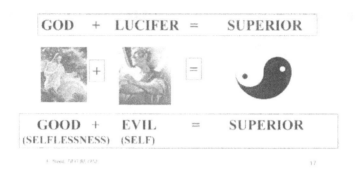

Figure 7. Christ and Satan

The degree of influence this "pinch" of evil had become after more than fifteen hundred years is revealed in the following verse.

> ...every imagination of the thoughts of his (man's) heart was only evil continually. (Genesis 6:5). God repented of making man and He covered the earth with a flood.

POST DELUGE–BABYLON–DISPERSION

Archeologists have discovered records and writings of past civilizations, which have been translated and studied. From these records, we get some knowledge of the concepts and beliefs of ancient times Cush was the son of Ham, and Ham the son of Noah. Of Cush it is said that he developed numerics, astrology, geometry, games of chance and hazard, and devised alchemy.[68]

From the Bible we learn that following the flood, Nimrod, a son of Cush, established the Mesopotamian civilization, and that Babylon was one of its cities.[69] Genesis 10: 8-12

The people of Babylon rejected God and attempted to build a tower that would reach to heaven, which they felt would protect them from another flood. God confounded the language of the people, so they could not understand each

---

68 Hislop, Alexander, *Two Babylons,* A.C. Black, Ltd., England, (1916), p. 95; Steed, Earnest, *Two Be One*, Logos International, PlainField, N.J., in Canada: G.R. Welch, Toronto, Ont., pp. 12–13.

69 *Genesis* 10:8–12; Hislop, op. cit., pp. 19–25.

other. From Babylon the people spread out over the face of the earth, carrying with them the religion that had developed in Babylon, that is, paganism/nature worship.[70]

ASTROLOGY–DUALISM–PAGANISM

The city of Babylon, "cradle of oriental civilization,"[71] located in the Mesopotamian Valley, was the origin of pagan religion. The Babylonians believed that a great power maintained the universe. However, they did not credit this power to God, but rather, to a power called "universal energy," "universal intelligence," "the creative principle," etc.

The universal energy was divided into *two parts* of supposedly opposing forces. These opposing "energies" termed *dualism,* were given various designations, such as good and evil, male and female, positive and negative, dominant and recessive, dark and light, yang and yin, etc. Every entity was determined to be either one or the other. This concept was applied to minerals, plants, and animals.

> From the Mesopotamian Valley the post diluvians spread out east, west, south, and north, carrying with them the same basic idea for the unification of opposites–the one great philosophy to achieve life's secrets–obtain all wisdom, and ultimate oneness. The ideas of Cush were carried into areas that are now Europe, China, and Asia. Except for those who worshiped the Creator God, their gods, few or many, were all allied to nature's opposites–the two most prominent being the *sun* and the *moon*. With the necessity for fire, and fire allied to heat and heat to the sun, sun worship predominated. Sympathy, they believed, existed between all forces; consequently, identification of similarities resulted. Therefore, the sun symbolized the male and moon, the female.

> Looking back, we detect how astrology of the past, with its relationship by mankind to sun, moon, and stars, became paramount, built on the basis of correspondences and sympathy; thus, occultism soon guided the major activities of life.[72]

---

70 Hislop, op. cit., p. 20; Garrison, Fielding H. , *History of Medicine,* W.B. Saunders and Co., Philadelphia, Penn.,(1929), p. 61.

71 *Ibid.*

72 Steed, Earnest, *Two Be One*, Logos International, Plainfield, N.J., in Canada G. R. Welch, Toronto, Ont., (1976), pp. 12-13.

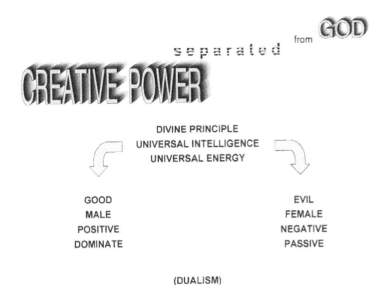

Figure 8. Creative power of God

In the Garden of Eden, Satan proposed to Adam and Eve the blending of good and evil to improve God's government. Earnest Steed, in the book *Two Be One,* p. 38, shares his perception of this principle used by Satan in his method of deception in the Garden of Eden, a pattern he has followed since. His mode of operation was not just introducing evil to counterbalance good. He blended *good* with *evil* so skillfully that evil was almost impossible to detect. It could be presented as follows:

(Selflessness)		*(Selfishness)*
Good	versus	Good and Evil
The Tree of Life	versus	The Tree of Knowledge of Good and Evil

It is this formula that has given Satan such power and success in his efforts.

> Satan himself was educated in the heavenly courts, and he has knowledge of good as well as of evil. He mingles the precious with the vile, and this is what gives him power to deceive.[73]

---

73   White, E.G., 8 *Testimonies*, Pacific Press Pub. Assn., Mountain View, CA, (1948), p. 306.

After the flood, man's great goal was to achieve a proper *balance* among the cosmos, earth, and man, as it was believed that a perfect balance would result in utopia. Thus the "knowledge of good and evil" involved not only a blending of good with evil, but the idea that harmony would only exist if this blending had universal application. This was, and is, the foundation of all non-biblical belief systems.[74]

On the back side of the covering for the book *Two Be One*, written by the publishers the following comment appears.

> In his studies, Steed has uncovered a startling discrepancy: the teachings of Christ as recorded in the Scriptures comprise the only philosophy that does not fit into the world's basic pattern for unity. For throughout the ages, mankind has seen oneness, the conjunction of all opposites, as being the culmination of all their dreams and imaginations, the way to eternal happiness. Christianity looks for *separation* to provide the sought-after peace.

It is not found by finding the proper blend with sin.

Having applied the concept of dualism to "universal energy," the great object then was to blend the divided energy back into *one,* covering every aspect of life. It became a supreme goal to blend opposites into proper balance to achieve life's secrets, obtain all wisdom, and ultimate oneness.[75]

The creation of the universe (macrocosm), and man (microcosm) was thus explained as being derived from this blending of opposites.

> We have created our own body, within the framework of certain universal and immanent laws, says the Buddhist.[76]

He refers to dualism. Actually, the doctrine of evolution is only a variant of dualism wherein the strong rises above the weak in the process of selection.

---

74   Steed, op. cit., p. vii–ix.

75   Steed, op. cit., p. 12–13.

76   Govinda, Lama Anagarika, *Foundations of Tibetan Mysticism,* Samuel Weiser, now Red Wheel Weiser, Newberry Park, MA, (1969), p. 159.

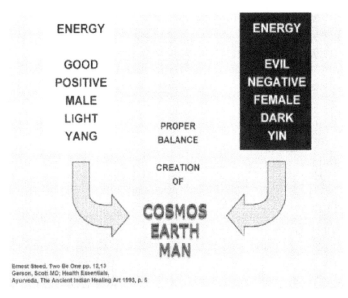

Figure 9. Blending together to create cosmos, earth

CORRESPONDENCE—ASSOCIATION—SYMPATHY

In this explanation for the origin of the cosmos, earth, and man, the belief was that there is close correspondence, association, and sympathy between the cosmos, earth, and man. In Maurice Bessy's book, *Magic and the Supernatural*, a figure of two circles is shown, one outer circle, and another inner circle, man, without stretched arms and legs is within the second circle. Surrounding the inner circle are the signs of the zodiac. Below this figure is the following explanation.

> A mirror of the world – "microcosm of the macrocosm." Man, as conceived in astrology, reflects the rhythms and structure of the universe in the same way as the universe mirrors the rhythms and the structure of Man himself. Everything is part of everything...[77]

It was believed that changes in man or the cosmos influenced the other. The planting of seed, the choice of food, all acts of life, in short, every action, it was believed, should be guided by the position of the planets.

This symbol of the circle around man is known as a "mandala," which in Sanskrit means circle. Though mandalas are of different designs they all represent the same idea–revealing the relationship of the cosmos to man. The outer circle represents the cosmos; the inner circle represents the earth, with

---

77   Bessy, Maurice, *Magic and the Supernatural,* Spring Books, NY, (1970), pp. 73-74.

the figure of a man in the inner circle representing the "at-one-ment" of the universe, earth, and man. This is a counterfeit of the "at-one-ment" with God that Jesus obtained for us on the cross. This symbol is often seen in New Age health literature. The lines drawn from the arms to leg, hand, and head form a five-pointed star (pentagram) which also represents the same belief.

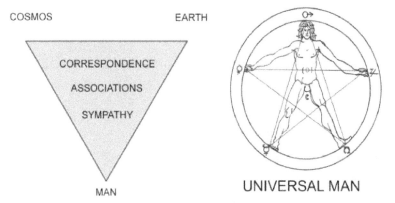

Figures 10. triangle of correspondence and circle with man

J.E. Cirlot, in his book *Dictionary of Symbols* under the title of "macrocosm-microcosm," makes the following comment:

> This relationship is symbolic of the situation in the universe of man as the "measure of all things." The basis of this relationship–which has occupied the minds of thinkers and mystics of all kinds in all ages–is the symbolism of man himself, particularly as the "universal man" together with his "correspondences" with the zodiac, the planets and the elements. As Origen observed: "Understand that you are another world in miniature and that you are the sun, the moon and also the stars."[78]

This implication is to be found in all symbolic traditions. Under the title "Man," the following statement is made,

Hence the pentagram (five-point star) is a sign of the microcosms,[79] and is a sacred symbol in neo-paganism. The ancient Chaldeans promoted the idea of unity of all things and applied it to every aspect of life. The *zodiac* was formed as a tool to apply this concept to life on earth and the practice of seeking guidance through the zodiac was referred to as reading ones *horoscope*.[80]

---

78   Cirlot, J.E., *A Dictionary of Symbols,* Philosophical Library, Inc., New York, NY (1962), p. 196.
79   *Ibid.*, p. 197.
80   Bessy, op. cit., pp. 67–74; Steed, op. cit., p.15.

In time, the zodiac system was consulted when making most of life's decisions.

> ...for astrology itself was based on an understanding and interpretation of these symbols in terms of the complexities of life and its origin and meaning. The zodiac was likened to a wheel with the changing times and seasons, but more so to the wheel of life. The Hindu sees it as the wheel of transmigration, the Buddhist as the wheel of completeness, and the Taoist of China, through the yang and yin and the circle of harmony; all visualize the correspondence or sympathy between opposites.[81]

The pagan religions originating in Babylon had their foundation in astrology and the zodiac, which are based on the belief of the existence of sympathy between the planets, earth, and man. The sun was the preeminent planet in the zodiac. To participate in a belief system that has the zodiac as a part of its beliefs is paying homage to Satan.

PAGAN'S STORY OF CREATION

> At first there was Chaos. From it pure light collected to itself and moved to create the sky. The darkness remaining moved and from itself formed the earth. From within this activity there arose two principles of yang and yin, light and dark, sky and earth. From this movement of like to like a balancing of forces occurred and growth and increase brought forth the beginning and the ten thousand creation, all of which take the sky and earth (yang and yin) as their mode. The yang (positive) is transformed by contact with the negative (yin) and so water, fire, wood, metal, and earth are produced. These five elements diffuse harmoniously and evolve into four seasons which proceed on their course. The two forces of maleness and femaleness reacting with and influencing each other bring myriad things into being. Generation follows generation, and there is no end to changes and transformations.

> *Insight Northwest* "The Healing Transformation, Some Lesser God, Keep The Hindu Creation Story:

> From this self, verily, space arose, from space, air, from air, fire, from fire, water, from water, earth, from earth, herbs, from herbs, food, from food, man.

> Taittiriya Upanishad 2:1 Reported in Ayurveda, Scott Gerson

---

81   Steed, op. cit., pp.15–16.

The Buddhist says:

"We have created our own bodies."

Foundations of Tibetan Mysticism, Govinda p. 159

These names of the basic elements, (water, fire, air, earth, metal, and/ or space) are not to be understood literally. They are words/synonyms of five planets, Jupiter, Saturn, Mars, Venus, and Mercury which are believed to be a continuing creative force in the cosmos and earth. There are no English words to adequately explain the concept.

Since the belief is that creation of all substance, animate and inanimate resulted from the balancing and proper mingling of the two aspects (good and evil, positive and negative, male and female, etc.) of so-called universal energy, it was felt that disease and illness were a result of an *imbalance* of these energies.[82] This energy, considered "god," is pantheism. "All is one and one is all,"—thus the belief that disease is a spiritual imbalance manifesting as physical disease.

It followed, then, that if an imbalance of energy caused health disorders, balancing would restore health. This led to a multitude of acts and practices designed to prevent and treat illness. As already noted, to treat an imbalance of energy, a myriad of methods were developed, which depended upon everything being categorized as good or evil, positive or negative, and yang or yin, etc. This approach to disease does not focus on following God's laws of health, nor recognizes disease as the body's response to violation of those laws.

Examples of substances used to restore balance are: herbs, minerals, climate and temperature, spells, dances, animal matter of all types, stones, liquids, relics, spoken words, written words, colors, flowers, zodiac influences, charms of all types, psychotherapy, magnetism, acupuncture, moxibustion, meditation, divination, numerology, music, sound, spirits, pictures, aromas, talismans, crystals, alchemy, foods, etc. All were labeled as being either positive or negative in their influence. Medical historian Garrison tells us that medicine did not progress as long as it was founded in the supernatural.[83]

The Scriptures teach that *separation* from evil, *not blending* with evil is God's way.

WORLDWIDE BELIEF IN ENERGY BALANCING

In the United States, many of the Native American Indians believe in dualism, and it is a principle they may apply in health and healing. Their

---

82   Steed, op. cit., p. 100; Garrison, op. cit., pp. 74, 88.
83   Garrison, op. cit., p. 24.

practices involve balancing animal spirits and/or energies. Navajo sand paintings are used to correct the believed imbalanced energies of those who are ill.[84]

The sand paintings are formed on the ground, and may take an entire day to make. A variety of plants, seeds, and other natural substances are used in forming the painting. There are hundreds of varieties of sand paintings, and are said to be kept in the head of the shaman. A sick person sits on the painting for several hours. Then the painting is scooped up, taken up and buried, as it is believed to have absorbed the excess spirit or energy of either the good or evil influence.[85] The sand paintings are made with colors and patterns representing dualism by containing contrasting objects, colors or positions.

The shaman, or medicine man, may also use dances, "sings" (groups of people singing about the sick person), or a bag containing various objects, as well as certain sounds to influence the spirits and powers that cause sickness. These methods are used as sympathetic remedies.

In the past, Europeans associated particular organs of the body with the specific houses of the zodiac. The symbols of animals taken from the zodiac were assigned to the organs. Aries the ram pertained to the head, while Pisces the fish was for the feet. When doctors determined an organ had an energy imbalance they chose a treatment that supposedly would influence the correspondence between that organ and its zodiac house.[86]

---

84   Bahti, Tom, *Southwestern Indian Ceremonials,* K.C. Publications, Las Vegas, NV, (1987), p.10.

85   *Ibid.*

86   Bessy, op. cit. pp. 73-74; Garrison, op. cit., p. 37.

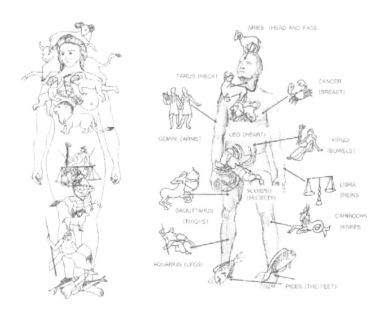

Figures 11. Man covered with animals representingassociation of man with zodiac

Remember that the zodiac is based on the planets with the sun as chief, and sun worship is Luciferic (Satanic) worship.

> His (Satan's) arts and devices are received as from heaven and faith in the Bible is destroyed in the minds of thousands. Satan here receives the worship which suits his satanic majesty...Satan uses these very things to destroy virtue and lay the foundation of spiritualism.[87]

THREE WORLD CENTERS OF MEDICAL INFLUENCE

In the old world, there were three great centers of learning that influenced the concepts in medicine over the last thirty-five hundred years. The *first* was on the Island of Kos where Hippocrates lived and practiced.[88] The *second* was the Indus River valley in India from where came Ayurveda. It is also where the

---

87   White, E.G., I *Testimonies,* Pacific Press Pub. Assn., Mountain View, CA, now Nampa ID, (1948), pp. 296.

88   Lyons, Albert S. M.D., Petrucelli, R. Joseph M.D., *Medicine an Illustrated History,* Harry N. Abrams, Inc., Publishers, New York, NY, (1978), p. 207.

Hindu religion had its roots.[89] The *third* was in China, the place of origin of Traditional Chinese Medicine.[90]

The ancient Vedas, written in the Sanskrit language, contain the story of the origin of Hinduism and its health and healing concepts. These writings are thirty-five hundred years old and were written by "Sages" (holy men) who retired into the foot-hills of the mountains and there:

> ...produced India's original systems of meditation, yoga, and astrology.[91]

This healing system is called *Ayurveda, the Ancient Indian Healing Tradition*. The Ayurvedic approach to health is not separate from Hinduism; *it is* Hinduism.

The *foundation* of all treatment for health and healing in Ayurveda is the *practice of meditation*. In fact, there is little help to be gained in other health and healing methods in Ayurveda without the use of meditation and yoga.[92] The practice of meditation is said to bring the inner self, the universal energy, the prana (air, breath), the *god* within us, to such a level that it would allow us to interact with the spirit entities, and eventually enter that same spirit state.[93]

The whole religious conquest of the Hindu is to escape this life and move into the spirit world. There is no separation between spiritual and physical in health and healing in Hinduism. It is said by an ex-Guru, who is now a Christian, that you cannot take Hinduism out of yoga and meditation, and you cannot have yoga and meditatin without Hinuism.[94]

Turning our discussion now to Chinese traditional healing, a common symbol represents the summation of their Tao beliefs. The *pa kua*, or circle of harmony, also showing eight syndromes of disease, (see chapter 8, Acupuncture and Chinese Traditional Medicine) represents constant transformation in order to achieve harmony and balance. It is a symbol of how another system of universal energy, called *chi* by the Chinese, relates to our bodies.[94]

There seems to be no contention between the different groups—European, Indian, or Chinese—over the different explanations of the supposed manner of distribution of "universal energy" within the body.

---

89   Gerson, Scott, *Ayurveda the Ancient Indian Healing Tradition* Shaftesbury, Dorset, (Element Books) Rockport, MA, (1993), p. 3; Lyons, op. cit., p. 105.

90   Lyons, op. cit., p. 121.

91   Gerson, op. cit., p. 3.

92   *Ibid.*, p. 78.

93   Willis, Richard J.B., *Holistic Health Holistic Hoax,* Stanborough Press Ltd., Alma Park, Grantham, Lincolnshire, England, (1997), Chapter 13.

94   Lyons, op. cit., p. 125; Steed, op. cit., p. 46.

Satan may use certain healing methods that may have some physiological basis, but it is wrapped up in his dogma. Those who believe in these concepts do not look to God as the restorer of health. Ellen White wrote:

> Angels of God will preserve His people while they walk in the path of duty; but there is no assurance of such protection for those who deliberately venture upon Satan's ground. An agent of the great deceiver will say and do anything to gain his object. It matters little whether he calls himself a "spiritualist," an "electric physician," or a "magnetic healer."[95]

> Satanic agents claim to cure disease. They contribute their power to electricity, magnetism or the so-called "sympathetic remedies," while truth they are but channels for Satan's electric currents. By these means he casts his spell over the bodies and souls of men.[96]

ENERGY BALANCING METHODS OF HEALING

The American Medical Association Committee for investigating alternative therapies has listed more than one hundred different methods of healing used and promoted today. The *Alternative Health Dictionary* lists more than four thousand names of various therapies of energy balancing. I list here some of the commonly used techniques. An alternative therapy would be defined as a therapy that does not have scientific evidence of effectiveness and usually has a history of use as a "folk medicine" therapy.

PSYCHIC THERAPY	AROMATHERAPY
ACUPUNCTURE	ESSENTIAL OILS
ACUPRESSURE	SONOPUNCTURE
MOXIBUSTION	LASERPUNCTURE
HOMEOPATHY	IRIDOLOGY
REFLEXOLOGY	POLARITY
MARTIAL ARTS	MARMA POINT MASSAGE
ROLFING	CHAKRA BALANCING
MAGNETIC HEALERS	REIKI
SOMA BODY WORK	COLOR THERAPY
RADIONICS	MERIDIAN THERAPY
MEDITATION	SOUND THERAPY
YOGA	GUIDED IMAGERY

---

95   White, E.G., *Evangelism*, Pacific Pres Pub. Assn., Mountain View, CA, (1946) p. 607.
96   *Ibid.*, p. 609.

TONING	VISUALIZATION
BIOFEEDBACK	ENERGY HEALING
TOUCH FOR HEALTH	VIBRATIONAL MED.
THERAPEUTIC TOUCH	ABSENT HEALING
PENDULUM USE	MAGNETS
FLOWER ESSENCES	PAST LIFE REGRESSION
CRYSTALS	ORTHOMOLECULAR
SOUND THERAPY	MEDICINE
TRANSCENDENTAL	CHANNELING MEDICINE

In the following chapters of this book, we will look carefully at several of these different healing methods. They all have the same basic foundation, that of being involved with moving and balancing a non-measurable, non-demonstrable vital force, energy, prana, chi, etc.

Why so many therapeutic approaches to balancing energy? Because none of them are based on true physics and science, but on the paranormal or psychic. It really matters little as to the physical method of therapy. It has a lot more to do with the mental attitude, and acceptance of the theory of *universal energy* or *intelligence*. It also strongly depends on the person administering the therapy and his connection to this unseen power. This *energy* has been given at least ninety different names, yet they all refer to the same thing. Of the men who gave so many names to this *energy,* it was found that the first fifty of them reviewed were channelers and psychics, and it may be that nearly all were.[97]

The rise and renewal of these ancient healing practices has been rapid, with no evidence of slowing. In the United States and other countries of the world, many of the medical teaching institutions have incorporated some of these practices in their curriculum. Physicians from around the world travel to China to take courses in Traditional Chinese Medicine. I have visited with medical students from Europe who were in China for a three-month rotation training in Chinese medical schools, with the primary interest in learning traditional Chinese medicine. Probably near fifty percent of hospitals in the United States have made available some type of *alternative therapy* because it is popular and the hospitals are competing for business.

The interest in alternative therapies is strong among the people of the Western nations, partly because it is marketed as *natural* therapy (without the use of drugs). People do not know the history of these treatment methods, and many believe that new knowledge has led to their use. Others believe that old

---

97   Wilson & Weldon, Occult Shock & Psychic Forces, Master Books division of CLP, San Diego, CA (1980), p. 247.

beneficial healing methods have been lost and are now being resurrected to our benefit.

A careful review of medical history will reveal that much of the philosophy behind alternative therapies comes from the ancient Indian healing methods called Ayurveda, from early European concepts of healing, and also from traditional Chinese medicine therapies. Earnest Steed, in his book, *Two Be One*, chapter 4, traces the influence of astrology via the zodiac upon the above-mentioned ancient systems.

Historically, there is no evidence that the nations that depended on these therapies benefited from them. Following are quotes from some medical history books:

> It follows that, under different aspects of space and time, the essential traits of folk medicine and ancient medicine have been alike in tendency, differing only in unimportant details. In the light of anthropology, this proposition may be taken as proved. Cuneiform, hieroglyphic, runic, birch-bark, and palm-leaf inscriptions all indicate that the folk-ways of early medicine, whether Acadian or Scandinavian, Slavic or Celtic, Roman or Polynesian, have been the same–in each case an affair of charms and spells, plant-lore and psychotherapy, to stave off the effects of supernatural agencies. Where this frame of mind persists, there is no possibility of advancement for medicine.[98]

> Until recently Chinese medicine has been what our own medicine might be had we been guided by medieval ideas down to the present time, that is, absolutely stationary.[99]

Where these therapies were used as the main method of medical treatment there was no improvement either in the incidence of disease or in longevity. China had an average life span in 1949 of 35 years. The approach in China toward the cause of disease changed and a scientific approach was instituted, with the establishment of hygienic and basic disease prevention methods based on present-day science. The average life span increased to 70 by the year 2000. (World Health Organization). This is considered one of the great medical events of the past century.

We are warned in the Scriptures of the devil's attempt to deceive God's people and that at the close of earth's history he will deceive all the nations.[100] In health and healing, his power will be especially strong, and those who are not diligent Bible students will find it very difficult to tell the real from the

---

98   Garrison, op, cit., p. 18.
99   *Ibid.*, p. 73.
100 Revelation 16:13, 14.

counterfeit. The true power of healing will come from God, the author and sustainer of our lives.

The counterfeit teaches that the origin and power that sustains us is from within. Accessing this power from within is said to affect health and healing. The majority of alternative therapies today are ways of attempting to access power from within, to balance good and evil characteristics, and bring about change and healing. Accepting these methods of treatment effectively means separation from God.[101]

This is the issue: Will we choose to follow God and have *eternal life,* or follow the devil and have *eternal death*? In the next chapter we take a more in-depth look at this so-called universal energy that has been divided into two parts resulting in the worldwide belief in dualism.

---

101   White, E.G., *The Ministry of Healing,* Pacific Press Pub. Assn., Mountain View, CA, (1909), pp. 428–429.

CHAPTER 5
UNIVERSAL ENERGY

False science is one of the agencies that Satan used in the heavenly courts, and it is used by him today. The false assertions that he made to the angels, his subtle scientific theories, seduced many of them from their loyalty to God.[102]

Satan presented the same temptations on earth that he had used in heaven.

The field into which Satan led our first parents is the same to which he is leading men today. He is flooding the world with pleasing fables.[103]

We are living in an age of great light; but much that is called 'light' is opening the way for the wisdom and arts of Satan. Many things will be presented that appear to be true, and yet they need to be carefully considered with much prayer; for they may be specious devices of the enemy. *The path of error often appears to lie close to the path of truth. It is hardly distinguishable from the path that leads to holiness and heaven.* But the mind enlightened by the Holy Spirit may discern that it is diverging from the right way. After a while the two are seen to be widely separated.[104]

Satan desired the worship of man, and to obtain such, he subverted the Biblical story of creation. He deceived man into worshiping the power and works of God but not God. Before the flood, man worshiped nature.[105] Shortly following the flood, nature worship again appeared as the dominant form of worship. God is proclaimed as an *essence, an actuating energy,* pervading all nature.

If God is an essence pervading all nature, then He dwells in all men; and in order to attain holiness, man has only to develop the power that is within him.... These theories, followed to their logical conclusion, sweep away the whole Christian economy. They do away with the necessity for the atonement and make man his own savior. These theories regarding God make His word of no effect.[106]

---

102   White, E.G., *Testimonies* Vol. 8; Pacific Press Pub. Assn., Mountain View, CA (Now in Nampa, ID), (1904), p. 290.
103   *Ibid.*, p. 290.
104   *Ibid.*, pp. 290–291.
105   *Ibid.*, pp. 293–294.
106   *Ibid.*, p. 291.

The essence, the *actuating energy* from which the universe, earth, and man are made, according to pantheistic theories, is called by many names. Different languages, cultures, religions, and leaders in pantheistic doctrine have created a large variety of terms which refer to the same theoretical power. Nearly one hundred of these different names have appeared in print. Listed below are some of the more commonly used terms

PRANA	HINDUISM
CH'I [KI, QI]	TAOISM [TCM]
LOGOS*	GREEK
MANA	POLYNESIAN
ORENDA	AMERICAN INDIAN
ANIMAL MAGNETISM	FRANZ MESMER
THE INNATE	CHIROPRACTIC
ORGONE ENERGY	WILHELM REICH
VITAL ENERGY	HOMEOPATHY
ODIC FORCE	OUIJA BOARD
BIOPLASMA	RUSSIAN PARAPSYCOLOGY
THE FORCE	STAR WARS [GEORGE LUCAS]

Many English synonyms are used to refer to this supposed power. "Universal Intelligence" is a name commonly used, as is the term "energy." I suspect each language likewise has many synonyms for this power. Listed below are several English synonyms.

ONE
SELF, HIGHER SELF, SUPREME SELF, DIVINE SELF, PURER CONSCIOUSNESS, HIGHER POWER
CREATIVE PRINCIPLE, SOURCE, "I AM"
ESSENCE
VITAL FORCE, VITALISM, LIFE FORCE
VIBRATIONAL FORCE
MONISM
ULTIMATE UNIFIED ENERGY FIELD
UNIVERSAL INTELLIGENCE, ENERGY
SUPREME ULTIMATE

In the world of pantheism there are varying descriptions as to how the *energy* (of which they say man is made) exists within man. The system of Ayurveda (ancient Indian healing art) describes the energy as localized in seven centers within man. These are called *chakras*. Man is said to have an "aura," produced by the chakras, which is *Life Force*, *Universal Energy* (*electromagnetic force* to some New Age scientists) and extends *outside* the body. It is to this perceived energy force that many alternative healing modalities direct their focus.[107]

> Two key words, microcosm and macrocosm, are used to portray the primary opposites, heaven and earth, thought to be in correspondence or sympathy.[108]

Macrocosm stands for the sun, moon, and stars, while microcosm stands for man. In pantheism, these two opposites, macrocosm and microcosm, must harmonize. The use of the "zodiac" was established in Chaldea to guide in achieving this harmony.[109]

UNIVERSAL ENERGY'S SEVEN DIVISIONS

In the Oriental view of universal energy there are *seven divisions* or levels of energy. This Eastern concept is accepted by neo-paganism (New Age Movement) of today. Understanding a little about this belief of divisions or levels of universal energy will be of value in comprehending the explanations of presumed power of various techniques applied in health and healing. At the same time, we will get a glimpse of some of the theology of the Eastern religions, making it increasingly clear that involvement in their techniques in health and healing might unsuspectingly lead to acceptance of their religious precepts.

---

107   Hill, Ann, *A Visual Encyclopedia of Unconventional Medicine,* Crown Pub. Inc. NY (1978), p. 46.
108   Bessy, Maurice, *Magic and the Supernatural,* Spring Books, NY, (1970), p. 74 Jaggi, O.P.; *Yogic and Tantric Medicine,* Atma Ram and Sons, Delhi, India, (1973), p. 96.
109   Bessy, op. cit. p. 67.

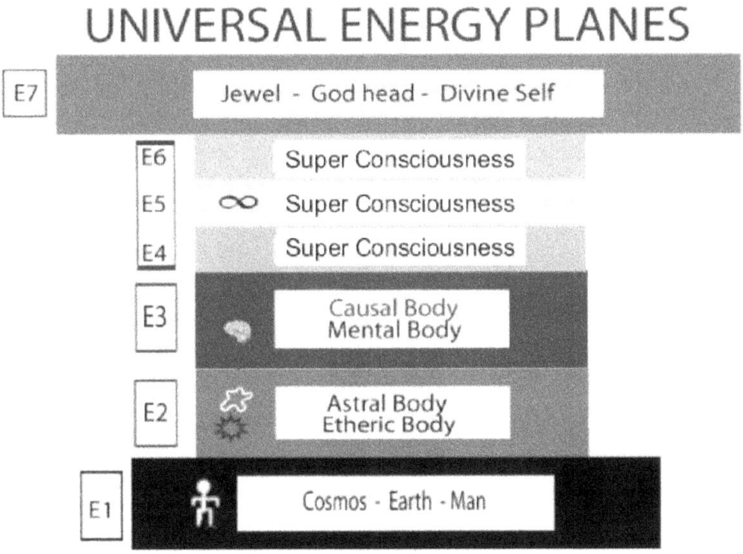

UNIVERSAL ENERGY PLANES

E7	Jewel - God head - Divine Self
E6	Super Consciousness
E5	∞ Super Consciousness
E4	Super Consciousness
E3	Causal Body / Mental Body
E2	Astral Body / Etheric Body
E1	Cosmos - Earth - Man

Figure 12. 7 frequency levels

Universal energy—life force energy is said by the New Age healers to be of seven levels or planes in distribution and function. Of late, an occasional New Age scientist will call this perceived energy, *electromagnetic energy*, which he believes to have specific vibrational frequencies at various levels. In this concept the bottom level frequency of energy has *materialized* and formed the cosmos, earth, and man. Dr. Gerber, a medical doctor, who is a very prominent New Age author, tells us in his text *Vibrational Medicine* that the other levels of universal energy have different and increasing frequencies above the speed of light.[110] The different levels of energy are believed to have specific progressive influences, first on the physical body, then on the spiritual path to godhood. The second and third levels are spoken of as having *subtle bodies*. In the days before the development of the science of physics, universal energy—life force energy was explained by the term, *spiritual power*, and different frequencies of light energy (not demonstrated by science) were not a part of their explanation.

The concept is that frequency level <u>one</u> contains the materialized cosmos including man, and is believed to be composed of energy traveling at the speed of light. The <u>second</u> level of frequencies involves *"subtle bodies"*. These hypothesized bodies surround the physical body and are even supposed to be of different colors. The first body, *etheric body,* or energy plane, is said to have

---

110 Gerber, Richard M.D., *Exploring Vibrational Medicine*, Sounds True, Boulder, CO, (2001), CD's discs 1 & 2.

the function of being an "electromagnetic" template of our physical body, and is believed to be the controlling influence in the function of our physiology. When imbalance is present in the etheric body, eventually the physical body will present with malfunction or disease. Many healing techniques are aimed at correcting or balancing the status of the etheric body. The next higher body is called *astral body*, which functions in the "out of body," "light in tunnel,"

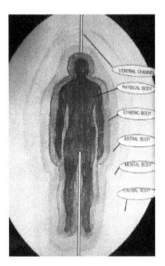

Figure 13. 7 multiple bodies

and "astral travel apart from body" experiences. The <u>third</u> level of frequency involves the *mental body,* and is said to deal with higher thought processes: We then come to the *causal body,* which functions in re-incarnation beliefs. It is said to store life experiences from *past and future lives*.

Death involves the physical body and it disappears, yet the "subtle" bodies continue on and receive the new re-incarnated body in whatever form it presents, animal or human, possibly in a lower caste, or hopefully, at a higher status.

Levels 4–7 of universal energy frequencies deal with increasing levels of "consciousness" and at the top, level 7 symbolized by the *lotus flower or* the *Jewel*, immortality— eternal life, is attained. This top level is said to interconnect with the energies of all the universe, and thus the expression *all is one and one is all, or as above so below*. It is at this level that immortality and *godhood* is said to take place."[111]

111   Green, Elmer and Alyce, *Beyond Biofeedback,* Knoll Pub. Co. Inc., Ft. Wayne, IN, (1977), pp. 299– 315.

A point of interest is the belief that plants contain higher frequency levels of energy. By consuming plants as our diet, we can obtain from them higher levels of consciousness. This is one of the reasons vegetarianism is common within neo-paganism.

The goal of neo-paganism of the West and the religions of the East is to attain to the energy frequency level of the lotus and the jewel attaining godhood and escaping reincarnation. All religious activities are directed to this concept. *Universal energy* as described in this chapter is the core foundational belief of Eastern religions and in Western occultism. The religious activities are for the purpose of raising energy frequency levels from the material, speed of light level, up through the higher frequency levels and eventually reach to the Ultimate level. Illness is considered a burp, a blurb in the progress of ascending to higher frequency planes and to godhood. A multitude of acts and practices in these religions are designed with the idea that they will raise a person to the experience of nirvana.[112],[113]

PANTHEIST'S EXPLANATION FOR CAUSE OF DISEASE

Illness and disease are explained in the pantheistic viewpoint as resulting from imbalance or blockage of the presence, and flow through the body, of universal energy. Therapies are designed to balance, unblock, restore, infuse, or otherwise manipulate invisible energies which allegedly exist or circulate within the human body.[114]

On the other hand, Divine energy does not circulate within the body through psychic pathways whose imbalance causes disease. We cannot manipulate the power of God by putting needles in our skin, by massaging pressure points, sitting in the yoga position, or by breathing exercises.

E.G. White wrote the following concerning *universal energy:*

The mighty power that works through all nature and sustains all things is *not*, as some men of science claim, merely an all pervading principle, *an actuating energy*. God is a spirit; yet He is a personal being, for man was made in His image. As a personal being, God has revealed Himself in His Son. Jesus, the outshining of the Father's glory, "and the express image of His person" (Hebrews 1:3), was on earth found in fashion as a man. As a personal Savior He came to the world. As a personal Savior He ascended on high. As a personal

112 Gerber, op. cit., discs 1, 2.
113 Prophet, Elizabeth Clare, *Djwal Kul Intermediate Studies of the Human Aura,* Dictated by Djwal Kul an ascended master also known as the Tibetan Master; Summit University Press, Colorado Springs, CO, (1974), pp. 27–31.
114 Ankerberg, John, Weldon, John, *Can You Trust Your Doctor?,* Wolgemuth & Hyatt, Brentwood, TN, (1991), p. 67.

Savior He intercedes in the heavenly courts. Before the throne of God in our behalf ministers "One like the Son of man." Daniel 7:13.[115]

Mrs. White often used the term *vital force* or similar expressions in her health writings. She was in no way expressing the same concept as that of *universal energy*. She referred to the normal metabolism and functioning of our body that depends upon being in harmony with the laws of health, and the proper association of our systems to pure air, sunshine, water, exercise, rest, proper diet, avoiding injurious substances, using with moderation beneficial foods and placing our trust in God by keeping His physical and spiritual laws. Under these conditions, our system will function at its best.

We have learned in chapter 4 of the foundational teaching of pantheism's explanation of our origin, that of blending two opposing parts of an imaginary universal energy. In this chapter we have looked at the many different names given to this energy. The concept is that illness and disease result from the imbalance of the two parts (yin-yang) of energy in our system. Treatment of disease in Satan's system is an act of attempting to rebalance the energy. In following chapters we will look at various methods devised to affect balance and/or correct the vibration of universal energy in order to bring about health and healing.

That which takes our allegiance away from a Creator God and directs our allegiance to His counterfeit, will make void the grace of Christ toward us. It makes His word of no effect.[116]

115   White, E.G., *Education*, Pacific Press Pub. Assn., Nampa ID,, (1903), pp.131–132.
116   White, E.G., *The Ministry of Healing,* The Pacific Press Pub. Assn., Nampa, ID, (1905), pp. 428–429.

CHAPTER 6

BABYLONIAN SPIRITUALISTIC MYSTERIESIN THE CHRISTIAN CIVILIZATION

An employee of a Christian publishing establishment in Russia missed work intermittently because of abdominal pain. Physicians could not discover the cause and eventually, this person was unable to work. He then sought the services of an alternative medicine practitioner. By feeling the ear of this employee, the practitioner diagnosed an infestation of round worms in the stomach and intestines. Medicine was prescribed, which caused the worms to be eliminated. The pain ceased and the employee returned to work.

A few months later, another employee developed abdominal pain. This individual heard an announcement on television about a certain healing technique and decided to try it. He sent to the TV healer a month's wages in rubles. He then taped one of his own coins to the monitor of his television, and a healing current was supposed to be transferred to the coin. In turn, the coin was then taped to his abdomen. The coin was to transfer healing energy to cure his abdominal pain, even though no diagnosis had been established.

The above two incidents initiated my receiving an invitation in 1998, to organize a seminar on Mystical Medicine. The seminar was to be presented to Health Educators of the Conferences of the Euro-Asian Division of Seventh-day Adventists. This division encompasses all of the countries of the former Soviet Union. Many of the health educators were nurses, dentists, and physicians.

The use of pagan healing methods in this part of the world was so endemic that it was considered regular medical practice; so much so, that these methods were incorporated into the practice of some physicians who had recently joined the church as well as a few who had been in the church for years.

It was a sobering task for us, as foreign doctors who did not use pagan healing techniques, to attempt to convince the Eastern European doctors that these pagan methods were wrong, especially since they used, believed in, and derived some income from use of these methods. We needed to demonstrate the intimate connection between the healing techniques and the doctrines of paganism. The previous chapter, combined with this chapter, is the result of that study. This information has proved to be a powerful influence in convincing individuals of the source of power in most non-conventional healing techniques.

To understand the rise, growth, as well as the coming out into the open, of mystical medicine in our day, we have to understand its past, and have a true understanding of its origins and author.

The pagan civilization continued the philosophy of the zodiac with its mystical concepts, and the doctrine of "dualism," since the dispersion from Babylon. Satan, the great Counterfeiter, was able to influence the people of Israel through the Canaanites, who were idol worshipers and practiced the mysteries of Babylon. For over 900 years Israel was harassed and intermittently succumbed to the influence of its pagan neighbors. Israel's captivity in Babylon in 606 B.C. effectively ended their idol worship.

Books covering medical history chronicle from the earliest civilizations, the advancement (or lack of it) during each succeeding civilization. It is interesting to note that information concerning the Jewish civilization is very brief, and no mention is made of any outstanding advancement in treatment methods. But there is one distinct difference. It was the only nation that practiced prevention and hygiene in dealing with disease. Careful study of the Bible will show that the health information God gave to Israel during the exodus focused on proper health habits and hygiene. No other civilization presented prevention as an approach to its health problems.

When the Jews returned from the Babylonian exile Satan devised another plan of attack whereby he could usurp their loyalty to God. This he accomplished by the infiltration of the Babylonian mysteries into their religion by way of a secret society.

SECRET SOCIETIES

Sometime following the return of the Jews to their homeland after seventy years of captivity in Babylon, a secret society began in Israel. No one knows for sure when this occurred, but it is believed by researchers that some of the Jewish priests, while in Babylon, probably began mixing their religion with Babylonian mysteries (the hidden knowledge based on astrology) and Zoroastrianism (religion of Persia). They carried back home with them this mixture in a society called the "Cabala" ("Cabbala" or "Kabalah" and "Kabbalah"), which is based on dualism.

> But esotericism again presents a dual aspect. Here, as in every phase of earthly life, there is the 'revers de la medaille' white and black, light and darkness, the Heaven and Hell of the human mind.[117]...

---

117   Webster, Nesta, *Secret Societies and Subversive Movements,* (Christian Book club of America, Hawthorne, CA, (1924) p. 3, Available through Emissary Publications, 0205 SE Clackamas Rd., # 1776, Clackamas, OR 97015, (503-842-2050).

Over time, the doctrine of the Cabala infiltrated and blended with Judaism, to such an extent that one author described it as:

...the heart and life of Judaism.[118]

The modern Jewish Cabala presents a dual aspect, theoretical and practical; the former concerned with theosophical speculations, the latter with magical practices.[119]

The Cabala uses a mystical approach to illness and its treatment. One method uses numbers and letters on "talismans" applied near the bed of the sick.

In the hill country of Israel, north of Galilee, is a small Palestinian town with a Jewish section, located at the peak of a small mountain.

The Sea of Galilee can be seen in the distance. This is Safed, considered one of the "holy" cities in Israel today. As you enter the town, a sign will tell you that this is the location of the school of the Cabala.

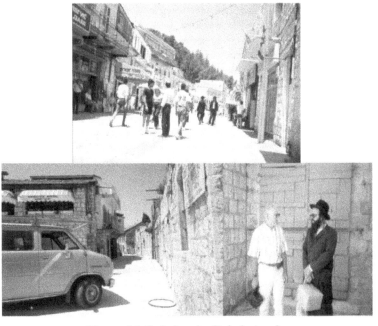

Figure 14. Safed and a Kabala teacher

118   Franke, Adolph, *La Kabbalah,* p. 288 (reported in Secret Societies, by Nesta Webster p. 9); Stehelin, J.P.; The Traditions of the Jews, p. 145 (printed for G. Smith in London 1742-43) (Above reference reported in Webster,(1922), op, cit., p. 9).

119   Webster, op. cit., pp. 12–13.

From the Cabala came the Gnostics, that sect which greatly opposed the Christian movement in the days of Paul and the Apostles.

> The Freemason, Ragon, gives the clue in these words: "The Cabala, is the key of the occult sciences, The Gnostics were born of the Cabalists."[120]

Simon Magus, whom Peter rebuked because he tried to buy the power of the Holy Ghost for the laying on of hands (Acts 8), is known in secular writings as the founder of Gnosticism. He was also a magician and was involved with mystical medicine. Legend has it that he became sorcerer to Nero, who had a statue made in his (Simon Magus) likeness and placed in Rome.

> In the *Dictionary of Christian Biography*, Vol. 4, p. 682, we read that "when Justin Martyr wrote his Apology (152 A.D.), the sect of the Simonians appears to have been formidable, for he speaks four times of their founder, Simon...and tells that he came to Rome in the day of Claudius Caesar (45 A.D.), and made such an impression by his magical powers, that he was honored as a god, a statue being erected to him on the Tiber, between the two bridges, bearing the inscription "Simoni deo Sancto" (i.e., the holy god Simon).[121]

The heart of the doctrine of these secret societies was pantheism, God in everything and everything God. The deification of humanity became a supreme doctrine of the secret societies. Nature worship, too, was an end result.

A major reference book of the Masonic order, *Morals and Dogma of the Ancient and Accepted Scottish Rite of Freemasonry* by Albert Pike, has a forty-page discussion of Gnosticism and its connection to Freemasonry. Of Gnosticism, Pike wrote:

> The Gnostics derived their leading doctrines and ideas from Plato and Philo, the Zend-avesta and the Kabalah, and the Sacred books of India and Egypt; and thus introduced into the bosom of Christianity the cosmological and theosophical speculations, which had formed the larger portion of the ancient religions of the Orient, joined with those of the Egyptian, Greek, and Jewish doctrines, which the New-Platonists had equally adopted in the Occident.[122]

---

120   Ragon, *Maconnerie Occulte*, Emile Nourry, Paris, (1853), p. 78; Reported in *Secret Societies* by Nesta Webster, p. 28.

121   Griffin, Des, *Fourth Reich of the Rich*, Emissary Publications, Clackamas, OR, (1989), (503–824–2050) p. 33.

122   Pike, Albert, *Morals and Dogma of the Ancient and Accepted Scottish Rite of Freemasonry*, Kessinger Publishing Co., Kila, MT, (1925), p. 248 (original publication 1871 In Charleston, South Carolina).

Pike, a past Sovereign Pontiff of Universal Freemasonry, traces the chronological growth and spread of the Mysteries over the face of the earth from ancient Babylon to the present-day Masonic Order. In reference to the esoteric doctrines of the Mysteries, he states.

> The communication of this knowledge and other secrets, some of which are perhaps lost, constituted, under other names, what we now call Masonry, or Free or Frank-Masonry. ...The present name of the Order, and its titles, and the names of the Degrees now in use, were not then known. .But, by whatever name it was known in this or any other country, Masonry existed as it now exists, the same in spirit and at heart, ...before even the first colonies emigrated into southern India, Persia, and Egypt, from the cradle of the human race (Ancient Babylon).[123]

These doctrines were preserved among the Christian civilization over the ages within the societies of the Kabbalah, Gnosticism, Manichaeism, various secret orders of the Islamic countries, Sufis, Knights Templars, Rosicrucian's, and Freemasonry. Notice the following conclusion by an author and researcher in this subject.

> Luciferian Occultism controls Freemasonry—Luciferian Occultism—is therefore not a novelty, but it bore a different name in the early days of Christianity. It was called Gnosticism and its founder was Simon the Magician.[124]

Satan's goal is to pervert Christianity with these concepts, and *counterfeit healing* is the right arm of his message. So it continues to this day. From the time of the early church through the ages to our day, these spiritual and healing mysticisms have been kept alive in the Christian community via secret societies with the aim of promoting, in disguise, the worship of Lucifer. Healing modalities are used to attract people, progressing on to the philosophical and spiritual teachings of their *theosophy*—pagan theology, see glossary.

The Babylonian mysteries were the basis of paganism and nature worship of the people who dispersed from Babylon, which today we recognize as the old religions of Egypt, Persia, Greece, India, Oriental countries, Americas, etc. The common core philosophy is *pantheism*. Their cosmological beliefs and teachings through time are reflected in their approach to medical care.

From French Freemasonry (Grand Orient lodges), greatly influenced by Illuminism at the end of the 18th century, arose various American and

---

123 *Ibid.*, pp. 207–208.
124 Miller, Edith Starr, *Occult Theocracy;* printed in France and no Publishing companies name given in the book, (Originally Published in 1933, not printed for general sale, reprinted in 1980, Hawthorne, CA. by The Christian Book Club of America, p. 33).

European secret political societies, the international banking elite, Marxism, and eventually the World Council of Churches. Nesta Webster in her book *Secret Societies,* reveals that the Freemasons of France gave support to the establishment in 1875 of the Theosophical Society in New York.[125]

NEW AGE MOVEMENT

In the 1970's the influence of all of the above-mentioned and other pantheistic societies came together to bring about what is now known as the New Age Movement. The expression East–West refers to the joining of Western occultism with Eastern mysticism.

With reference to the teachings of these societies, Albert Pike made the following statement July 14, 1889, to the twenty-three Supreme Councils of the World (His answer was recorded by A.C. De La Five in *La Femme et L'Enfant dans la Franc–Maconnerie Universelle* p. 588):

> If Lucifer were not God, would Adonay (the God of the Christians) whose deeds prove his cruelty, perfidy, and hatred of man, barbarism and repulsion for science, would Adonay and his priests, calumniate him? Yes Lucifer is God, and unfortunately Adonay is also God. For the eternal law is that there is no light without shade, no beauty without ugliness, no white without black, for the absolute can only exist as two Gods: darkness being necessary to light to serve as its foil as the pedestal is necessary to the statue, and brake to the locomotive. ...Thus, the doctrine of Satanism is a heresy: and the true and pure philosophic religion is the belief in Lucifer, the equal of Adonay; but Lucifer, God of Light and Good, is struggling for humanity against Adonay, the God of Darkness and Evil.[126]

In Revelation 11, we find a prophecy about a *Beast* that comes out of the bottomless pit. Adventists have understood this to refer to the spiritualistic power that was behind the French revolution in 1789- 1799, which brought in the Reign of Terror in 1793, and which controlled the country for three and one half years. Nesta Webster, in her book *Secret Societies and Subversive Movements,* credits the secret societies, more specifically the Masonic lodge of Paris called Grand Orient, controlled by the Illuminist, as the primary force behind the rise of radicals, anarchy, philosophy, encyclopedists, atheism, and the French revolution.[127]

125　Webster, op. cit., pp. 297–310.
126　Miller, op. cit., pp. 220, 221; Reported in Kah, Gary; *En Route to Global Occupation,* Huntington House Pub., Lafayette, LA, (1992), p. 124.
127　Webster, op. cit., p. 150.

Napoleon's rise to power in France lessened control of the government by this spiritualistic power but its influence continued "underground," and has grown worldwide in such movements as humanism, socialism, communism, etc. From the atheistic and spiritualistic movement of the French revolution sprang different organizations. Not all of them were atheistic; some were Deists, others were guided by ancient pagan doctrines somewhat similar to those taught by the modern Theosophy Society, which was started in New York in 1875. This society had great influence and ultimately helped usher in the *New Age Movement,* with all its mystical medical practices.

E.G. White frequently places the word *spiritualism* in conjunction with the word *theosophy* as she discussed this term. She wrote to a man entrapped in such:

> There is danger in having the least connection with Theosophy, or Spiritualism. It is Spiritualism in essence, and will always lead in the same path as Spiritualism. These are the doctrines that seduce the people whom Christ has purchased with His own blood. You cannot break this spell. You have not yet broken it.[128]

In the book *Education*, (by E.G. White) , it is stated that the fundamental doctrinal teachings of:

> Spiritualism asserts that men are unfallen demigods; that "each mind will judge itself;" that "true knowledge places all men above the law;" that "all sins committed are innocent;" for "whatever is, is right," and "God doth not condemn."[129]

We are admonished that the same spirit that prevailed leading into the French revolution of 1789 will return:

> ...the world wide dissemination of the teachings that led to the French revolution–all are tending to involve the whole world in a struggle similar to that which convulsed France.[130]

The Theosophical Society was founded in 1875 by Helen Blavatsky and Henry Olcott. Mrs. Blavatsky stated that she came from Tibet where she said she had been initiated into esoteric doctrines. Annie Besant, an English lady, was Blavatsky's successor in leadership of the Theosophy Society. She, (Annie Besant), became Vice-President of Co-Masonry (In France women had been

---

128 White, E.G., *Manuscript Releases,* Vol. 13 (nos. 1000–1080), (1990), No. 1000.
129 White, E.G., *Education,* Pacific Press Publishing Assn., Nampa, ID, (1903), pp. 227–8.
130 *Ibid.*

allowed to enter the Masonic Order in this branch called "Co-Masonry"). Mrs. Besant led the movement for three decades.[131]

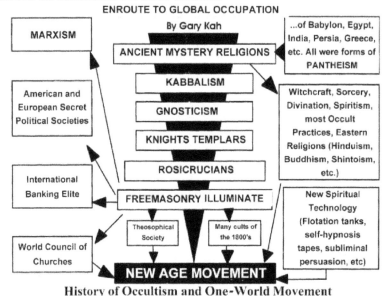

Figure 15.Graph of secret societies

Cardinal Caro Y. Rodriguez, Archbishop of Santiago, Chile, in exposing the Masonic Order, wrote:

> Madame Blavatsky, the promoter or founder of Theosophy in Europe, was also a member of the Masonic Lodge; her successor, Annie Besant, President of the Theosophical Society in 1911 was Vice President and Great Teacher of the Supreme Council of the International of C0-Masonry—and among us, in our city the brother masons are the ones that contribute mostly to the spread of the Theosophical Society.[132]

He summarized his comments on Co-Masonry as follows:

> It is understood: The theosophical doctrines on the nature of God and the soul, are the same doctrines as taught in masonry, it is enough to read of the International Order of Co-Masonry–and among us, the books dealing with the history of Theosophy to see that each theosophical center is founded, almost without a doubt by members of the Lodge.[133]

---

131 Kah, op. cit., pp. 89.
132 Rodriguez, Cardinal Carl Y., *The Mystery of Free Masonry Unveiled,* Haw thorne, CA, Christian Book Club of America, (1971), pp. 336, 238. Reported in Kah. op. cit., p. 90.
133 *Ibid.*

Nesta Webster, in *Secret Societies* and *Subversive Movements*, pp. 297-310, discusses the association of theosophy with the Grand Orient lodges of France.

The third leader in this movement was Alice Bailey who lived in the U.S. Under the guidance of a spirit guide (Djwhal Khul, also known as The Tibetan Master), she wrote more than twenty books from messages channeled from this spirit guide and which have been the foundation and guide for the New Age movement.[134] This movement is the major promoter of "mystical medicine" in the United States and around the world. It also has been very effective in drawing millions of people to the belief of theosophy.

Alice Bailey was closely connected to the Masonic Order. The following excerpt from her book *The Externalization of the Hierarchy*, states:

> The Masonic Movement—it is the custodian of the law; it is the home of the mysteries and the seat of initiation. It holds in its symbolism the ritual of deity, and the way of salvation is pictorially preserved in its work.[135]

Constance Cumbey, in her book *The Hidden Dangers of the Rainbow*, on p. 46, states that from her research she learned that the Theosophical Society, in 1875, received orders from "spirit messengers" that the organization was to remain secret for one hundred years. They worked quietly but were still able to spread their dogma to the world. In 1975 they went public with their presence and programs.[136]

EAST—WEST

In 1989, I began receiving at my medical office a journal called *New Age*. It contained only holistic-type medical articles. All of its advertisements were for products relevant to holistic health practices (techniques based on pantheistic concepts). I had no idea who sent it to me (it was an expensive magazine). In 1992, I read in a book, *Enroute to Global Occupation,* by Gary Kah, that someone had been able to make contact with the publishers of this journal (*New Age*) and inquired about advertising. They received a letter in return and on the letterhead these words identified the source of this journal, *"Ancient and Accepted Scottish Rite of Free Masonry."* Finally, I had the

---

134 Cumbey, Constance, *The Hidden Dangers of the Rainbow,* Huntington House Inc., Shreveport, LA, (1983), pp. 49–50.

135 Bailey, Alice, *Externalization of the Hierarchy,* Lucis Publishing Co., New York, NY (1983), p. 511. Reported in Kah, op. cit. p. 89.

136 Cumbey, op. cit., p. 46.

answer as to who was sending the journal to my office. The magazine soon thereafter changed its name to *East–West*.

Ellen White gave warnings about theosophical teachings.

> There are many who shrink with horror from the thought of consulting spirit mediums, but who are attracted by more pleasing forms of spiritism, such as the Emmanuel movement. Still others are led astray by the teachings of Christian Science, and by the mysticism of Theosophy and other Oriental Religions.[137]

In 1904 Mrs. White wrote:

> A power from beneath is working to bring about the last great scenes in the drama–Satan coming as Christ, and working with all deceivableness of unrighteousness in those who are binding themselves together in *secret societies.*[138]

> Today, the mysteries of heathen worship are replaced by the *secret associations* and séances, the obscurities and wonders of spiritualistic mediums. The disclosures of these mediums are eagerly received by thousands who refuse to accept light from God's Word or through his Spirit. Believers in spiritualism may speak with scorn of the magicians of old but the great deceiver laughs in triumph as they yield to his arts presented in a different form.[139]

Michael Howard (who is not a critic but a sympathizer of this pantheistic theology), writes the following:

> A very important work of the *secret societies* has always been the *ultimate unification of the world religions*. This aim was based on the restoration of the pre-Christian Mystery Tradition, which had been persecuted by the early Church and forced to go underground in medieval Europe, and the recognition that all religions had originated in a universal spirituality referred to as the *Ancient Wisdom*.

> ...It forms the basis for the ancient Egyptian Mysteries, Gnosticism, esoteric Christianity, the Cabbala, the Hermetic Tradition, Alchemy and societies such as the Templars, Freemasons and Rosicrucians, the occult doctrines of Geomancy, Alchemy, Astrology and sexual magic taught by these secret societies were

---

137   White, E. G., *Evangelism*, Pacific Press, Pub. Assn., Mountain View, CA, (1946), (now in Nampa, Idaho) p. 606.

138   White, E.G., *Testimonies for the Church* Vol. 8, Pacific Press Pub. Assn., Nampa, ID, (1948), p. 28.

139   White, E.G., *The Review and Herald,* The Fall of the House of Ahab, Jan 15, (1914), Review and Herald Publishing. Assn., Silver Spring, MD.

used as symbolic metaphors illustrating the progression of the individual from material darkness to the spiritual light of understanding.[140]

It is these organizations that are the powers behind the New Age Movement and its pagan system of health and healing has been the right arm of their missionary endeavors.

---

140   Howard, Michael, *The Occult Conspiracy, Secret Societies–Their Influence and Power in World History;* Destiny Books, Rochester, VT, (1998), p.170, 171.

CHAPTER 7

MEDITATION—AYURVEDA THE ANCIENT HEALING TRADITION OF INDIA- PART I

THE GREAT WISDOM OF THE EAST?

While attending a mini seminar on alternative medicine, I was impressed by the enthusiasm of those putting on this demonstration. When asked how these treatments work, the answer was "we do not know but it works." There was comment about the "great wisdom from the East." It was insinuated that great knowledge of healing from the past had been abandoned, but it was being resurrected and we were being recipients of it.

This comment brought to memory that which I had learned of the healing methods of the past, from the West and East, but I could not recall any knowledge in the history of medicine that we were neglecting. In fact, I could only give thanks that we had left most of the old knowledge to the past. This was especially true of the basic concepts of anatomy, physiology, and disease including the old concept of its cause. The old world view explaining man's existence, his purpose in life, and his future, is definitely not in harmony with the Biblical world view.

Therefore, I determined to prepare a presentation about the ancient healing methods of the East. The West has its own history in occult healing modalities, and today we see a blending of the two, hence the expression *East–West*.

Outside of God's original plan for health and healing, the oldest continuous system of medicine is called *Ayurveda*. It had its beginning in the Indus River valley in northern India sometime before 1700 B.C.

> ...It was established by the same ancient sages (holy men) who produced India's original system of meditation, yoga and astrology. Ayurveda has both a spiritual and practical basis,[141]

The word "Ayurveda" is derived from two words of the Sanskrit language. "Ayus" and "vid," meaning life and knowledge respectively. Ayus, or life, represents a combination of the body, the sense organs, the mind, and the soul.

---

141   Gerson, Scott M.D., Ayurveda, *The Ancient Indian Healing Art,* Element Inc., Rockport, Mass, (1993), p. 3.

The Ayurveda healing tradition is an integral part of the Hindu religion. *Vedas* are ancient Hindu books of knowledge said to have been "divinely revealed" to ancient sages (holy men). The Vedas, written in Sanskrit, were started more than 3500 years ago.[142]

The Vedas are believed to embody the rhythm, knowledge, and arrangement of the universe, the secrets to sickness, health and healing. As the living sage of astrology in India, Dr. B.V. Raman has written,

> The influences of planets on human diseases appear with such persistence that it is impossible to ignore their effect. The sun and the moon provide the strongest influence on human healing, and their movements indicate changes not only in the seasons but also in human health and behavior.[143]

> According to Ayurveda, everything in the material creation is composed of combinations of the five elements: space, air, fire, water and earth. These five elements derive from, and are the manifestations of, an unmanifest and undifferentiated *Creative Principle*, which is One. (universal energy).[144]

The *Creative Principle* is believed to manifest throughout the universe as *two great antagonistic forces* which continually create, sustain, and destroy all that exists in the universe. These forces (in Sanskrit) are called *rajas* and *tamas,* to the Chinese, yin and yang, (dualism). In Ayurveda, there is a belief that three psychic forces govern the mental and spiritual health. This system is derived from astrology.

> The basis of all treatments in the Ayurvedic system is the balancing of the life energies within us.[145] Meditation is a primary and fundamental tool in this balancing therapy which uses diets, herbs, mineral substances, and aromas as well.[146]

Ayurveda teaches that the "mind-body" has the intelligence and ability to heal itself. This intelligence is believed to operate in the macrocosm (cosmos) which also directs the yearly migration of birds, seasons and their changes, the movement of tides, the positioning and movement of the planets and stars in the universe, and also the human physiology referred to as the microcosm.

---

142 Lyons, Albert S. M.D., Petrucelli, II, R. Joseph M.D. , *Medicine, An Illustrated History;* Harry N. Abrams, Inc., Publishers, New York, (1978), p. 105.
143 Warrier, Gopi; Deepika Gunawan M.D., *The Complete Illustrated Guide to Ayurveda,* Barnes and Noble Books, (1997), p. 170.
144 Gerson, op. cit., p. 3.
145 *Ibid.,* p. 5.
146 *Ibid.*

It is the sole function of Ayurveda to promote the flow of this great intelligence (universal energy) through each and every human being.[147]

In the Hindu thought and in Ayurveda healing tradition, the *Creative Principle,* as an indescribable force, might be referred to as the unified energy field which underlies all of creation. Ayurvedic physicians see man simultaneously as energy and matter and view diseases in the same way.

The previous paragraphs have given very briefly the basic astrological—cosmological foundation from which Ayurvedic medicine is derived. We will now look at how it is applied. The dominant healing practice of India was Ayurveda. It is interesting that there was also conventional medical care. India was known for its advanced surgical skills during the dark ages, while Europe lost its skills and knowledge. So we had alongside each other, without apparent conflict, astrological—based practice of healing, as well as medical practice that was not based on the Hindu religion and cosmology. The basic therapeutics developed in Ayurvedic medicine gradually spread to the world: first to Tibet, then on to China, Japan and to the rest of the East. It also spread to Persia and the Arabian Empire in the eleventh century. In the middle ages it showed up in Europe,[148] and it is evident that in the United States its influence was present in methods of treatment in the 1700's and early 1800's.

In Ayurvedic medicine, two forces make up these supposed divisions of energy, together called *life force.* A third division of energy is added and is made up of parts of the other two.

Man is said to have had his *origin* from the mingling of these forces in a proper balance. In Ayurvedic teachings, health depends upon the perfect balance among the three forces.

When imbalance is present in these energy divisions, called *doshas,* dysfunction or disease supposedly occurs. It is believed that balancing the doshas will restore health. Ayurvedic medicine has as *its goal the balancing of doshas*, these divisions of energy.

The doshas are identified with the three supposed universal forces: sun, moon, and wind.[149]

---

147 *Ibid.,* p. 6.
148 Lyons, op. cit., p.105.
149 Raso, M.D., R.D., *Mystical Diets,* Prometheus Books, Buffalo, NY, (1993), p. 87.

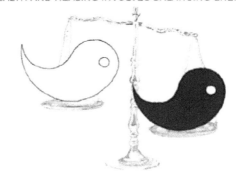

Figure 16. scales with yin and yang

CHAKRAS–AURA

Ayurveda teaches that there are *seven* centers of concentrated, focused, universal energy in the body, which collectively form an *aura*, an invisible light to the "non-sensitive," which surrounds a person. There are *sensitives* who say they can see the colored light of the aura. These energy centers start at the coccyx area and then are said to be located in the sacral, mid-abdomen, heart, throat, behind the eyes, and on the top of the head, all having connection to or close association with the spinal cord. A center is called "c*hakra,*" meaning "wheel," which can be considered a "whirling vortex" of energy. Think of a cyclone as a vortex of swirling cone shaped energy powered by hot air beneath and cold above, representing dualism. Dualism is incorporated in the explanation of the swirling energy of the chakra as being powered by doshas (rajas & tamas) to bring energy balance. Dualism is a foundational concept in Ayurveda and Oriental religions.

Chakras are supposed to promote and regulate the spread of universal energy to the organs of the body, each center focusing on distributing energy to certain organs in its anatomical area. The energy is distributed from the chakras via "nadis," which are invisible non- anatomical channels proceeding out from the chakras to carry energy. There is said to be 72,000 nadis.

Ayurveda is founded upon belief in the universal energy theory and postulate that all living objects have an energy field outside of, and surrounding the body, which is said to influence other energy fields. Seven rays of colored lights constitute this energy field, believed to represent seven endocrine glands. The harmony and energy balance of the individual can be ascertained by observing this aura. Ayurveda also teaches that:

> Every animate and inanimate substance, provided its function is not impaired, has an "aura", which exists because of the life forces inherent in the natural constituents of its form. This life force, whether from mineral, vegetable, animal or human sources, creates a common auric realm or plane, which is a storehouse of pure, untapped energy. On this plane the mineral and vegetable kingdoms are constantly engaged, through their own channels of communication, in transferring their particular life force to the more subtle natures of animals and humans. Thus the aura depicts the sum total of all these qualities and presents a complete and whole picture of the subject.[150]

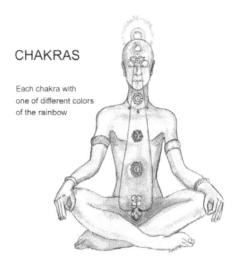

CHAKRAS

Each chakra with
one of different colors
of the rainbow

Figure 17 Chakras

Ann Hill, in her book *A Visual Encyclopedia of Unconventional Medicine*, describes the *aura* as seven rays of the *presumed* human unified energy field, forming seven colors. Each individual is said to have different frequencies of these rays. She tells us that the aura can be drawn by a trained *sensitive*, viewing the aura, or by observing some object an individual has handled. A *sensitive* of special skills is said to be able to determine a person's mental and spiritual state as well as to diagnose illness if present, by inspection of the aura. The nature of the color, bright or dull, reveals and determines the physical condition and/ or health, and also a person's spiritual status.

---

150   Hill, Ann, *A Visual Encyclopedia of Unconventional Medicine,* Crown Publishing Inc. NY, (1978), p. 46.

This *aura* or *magnetic energy field* cannot be demonstrated by science. It can be perceived only by persons who are *sensitives* or *mediumistic*.[151]

In the chapter on universal energy we learned about the hypothesized concept of the division of universal energy into seven electromagnetic frequency levels. The lowest frequency level is at the speed of light and all other levels are at a greatly increased frequency speed. This concept is not in harmony with known laws of physics that are understood today. The subject of the seven chakras is not the same as seven frequency levels. The lower chakras in their anatomical positions are said to handle and process energy at low levels of frequency and that higher chakras handle high frequency levels. Chakras are supposed to be able to act as transformers and convert low frequency levels of energy to higher levels, passing the energy up the chain of chakras and vice versa with the top chakras transforming high frequency energy into lower levels, passing it downward to the lowest chakra which is able to pass this energy into the physical body.

The higher frequency levels of energy are believed to come from the cosmos through the top chakra at the top of the head to be passed down the other chakras and eventually throughout the body. As a person is able to raise, by meditation and yoga, his *subtle energies* to the level of the top chakra those energies are interchanged with the energies of the cosmos. Also, plant food is believed to possess mid-level frequencies of energy; this, in turn, influences the middle level chakras. Universal energy also comes to the body via the air (prana) we breathe, which is believed to be a major source of subtle energy. The *aura* which is supposedly produced from the sum total energies of the seven chakras and emanates light outside of the body can be felt, seen, and influenced by an *aura* of another, by coming into close proximity, by application of hands, and with special procedures of sending energy over a distance to another.

---

151 *The New Age Movement and Seventh-day Adventists*, (1987), Biblical Research Institute
     of General Conference of Seventh-day Adventists, Hagerstown, MD, p. 9.

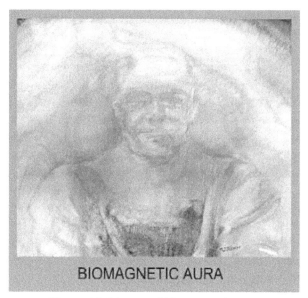

BIOMAGNETIC AURA

Figure 18. Picture of bio magnetic aura

The root chakra (chakra # 1 at the coccyx) is also regarded as the seat of *kundalini*. The *kundalini* is symbolized as a coiled serpent within the sacral/coccygeal region. The coiled serpent represents a powerful subtle force that is poised and waiting to spring into action. Only when the proper meditative and attitudinal changes have occurred does this force become directed upwards through the appropriate spinal pathway and activate each of the major chakras during its ascent to the crown. The kundalini is the creative force of manifestation which assists in the alignment of the chakras, the release of stored stress from the bodily centers, and the lifting of consciousness into higher spiritual levels.[152]

The chakras are said to be in the colors of the rainbow, with each chakra having a specific color. Each aura has a frequency of resonance or vibration and emits a fine electrical current and in turn can receive vital energies from external influences. This is the source of belief in *vibrational medicine.*" The human body is said to be a symphony of color, including the skeleton. The various colors we apply to the body with:

(a) ...clothing, walls, illumination, or (b) by mental image-making, counseling and guided meditation, (c) through projection, on the spiritual level, to any

---

152   Gerber, Richard M.D., *Vibrational Medicine, The # 1 Handbook of Subtle-Energy Therapies,* Bear and Co., Rochester, Vermont, (2001), p. 389.

person anywhere, is believed to build the forces and strength of the chakras and the aura to effect healing.[153]

When *magenta* an eighth color is added, an octave is produced and then music is also able to influence the chakras. Gems are known to refract light, dividing it into different colors. Sunlight consists of seven colors of the rainbow, so it is believed these refracted sunrays from gems can increase the energy (vibrations) of the chakra specific to each hue of sunlight.

The seven natural colors, with the added eighth *magenta*, are used in therapy when there is an energy imbalance. The colors are red, orange, yellow, green, turquoise, blue, violet, and the added eighth color, magenta. It is believed that these colors correspond with three musical octaves and with twenty-four vertebrae of the spinal column. Two additional octaves have been added, so that infra-red can be applied to the sacrum and ultraviolet to the skull.

> ...The colour therapist uses the spinal chart which is also employed by the music therapist and astrologer *to dowse* (use the pendulum) out the problem areas of a patient and thus determine which colour is to be used in treatment.[154]

Color therapy can be performed by placing water in a colored glass vessel and letting the sun shine through it. The water is then ingested, thereby applying color therapy to correct imbalances in the aura. This type of treatment is still practiced. It is not necessary to visualize color, as therapy can be administered even to blind people with equal benefit; it is believed, by having them drink the sunlight-exposed water.

Nutrition and dietetics figure importantly in many of these healing systems. For example, in the yoga-oriented *Spiritual Nutrition and the Rainbow Diet* (1986), Gabriel Cousens, M.D. , states:

> By putting foods of various colors over each chakra (spiritual center of the human body), I was able to determine which colors were most enhancing for each chakra.[155]

The aura (composite energy) of a person is also believed to be influenced by sound and/or music. Music therapy is another method of restoring an imbalanced aura.

Each animate and inanimate object is also believed to have a specific energy frequency or vibration. (Not all believers in the aura accept that

---

153   Hill, op. cit., p. 219.
154   *Ibid.*, p. 218.
155   Raso, op. cit., p.13.

inanimate objects have an aura.) These vibrations are altered when disorder is present in the body. It is claimed that detection of altered vibrational forces can be done by the hands, Kirlian photography, or by Radiaesthesia using electronic instruments. Energy therapies and vibrational therapies, of which there are many varieties, seek to understand this continuous energetic aura, and to interact with it in order to facilitate health and healing.

The above-described beliefs and teachings of Ayurvedic medicine form the foundation of many ideas that are widespread in the field of alternative therapies today. I wish to make it clear to the reader that the above-described beliefs are not accepted in the sciences of medicine, physics and physiology. The detection of the basic energy, which is the center core belief of alternative therapy, cannot be found or measured by even the most sensitive instruments, a discrepancy that cannot be explained by its adherents.

I recommend an article found on the Internet, *Human Auras and Energy Fields* by Don Lindsay,[156] which discusses the subject of auras and whether or not science can demonstrate such. The following is his summary:

Humans do not have auras. There is no kind of 'energy field' consistently found around humans. I say this for a bunch of reasons:
- It is the consensus of the scientific and medical communities.
- Proponents have had a lot of years to produce positive evidence.
- Negative evidence from equipment.
- Negative evidence from photography.
- Negative evidence from those who see auras.
- Negative evidence from those who feel auras.

For those readers who might wish to further investigate the argument that there is proof of auras, I suggest the following specific article that claims there is scientific proof.

Spring Wolf's Spiritual Education Network
CHAKRAS & MAGICThe Aura the Colors of Life[157]

It is important not to confuse the claimed energy of the chakra and aura of Ayurveda, with the bio-electrical activity of living matter. There is certainly electrical activity within our bodies as is demonstrated by electrocardiographs, electroencephalographs, electromyography, etc. To do any of these tests it is necessary to either place needle probes into and under the skin, or to prepare the skin by sanding the outer layer of cells free to make good electrical contact

---

156   http://www.don–lindsay-archive.org (Q-auras)
157   http://sacredwicca.jigsy.com/chakras

on the skin. With the proper contact, electrical activity is then demonstrated in muscles and nerves. No electrical machines have shown electrical activity of a chakra, or of an aura inside or outside of the body. There is instrumentation that is one million times more sensitive than the living tissue of our bodies.

However, these electrical measuring instruments do not show evidence of Chakras—inside, or auras—outside the body. Not all practitioners of Eastern mysticism accept the explanation that universal energy can be explained by conventional physics and object to the term *electromagnetic* in describing such. They believe that universal energy is a spiritual entity, and that it cannot be described by common scientific terminology. Many modern scientists who are believers of Eastern mysticism do, however, attempt to explain their beliefs by scientific terms. Some psychics claim to be able to see the aura in color around individuals. When put to the test on these claims, they failed. If light from the believed *aura* did surround our bodies we might see rainbows about us when we are in the rain and the sun shines through the clouds. It would be very easy to demonstrate the colors of the rainbow by an optical prism held near the body if light was flowing from us, but this does not happen. The colors of the rainbow are light wave frequencies that are detected by the eyes of all of us, not just psychics or sensitives.

Dr. Elmer Green, who has his doctorate in physics and is a lifetime believer in Eastern mysticism, explains this concept: This universal energy, which is in question with science, exists in seven levels or degrees. The first level is the materialization of the energy and that is the material world around us. The other six levels are not measurable by instruments because those levels are beyond instrumentation detection. Only the human body is capable of detecting such (see chapter 19 on biofeedback). It is taught that these different levels of energy can exist simultaneously within the human body.

Oriental religions have as their purpose and goal in life to escape the cycle of reincarnation in which they believe they are caught up and to join the spirit world. They do this by a lifelong pursuit of raising the energy levels in the body up through the chakras to bring it to its peak performance at the seventh chakra on top of the head. The religious activities of the Hindu and other oriental religions are all for the purpose of maintaining an unhindered flow of universal energy, so as to raise the energy level to its zenith at the top chakra. Meditation and yoga are believed to raise kundalini and clear the chakras to allow the rising of universal energy, and their existence is solely for this purpose. When the universal energy comes in full power to the top chakra, a person's energy level has meshed with the energy of the universe and one experiences enlightenment, the Supreme Self, Lotus, Jewel, *Godhood* status. The reincarnation cycle is then broken and at death of the physical body the soul will assume its position with the spirit world of nirvana.

During the pursuit of immortality status described above, disorder or illness of the physical body may occur. This is understood simply as an interruption of flow of universal energy through the body and corrective measures have been invented to correct and bring about the continued free flow of energy. It is those therapeutic methods that constitute many of present day alternative medical therapies. It is vital to have understanding of the foundational doctrine of the Oriental religions so as to recognize their counterfeit of God's healing system and the false science proclaimed.

Meditation and yoga are simple, yet powerful techniques believed to open, activate, and cleanse congested or blocked flow of energy in chakras. Their most common use in America is for "relaxation," however, meditation is far more than that. It opens the mind to connect to the cosmic energies, the universal mind, the *Higher Self,* (*the pantheistic god*). We are told that the Higher Self holds the solutions to many of our problems.[158]

Understanding the tenets of Ayurveda and Hindu's basic dogmas is critical to understand therapeutic methods to be exposed later in this book. A vast amount of New Age doctrines and therapies are based upon the principles of what has been presented.

MEDITATION

Ayurveda uses meditation as a primary and fundamental tool for healing. It also promotes yoga, diet, herbs, mineral substances, cleansing practices, and aromas for maintenance or restoration of energy balance. Meditation and yoga are fundamental *tools* of Hinduism for progression to a higher spiritual plane, with the goal of leaving this life on earth and moving on into the spirit world. In Ayurvedic medicine, meditation is fundamental to accessing the powers of the cosmos in order to bring increase and balance of the energies within a person. It is also a process, physically and mentally, of trying to elevate the believed *divine* attributes within self and connect with the god of the cosmos, *Brahman*, the ultimate deity of Hinduism. Meditation, whether for health or spiritual reasons, is a way of *connecting with the spirit world*. It is through meditation that blending of the sun and moon energies are said to occur. When a perfect blend is achieved, immortality is said to be the result. Immortality is believed to bring perfect harmony with Brahman, the ultimate Hindu Deity.

The above is the Hindu plan of salvation (counterfeit of God's plan), the journey to nirvana, their heaven. It is centered in the dogma of *Self—Divine within*. By physical and mental acts it is believed that the divine within can be manipulated, resulting in progression to immortality, nirvana, and godhood. Physical disorders are considered simply a spiritual malady. Therapy is

158   Gerber, op. cit., p. 394.

anticipated not only to relieve physical and mental distress but to restore the individual to the path of progression to godhood.

Ayurveda declares the *essence* of the human being to be the *One*, the *Creative Principle, The Eternal Essence*. A Hindu physicist might describe this essence as the *ultimate unified energy field,* which Ayurveda says underlies all of creation. Humans are seen as energy converted to matter, and disease as deranged energy. This life energy, also called *prana,* is believed to be enhanced through meditation, yoga, deep breathing, herbs, cleansing, and foods. Life energy (prana) is proclaimed to increase with deep breathing of air *through the nose.*

> Of all the many forms of treatment described in the Ayurvedic texts, there is one which holds a pre-eminent position–*the practice of meditation.* This is the fertile soil upon which all other forms of therapy take root. Strictly speaking, without meditation the true healing potential of Ayurvedic medicine cannot be realized.[159]

The English word *meditation* has two definitions

1. Study, contemplation, pondering, on or about a subject by an active thought process.
2. Putting the mind into a passive, neutral—no thought mode, stilling the mind, ridding our mind of all thoughts, the silence, and so develop an altered state of consciousness.

In our discussion of *meditation* in the Ayurveda system we refer to this second definition. To enlarge upon the above definitions think of it in this way: study, contemplation, and pondering can be thought of as looking outward and upward, while the passive mode puts our thoughts inward and downward.

How does one bring about the non-thinking state? We find an answer in *Meditation as Medicine* p. 25 by Dharma Singh Khalsa M.D.

It is achieved by the powerful effects of:

1. the breath
2. a mantra (repetition of word or phrase)
3. focusing the mind
4. posture and movement including finger positions[160]

---

159   Gerson, op. cit. p. 78, 79.
160   Khaalsa, Dharma singh, M.D., Stauth, Cameron, *Meditation as Medicine,* fireside Rockefeller Center, New York, NY, (2001), p. 25.

Of the four acts given above in performing meditation the *two* most common and important are attention to *breath,* and repetition of a *mantra.* As the mind focuses on the breathing pattern, and at the same time on the repetitions of a word or phrase, a thoughtless state of the mind is triggered. The word *mantra* is from the Sanskrit language with the syllable "*man*" meaning "to think" and "*tra*" referring to liberation of thinking." By an act and process that stops the mind from thinking, the mind is *stilled.* The subject of movement will be explored further in the discussion of yoga. Meditation and yoga go together like a hand in a glove. Yoga will be presented later in the next chapter.

Meditation is practiced in many forms and by many names, some we probably have not recognized as being meditation. In his book *Meditation as Medicine,* Dr. Khalsa lists the following practices as being considered meditation using a common element—relaxation.

- Prayer—contemplative prayer, breath prayer, silence; (uses breath & mantra)
- Visualization—an *act of creation* by imagination, using god— power from within
- Sufi meditation—found in Islam, "whirling Dervishes," feverish dancing
- Guided Imagery—similar to visualization, minimizes thinking in words
- Mindfulness—Buddha type meditation, mind wanders as it focuses on breath
- The Relaxation Response—meditation, named so as to disguise, by Herbert Benson M.D.
- Transcendental meditation—with secret mantra, brought to USA by Maharishi Mahesh Yogi and popularized by the "Beatles"
- Zen Buddhist meditation—way to enlightenment, world view—one is all, all is one
- Native American meditation—drums, psychedelic herbs, crystals
- Movement meditation—tai chi, qi gong, martial arts
- Medical meditation—meditation combined with yoga and specific postures of body, limbs and fingers. Khalsa says--most powerful type of meditation.[161]

Continued practice of meditation over time causes gradual changes in the mystical subtle-energy flow through the chakras. They are slowly activated and cleared of any obstruction of flow, such as past traumatic emotional events, that of frustration, or anger, etc. Over time meditation will initiate a

---

161   *Ibid.,* p. 40

rise of *kundalini*—serpent power which is believed to be in the bottom chakra, forcing its climb up the subtle energy pathways (chakras) and within the spinal cord on its journey to the crown chakra and *enlightenment—godhood*.

Meditation and yoga are fundamental *tools* of Hinduism for progressing to a higher spiritual plane, with the goal of leaving this life on earth and moving into the spirit world. In Ayurvedic medicine, meditation is fundamental to accessing the powers of the cosmos in order to bring increase and balance of the energies within a person. It is also a process, physically and mentally, of trying to elevate the believed divine attributes within self and connect with the god of the cosmos, *Brahman*, the ultimate deity of Hinduism. Meditation, whether for health or spiritual reasons, is a way of connecting with the spirit world. It is through meditation that blending of the sun and moon energies are said to occur. When a perfect blend is achieved, immortality is the result. Immortality is believed to come from being in perfect harmony with Brahman, the Hindu Deity.

Transcendental meditation was brought to the USA by Maharishi Mahesh Yogi in 1957 and popularized by the Beatles music group, and is a slight variant style of meditation. A secret word is given to each initiate. Unbeknownst to the initiate, the word is a title or name of a Hindu god. Hunt and Weldon comment on this secret mantra in *America The sorcerer's New Apprentice* p. 31 stating that from authoritative texts, not only is the mantra the name of a Hindu god, but by reciting it over and over one is calling on that god to possess them. TM (Transcendental Meditation) worked its way into the New Jersey Public School system and parents sued saying that it was a religion, but TM lawyers argued that it was a science. The New Jersey Federal Court decided it was a religion and banned its presence in the schools. (Malnak V. Yogi, 440 F. Supp. 1284-1977) The decision was appealed, and on Feb. 2, 1979 the first court decision was upheld. TM thereafter took out every word in their written material that would indicate that it was religious, and it has since spread across the US as *science*. Below is the pledge to Maharishi that every teacher of TM has to sign.

"Serve the Holy Tradition and spread the light of God to all those who need it." Yet every TM teacher claims in his public lecture, "TM is not a religion."[162]

Dave Hunt in *Yoga and the Body of Christ* pages 12-16 exposes the planned and designed missionary movement of Hinduism that has spread to the world. He shares with the reader that the largest missionary organization in

---

162   Weldon, John, *The Transcendental Explosion,* Irvine harvest House, (1976), pp.23-4; reported in Wilson and Weldon, *Occult shock and Psychic Forces,* Master Books, a Division of CLP, p.35.

the world is Hindu—India's *Vishva Hindu Parishad* (VHP). Also, in January 1979, this organization sponsored a second "World Congress on Hinduism" in Allahabad, India, and with 60,000 delegates attending. This organization had first attempted their mission activities by promoting religion, but that was not successful. So they made a change by presenting it as science. A speaker at the 1979 congress made the following comment:

> Our mission in the West has been crowned with fantastic success. Hinduism is becoming the dominant world religion, and the end of Christianity has come near.[163]

The VHP organization has centers all over the world, with a branch in the USA called Vishwa Hindu Parashad of America, Inc.

We were warned long ago concerning mind therapies and spiritualism coming in as science:

> The sciences of phrenology, psychology, and mesmerism have been the channel through which Satan has come more directly to this generation, and wrought with that power which was to *characterize his work near the close of probation.*[164]

> In these days when skepticism and infidelity so often appear in a scientific garb, we need to be guarded on every hand. Through this means our great adversary is deceiving thousands and leading them captive according to his will. The advantage he takes of the sciences, *sciences which pertain to the human mind,* is tremendous. Here, serpent-like, he imperceptibly creeps in to corrupt the work of God.[165]

The practices of yoga and meditation are not without their dangers. Suicide is high among the instructors, demon possession, psychopathology, psychosis, epileptic seizures, hallucination, blackouts for hours, eyesight problems, extreme stomach cramps, mental confusion, sexual licentiousness, severe nightmares, anti-social behavior, recurrence of psychosomatic symptoms, and depression requiring psychiatric care. *America the Sorcerer's Apprentice* page 51, states so severe and so common are abnormal reactions to meditation and yoga that in 1980 John Hopkins University School of Medicine professor Stanislave Grof (expert in LSD) and his wife Christina (instructor

---

163   Hunt, Dave, *Yoga and The Body of Christ,* The Berean call, (2006), OR, p. 13.
164   White, E.G., *Messages to Young People,* Southern Publishing Association, Nashville, TN, (1930), p. 57.2.
165   White, E.G., 1 *Mind, Character, and Personality,* Southern Publishing Association, (1977), p. 19.

in Hatha Yoga) organized the "Spiritual Emergency Network" (SEN), now headquartered at California Institute Of Transpersonal Psychology in Menlo Park, California. By 1988 the organization (SEN) was coordinating 35 regional centers and utilizing 1500 professionals in attempting to handle psychological emergencies resulting from the mind altering practices of meditation and yoga.

Dr. Khalsa tells us in his book that the R*elaxation Response*, which Khalsa identifies as a *form of meditation*, was made popular by Harvard's Herbert Benson M.D.

> ...He [Benson] made meditation palatable to the medical community.[166]

The Office of Alternative Medicine, or OAM, which is a part of the National Institutes of Health has funded many studies on meditation. A 1994 report stated that:

> ... over a period of 25 years, Benson and colleagues have developed a large body of research." "meditation in general and the relaxation response in specific have slowly moved from alternative to mainstream medicine, although they are still overlooked by many conventional doctors.[167]

The techniques used in Benson's Relaxation Response are identical to those used in all other forms of meditation, namely concentration on breathing, posture or position of comfort, passive attitude, and use of a mantra. Unfortunately, there have been people who have not recognized the Relaxation Response for what it is, and using a Biblical term or verse as a mantra have felt it was just what its name speaks of, a simple measure to bring relaxation. Unfortunately it is much more than that. It, too, is a technique to still the mind, to bring in passivity to the thinking and allows an altered state of consciousness. There are physiologic changes in our autonomic nervous system when the relaxation response is used such as in the amount of oxygen consumed, and apparently many healthful changes can occur without use of drugs. Yet in that state we open our mind up to the possibility of contact with and control by powers of darkness.

These meditation or relaxation techniques have demonstrated decrease in oxygen consumption by the body, lower hydrocortisone blood levels, increase in immune factors (including increased leukocytes), and it calms brain wave activity. These benefits remain for several hours following meditation. Yes, these methods do have an effect on our physiology, however, we must determine what the source of this power is and influence upon our systems.

---

166 Khalsa, op. cit., p. 7.
167 *Ibid.*, p. 41.

Has there been a comparison of this apparently harmless technique with other forms of meditation? Yes, it was compared to Transcendental Meditation, the results of which are summarized in the following statement:

> Tests at the Thorndike Memorial Laboratory of Harvard have shown that a similar technique used with any sound or phrase or prayer or mantra brings forth the same physiologic changes noted during Transcendental Meditation: decreased oxygen consumption; noted during Transcendental Meditation: decreased oxygen consumption; decreased carbon-dioxide elimination; decreased rate of breathing. In other words using the basic necessary components, any one of the *age-old* or the *newly derived* techniques produces the same physiologic results regardless *of* the mental device used.[168]...

Are these changes from simple relaxation of our nerves, or is there another power apart from our Creator God at work? If another power, then from where? That is the question. Have I made accusation against innocent techniques? A question I have asked multiple times of myself. Well, I find that those involved in leading out and teaching in the field of meditation and yoga have included the Relaxation Response technique as one of their own, but simply changed to an acceptable name.

How an individual becomes interested in, or starts practicing yoga and/ or meditation has much to do with whether they continue. When a doctor recommends this practice to deal with certain medical problems the tendency to stay with it greatly increases. Frequent articles appear in medical literature proclaiming the medical benefits of yoga and meditation, so we see an ever increasing acceptance by the medical profession.

Herbert Benson M.D. , a Harvard University Medical School professor and president of the Mind/Body/Medical Institute in Chestnut Hill, Mass., tells in his book *The Relaxation Response* that his research group has studied all the forms of meditation used down through millennia by various religions. His research found certain essential acts paramount to reaching the altered state of consciousness and/or autonomic nervous system influences sought by the act of meditation. These are: comfortable position; muscular relaxation; deep rhythmic breathing; use of a mantra; all to bring the mind to a state of *passivity*. The mantra can be a word, phrase, sentence or even a Bible verse.

You may have been surprised to see "prayer" listed as one of the forms of meditation. How can that be? Is not prayer a dialogue with God? The Bible has recorded many prayers, and Christ prayed and taught his disciples to pray. Daniel chapter 9 reveals Daniel pleading with God to forgive Israel and fulfill

---

168   Benson, Herbert M.D., *Relaxation Response,* Wings Books, distributed by Outlet Book Company, Inc., Avenel, New Jersey, (1992), pp. 162, 163.

His pledge to return them to Canaan; John 17 contains a prayer that Christ prayed to His Father in heaven the night of his arrest. Are we to look at those prayers in the Bible as falling under the definition of "meditation" as we have previously defined it? The King James version of the Bible has fourteen places where the word meditate is used and six times for meditation. King David utilized that word the most, with Psalms 119 as the focus of its use:

> O how love I thy law! It is my meditation all the day.(Psalms 119: 97)

> But his delight (is) in the law of the LORD; and in his law doth he meditate day and night. (Psalms. 1: 2)

What is the real difference in the use of the words *meditate and meditation* as they are used in the Bible, in contrast to their meaning in the preceding paragraphs? Prayer, as found in the Bible, reveals man seeking God and opening his heart to him, inviting Him to be Lord of his life. The definition as understood in the use of meditation in previous paragraphs is the same definition as for a "mystic" that is.someone who uses rote methods to tap into their inner divinity.[169]

> Biblical style: But when ye pray, use not vain repetitions, as the heathen do: for they think that they shall be heard for their much speaking. Be not ye therefore like unto them: for your Father knoweth what things ye have need of before ye ask him. (Matthew. 6: 7, 8)

Few Christians would choose to be involved in the standard meditation and yoga practice, but is it possible that they might choose to do so when it has been given a new name and are told it is a way to come closer to God? Is that happening? Yes, it is sweeping through the Christian world community. The words of Paul ring out:

> Now the spirit expressly says that in later times some will depart from the faith, giving heed to deceiving spirits and doctrine of devils. (I Timothy 4: 1)

An early book to reach millions of people by promoting an apparently benign form of meditation was *Creative Visualization* in 1978 by Shakti Gawain. Ray Yungen tells us that this book could well be called the *mystics Bible.* This book promoted improved creativity, career achievements, relationships, health, relaxation, and peace. It caught on with the public as few

---

169 Yungen, Ray, *A Time of Departing,* Lighthouse Trails Publishing Company, Silverton, Oregon, (2006), p. 34.

books do and gained the attention of people that were not of the New Age community. Below is a quote from the book:

> Almost any form of meditation will eventually take you to an experience of yourself as source, or your higher self...Eventually you will start experiencing certain moments during your meditation when there is a sort of *click* in your consciousness and you feel like things are really working; you may even experience a lot of energy flowing through you or a warm radiant glow in your body. These are signs that you are beginning to channel the energy of yourself.[170]

(Emphasis authors)

Ray Yungen, an Evangelical minister has researched and followed for forty years the movement that is promoting a special type of prayer referred to as contemplative prayer, centering prayer, sacred space, silence, etc. The methods used in these prayers fit the criteria for mystic meditation. Youngen has written a book *A Time of Departing* which identifies and traces the origin, ancient history, recent history, and present influence and use of these mystical prayer techniques. He lists in his book authors who have written books promoting these prayer practices. These books have sold beyond belief. One set of authors sold fifty million copies, another author twenty million and a third seven million. Since then, there have been scores of books on the same topic by as many different authors.

What makes the practice of these special prayers so popular is that mediators using the prayer methods do get the *click* that Shakti Gawain spoke of. People are convinced they have been touched by the Holy Spirit and have experienced God. Eastern doctrine of *pantheism*—god *is* everything, has been altered a bit and made more deceptive to the Christian by teaching that God *is in* everything—*panentheism*. This becomes the world view of those using the mystical prayer practices. The Bible does not support these views.

> For in Him dwells all the fullness of the Godhead bodily, you are complete in Him which is the head of all principality and power. (Colosians 2: 9, 10)

> I am the Lord: that is my name: and my glory will I not give to another, neither my praise to graven images. (Isaiah. 42: 8)

Contemplative prayer (and synonym names) uses the basic principles of regular meditation that is, position of comfort, deep rhythmic breathing

---

170   Gawain, Shakti, *Creative Visualization,* Novato, California, National Publishing, (2002), back cover; reported in Yungen; op. cit., p. 19.

and use of mantra. This mantra may be some Bible name or verse but used in repetition. Then there is the emphasis on bringing the mind to a passive state, emptying of the mind, by concentration on the breath and mantra. This alters consciousness which is the key to all occult training, and can bring the individual to the *click* spoken of before, and now the individual is certain he has experienced the Holy Spirit and God.

Yungen traces the ancient history of the contemplative (meditation) movement to medieval monks known as the *Desert Fathers* living in the wilderness of the Middle East, who, in turn, most likely had borrowed the practice from the Far East. The Catholic mystics, *especially Ignatius Loyola,* over centuries kept the practice of meditation through prayer alive. It was picked up again in our age by Thomas Merton (1915—1968) a Catholic scholar who was to the contemplative prayer movement as was Martin Luther King to the civil rights movement. So too, Catholic scholar Henri Nouwen (1932-1996) had a strong part to play in promoting contemplation prayer to Catholics and mainline Protestants as well. The movement continued to pick up momentum as two monks joined in the fray, Thomas Keating and Basil Pennington. Yungen tells us that these monks blended their Catholic Christianity with Eastern mysticism and produced *centering prayer.*

The movement is also referred to as *Spiritual Formation.* One of its centers for spreading the contemplative prayer in this country is the Shalem Institute located near Washington D.C. and founded by Episcopal priest Tilden Edwards. Its purpose is to spread the practice of mystical prayer to Christianity. Thousands have taken training at this center, trained to be spiritual directors propagating mystical prayer. Another Episcopal priest, Matthew Fox, has influenced not only Catholics but also mainline Protestants, in promoting "God in everything." In his book *The Coming of the Cosmic Christ, Fox* makes the following comments: Divinity is found in all creatures.... The cosmic Christ is the "I Am" in every creature.[171]

> Without mysticism there will be no "deep ecumenism," no unleashing of the power of wisdom from all the world's religious traditions. Without this *mysticism* I am convinced there will never be global peace or justice since the human race needs spiritual depths and disciplines, celebration and rituals to awaken its better selves.[172]

Mysticism is leading many Christians into what is termed *inter-spirituality,* (a merging together of all faiths). It has as its basic tenet that divinity (God) is

---

171   Fox, Matthew, *The Coming of the Cosmic Christ,* (New York, NY: Harper- Collins Publishers, (1980), p. 154: reported in Youngen, op. cit., p. 68.

172   *Ibid.,* p. 68.

in all things, and the presence of God is in all religions and through mysticism this state is recognized. Once again let us consider the words of Ray Youngen:

> Former New Age medium, Brian Flynn, in his fascinating book, *Running Against the Wind*, explains it as a uniting of the world's religions through the common thread of mysticism. Flynn quotes the late Wane Teasdale (a lay monk who coined the term inter-spirituality) as saying that interspirituality is "the spiritual common ground which exists among the world's religions."[173]

In time, evangelical Protestants were infected with this movement. Richard Foster wrote a book *Celebration of Discipline* and is a prominent leader. He brought in *breath prayer*—that is, picking a single word or phrase and repeating it in conjunction with the breath. There have been scores of other ministers leading the charge and writing books, continuing its spread like a tsunami. The movement of mystical prayer has powered the formation of the *Emerging Church* which is an ecumenical movement including pagan, animist, Hindu, Catholic, protestant, Islam and all religions. The goal of the Emerging Church is to gather all religions under one banner. *Feelings,* not *thus saith the Word,* seems to be the measuring criteria in this movement.

If you consider carefully the above history of the development of the mystical prayer movement you will recognize that spiritual formation, contemplative prayer, centering prayer, silence, mysticism, and interspirituality have been introduced and promoted by clergy, not coming from the laity. The watchman on the wall will need to keep their eyes on fellow watchmen and sound the alarm when mysticism is recognized in the church.

I have only touched on this subject but that is enough to put out an *alert*. I suggest you obtain the book by Ray Yungen, *A Time of Departing,* and read it carefully. You will be shocked I am sure, but will gain a deeper understanding as to where we are in time. The words of the book *The Great Controversy* by E.G. White come to mind at this moment:

> ...Protestants of the United States will be foremost in stretching their hands across the gulf to grasp the hand of spiritualism; they will reach over the abyss to clasp hands with the Roman power; and under the influence of this threefold union, this country will follow in the steps of Rome in trampling on the rights of conscience....

> ...The line of distinction between professed Christians and the ungodly is now hardly distinguishable. Church members love what the world loves and are ready to join with them and Satan determines to unite them in one body and thus

---

173   Youngen, op. cit., p. 50.

strengthen his cause by seeping all into the ranks of spiritualism. Papists, who boast of miracles as a certain sign of the true church, will be readily deceived by this wonder-working power; and Protestants, having cast away the shield of truth, will also be deluded. Papists, Protestants, and worldlings will alike accept the form of godliness without the power, and they will see in this union a grand movement for the conversion of the world and the ushering in of the long expected millennium.

Through spiritualism, Satan appears as a benefactor of the race, healing the diseases of the people, and professing to present a new and more exalted system of religious faith; but at the same time he works as a destroyer.[174]

I will close this section with the following quote from Ray Yungen:

...Mysticism *neutralizes* doctrinal differences by sacrificing the truth of Scripture for a mystical experience. Mysticism offers a common ground, and supposedly, that commonality is *divinity in all*. But we know from Scripture there is one God and there is no other but He.[175]

---

174 White, E.G., *The Great Controversy,* Pacific Press Publishing Association, Nampa, ID, (1888), pp. 588,589.
175 Yungen, op. cit., pp. 196,197.

CHAPTER 8

Yoga—Yoga Exercises—cleansing Ayurveda the Ancient HealingTradition of India - Part II

Forty years in the past yoga was an activity that most Americans considered as Hinduism and associated with pagan idol worship. The Christian community tended to consider its practice as a denial of faith. In the intervening years many Americans have been conditioned to accept it as a healthy part of Christianity. The term "Christian Yoga" is often heard or read. Its practice has spread through clubs, sports, schools, television, businesses, churches, youth groups, medicine, entertainment industry, and for many individuals simply a practice at home. It has even been especially prepared and presented to the very young and promoted as a "family activity." Yoga has moved into wellness programs primarily through yoga exercises which have become popular in many churches, especially with young women.

Has the Christian community carefully analyzed yoga and found it to be an appropriate adjunct to the Judeo-Christian doctrines? Has there been any concern that it might be a "wolf in sheep's clothing?" Some pastors give warnings about its practice, while some others are encouraging its practice? We need to look carefully at the origin of yoga and its place and purpose in the Hindu worship for the past 3500 years. Then we need to answer the question, is its use safe for the Christian? Read carefully this chapter and learn more about this controversial subject.

YOGA

Yoga is an intrinsic part of Hinduism. Laurette Willis, who was led into New Age occultism through yoga and was then delivered through faith in Christ, and obedience to God's Word, explains:

> The goal of all yoga is to obtain oneness with the universe. That'salso known as the process of enlightenment, or union with Brah-man (Hinduism's highest god). The word "yoga" means "union" or "to yoke"...Yoga wants to get students to the point of complete numbness in their minds (to open them to this force).

God on the other hand, wants you to be transformed by the renewing of your mind through his Word.[176]

We read an opposing viewpoint:

Yoga is a science as well as a method of achieving spiritual harmony through the control of mind and body. The *asanas* (yogic postures) and *pranayama* (breath control) are practices that not only help us to acquire perfect health, but also develop the inner force that enables a believer to withstand stressful situations with a calm and serene mind.[177]

B.K.S. Iyengar, the founder of Hatha Yoga (used in the U.S.), makes the following statement regarding the goal of yoga,

...the means by which the human soul may be completely united with the Supreme Spirit pervading the universe and thus attain liberation (escape reincarnation)... *Yoga Journal,* May/June 1993, p. 69.

Yoga is an ancient physical practice of postures and movements established to *join* the mind, body, and spirit. Yoga means to hook up, to join, to unite. The primary purpose of posture and movement of yoga is to facilitate the flow of energy through the body and chakras, especially kundalini energy. As stated previously yoga is associated with meditation like a glove is with the hand. Dr. Khalsa tells us in *Meditation as Medicine* that he combines yoga with meditation to obtain a more powerful response in healing.

Swiss psychiatrist C.G. Jung, a spiritist and anti-Christian, brought yoga to the West nearly ninety years ago and was a devotee of it. He strongly emphasized that the spiritual cannot be taken out it, see quote below.

The numerous purely physical procedures of yoga (unite) the parts of the body... with the whole of the mind and spirit, as... in the pranayama exercises, where prana is both the breath and the universal dynamics of the cosmos... the elation of the body becomes one with the elation of the spirit.... Yoga practice is unthinkable, and would also be ineffectual, without the ideas on which it is based. It works the physical and the spiritual into one another in an extraordinarily complete way.[178]

---

176   Hunt, op. cit., P. 35.
177   Warrier, op. cit., p. 166.
178   Jung, C.G. , trans. R.F.C. Hull, *Psychology and the East,* Princeton Un. Press, (1978), pp. 80, 81: reported in Hunt, Dave, *Yoga and The body of Christ, The Berean Call,* Bend, Oregon, (2006), p. 9.

Later, Yogi Paramahansa Yogananda popularized yoga in this country in the latter part of the twentieth century by introducing it as science in the guise of health enhancement. Yoga was presented as a purely physical practice non-related to religion. Hatha yoga, often considered only as physical yoga, has for its center of instruction the "Temple of Kriya Yoga" in Chicago. Yogananda initiated approximately 100,000 people into Kriya Yoga (or Hatha Yoga) for the purpose of "self-realization" (to realize one's oneness with God). The leaders in this movement have been "Yogi's," or holy men.

> These techniques were all precisely developed over centuries to induce subtle changes in states of consciousness leading to "self-realization." They were not developed for physical benefits.[179]

Medical newspapers and journals frequently print articles reporting, yet another medical condition that improves with the use of yoga and/or meditation. A government survey of 31,000 adults revealed that eight percent of Americans use yoga as an alternative medical therapy. As of 2004, Wal-Mart web site listed 990, and Target's, 4235 yoga products for sale.[180]

Richard Hittleman a leader in the "physical yoga" movement in the USA makes the following comment:

> ...as yoga students practiced the physical positions, they would eventually be ready to investigate the spiritual component which is "the entire essence of the subject."[181]

Yoga is sweeping the West. Multiple millions practice yoga not intending to embrace Hinduism, yet using the fundamental tools of Hinduism and placing their minds under its influence. They do not contemplate on God while in yoga meditation. Instead, they try to empty their minds of all thought, or concentrate on a single thought so as to achieve mental rest or "passivity of mind". The end result, however, allows opportunity for Satan to control one's mind. We are to contemplate on God through prayer and study scriptures of the Bible, while inviting the Holy Spirit to direct our thoughts.

Yoga is also a commercial business. Consider the financial impact of this movement:

> Nationally, Yoga is a 22.5 billion dollar industry. Advertisements for yoga books, videos, clothes, wellness retreats and even yoga business training classes can be

179   Hunt, Dave, *Yoga and The Body of Christ, The Berean Call*, Bend, OR, (2006), p. 18.
180   http://www.letusreason.org/NAM1.htm
181   *Yoga Journal,* May/June, (1993), p. 68.

found in the back of magazines such as Yoga Journal, and the phenomenon in now reaching into the mainstream...35 million Americans who will try yoga for the first time this year. Once confined to New Agers with an interest in Eastern spirituality, yoga is catching on among young men, fitness fanatics, aging baby boomers and other unlikely enthusiasts who claim the mind body practice does everything from healing illness to tighten abs.[182]

Contrast yoga meditation with Christian meditation which really is best called *study*, or *contemplation*. The Christian attitude is that of allowing God to direct his thoughts and life. He does not look inward in an attempt to raise his divinity to godhood, but outward and upward to the Creator God as the source of power and redemption. This is directly opposite to Ayurvedic principles. Can one take a fundamental act and practice, physical and mental, from a pagan religion (Satan's ground) and make it Christian? The *Christian Yoga* term is an oxymoron. As the Hindu Holy men tell us we cannot take yoga out of Hinduism nor can you take Hinduism out of Yoga.

Reflecting upon the subject of meditation and yoga in the 1950's, I cannot remember that the subject was ever thought of or considered by people with whom I associated. In the 1960's a change was observed occurring on college campuses, such as style of dress, long hair on men etc. Standards were changing, and to one not involved in the culture change of the youth it was not well understood. Many influences were creating the outward changes we were seeing and most of us did not understand what was happening. One of the greatest influences for change came from the influence of psychedelic drugs and the popular music of the period. Timothy Leary is a name that comes to mind when *this subject of psychedelic drug* use is mentioned. He championed the use of LSD; other substances such as peyote, marijuana, amphetamine were easily available. The mind trips experienced with these substances blew away old norms and created a desire for ever expanding "consciousness." Drug using musicians; Presley, the Beatles, Rolling Stones, and many other music groups came on the scene captivating the youth and opening up the drug use as nothing else could do. This was a stepping stone to even more exhilarating practice of yoga and the "trips" that could be taken in this manner without purchasing drugs.[183]

The Beatles spent time in an *ashram* in India learning meditation and yoga then returned to the music performance circuit, promoting yoga. They had learned that mind trips, equal and beyond what drugs give, could be experienced by yoga without drugs. Yoga was now on a roll. Meditation and yoga is not a novelty any longer, it has gone "Main Street," even in many of our

182 http://www.letusreason.org/NAM1.htm
183 Hunt, Dave, McMahon, T.A., *America The Sorcerer's New Apprentice,* Harvest House Publishers, Eugene, Oregon, (1988), pp. 233-252.

leading hospitals. An altered state of consciousness (trance) is a prerequisite to experience mind trips and obtaining a *spirit guide*.

> In view of the nonphysical nature of consciousness, it is intriguing that those who practice divination techniques for initiating contact with *spirit* dimension all agree that the secret is in achieving the requisite state of consciousness through drugs, yoga (other forms of Eastern meditation), hypnosis, and mediumistic trance. It is not surprising, then, that this "altered state of consciousness" and the contact it brings with "spirit guides" has always been the traditional shamanistic method of achieving paranormal or psychic powers. It has also often opened the door to what has become known as possession.[184]...

YOGA EXERCISES

Yoga is an act whereby a person assumes a physical posture in Sanskrit called *asana*. There are more than fifty different postures in yoga. The purpose of yoga is to facilitate liberation from reincarnation (rebirth) as taught in pagan religions, and yoke (yoga) together the individual soul with a pagan Deity. By the practice of yoga the agitated mind is said to be brought under control. In the meditation-yoga system, the mind is controlled by focusing on obtaining to Samadhi, Lotus, Supreme Self, Godhood. At this level of attainment in meditation and yoga, the individual knows that he is a real entity having a life that will go on in spite of the destruction of the body. Meditation is an integral part of yoga practices and all that has been said about meditation is equally applicable to yoga. Szurko, an ex-yogic master, explains:

> The importance of asanas (physical postures), pranayama (breath control)... to the yogi pursuing liberation lies partly in the belief that the body is the microcosm of the universe; that is to say, whatever exists in the universe may be found in the body, which is a "universe in miniature." Thus the yogi finds within himself all bodies; all truth; heaven and hell; all the expanses of space and the whole of time as well as of eternity; spirit, the gods, and Deity itself. It follows in yogic theory that the person who masters this "universe within" will become, to the same degree, master of the cosmos.[185]

The knowledge of the universe is believed to be found in Self; and that all healing is to be found in Self. Yoga is less of a treatment for illness and more for preventative measures. The Hindu believes that yoga exercises decreases

---

184 *Ibid.*, p. 155.
185 Davies, Gaius, *Stress*, Kingsway Publication, Eastbourne, England, (1988), p. 241; reported in Willis, Richard J.B., *Holistic Health Holistic Hoax?*, Pensive Publications, 10 Holland Gardens, Watford, Hertfordshire, WD2 6JW, (1997), p. 231.

congestion and blockage of energy and facilitates its flow. Sitting straight during meditation or even without meditation, it is believed, will allow for release of the congestion and blockage of the universal energy making it flow smoothly through various organs. These exercises will supposedly stimulate the *chakras* (energy centers) which, in turn, allow the energy to flow freely and maintain health.

The above concept has been accepted by western mysticism and magic in whole and forms the philosophical basis of most alternative medical therapies yet to be discussed.

The positions of the yoga postures are important in its concept because each position is proclaimed to direct prana or universal energy to specific parts of the body. In Hatha yoga the spine is to be kept straight so that the latent kundalini, or *serpent force*, supposedly coiled up at the base of the spine from birth, will be able to ascend through the chakras (energy centers of Hinduism) toward the top chakra. All of these acts are directed at "stilling the mind." Hatha yoga is the most popular in the US. "Ha" means sun and "tha" is moon. Breathing through the nose in the left nostril will bring in the moon energy and in the right nostril the sun energy. Both sun and moon energy then travel downward through special (nonexistent) passages, one on each side of the body, and go to the bottom chakra at the coccyx area. This energy will then ascend up through the body by the help of yoga postures and exercises until the energy comes into full force at the top chakra, signifying that eternal life has been attained.

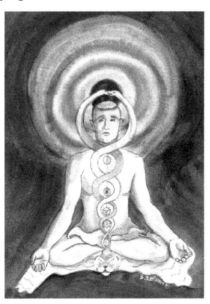

Figure 19. Kundalini -- serpent power

Let Us Reason Ministries placed an article about yoga on the Internet entitled "Yoga Today's Lifestyle for Health." The author of the article, once a practitioner of yoga, tells of becoming involved in yoga meditation as a result of practicing the yoga exercise positions. He cautions us that the physical yoga is not separate from the whole of Eastern Metaphysics.

How popular are yoga exercises? Let Us Reason Ministries' article on this gives just a glimpse of the interest.

> Hatha yoga exercises are taught as part of YMCA physical education programs, in health spas and given as physical exercise on TV programs. Eighty percent of clubs now offer yoga classes. Yoga is also incorporated into institutional and liberal churches on the assumption that these techniques are nothing more than benign physical exercises which condition the mind and body. It has come in under the guise of stress reduction. Touted as scientifically proven is more an assumption that is really at worst, a presumption.[186]

The response that so often comes from participants of yoga exercise is that they are only doing "stretching exercises." What could be wrong or dangerous with that? The answer is given by the author of the article submitted by Let Us Reason Ministries:

> The poses that they so diligently practice in their stretching are named after Hindu Gods, and what one is actually doing, is calling on them. In that worshipful pose, they are bowing and for all intents and purposes worshipping that god. Our God says: 'You shall not bow down to them or worship them; for I, the Lord your God, am a jealous God.'[187]

Another Yogic or Hindu mystic, Sri Aurobindo taught that all yoga, including Hatha yoga, "has the same goal-unity with the Supreme." Many people think they are just taking a physical fitness activity when they join a yoga exercise group. The Master mystics and the Yogis tell us you cannot separate the physical from the spiritual. Szurko an ex mystic says:

> When I taught yoga, it became apparent that for many people the spiritual dimension of the discipline was self-manifesting it could be ignored at first, but not for long.[188]

I quote Yogi Ramacharaka:

---

186 http://www.letusreason.org/NAM1.htm p.1
187 http://www. letusreason.org/NAM1.htm p. 6
188 Szurko, Christtian., *Can Yoga be Reconciled with Christianity?*, The Church Medicine and the New Age, (1995), p. 107; reported in Willis, op. cit., p. 232.

The beginner will also do well to study 'Hatha Yoga' in order to render his physical body healthy and sound and thus give the spirit a worthy Temple in which to manifest.[189]

Theos Bernard, states:

...Great Masters, through the potency of Hatha Yoga, breaking the scepter of death, are roaming in the universe.[190]

Combined with yoga exercise is the emphasis placed on breathing. In Eastern medicine this is paramount. Air (*prana*) is believed to carry the universal energy, (life force), into an individual, and breathing in a certain manner (through the nose) increases the amount of this universal energy, intelligence, consciousness, or Creative Principle in a person. Ramacharaka also tells us:

The Yogi practices exercises by which he attains control of his body, and is enabled to send to any organ or part an increased flow of vital force—prana, thereby strengthening and invigoration the part or organ...He knows that by rhythmical breathing one may bring in the unfoldment of his latent powers. He knows that by controlled breathing he may not only cure disease in himself and others, but also practically do away with fear and worry and the baser emotions.[191]

The Complete Illustrated Encyclopedia of Alternative Healing Therapies, tells us,

The exercises of yoga are *all* designed to direct the flow of 'prana' and to release the body's internal energy to create spiritual awareness. Yoga is thus a form of preparation of the mind, body, and spirit, which must be unified through conduct, right-thinking, and meditation, before the ultimate merging of the self with the universe, or the totality of all that is – the equivalent of God or the Hindu goal of *nirvana*. In this wider context, the postural and breathing exercises of *hatha* yoga are simply a means of promoting meditation and internal balance, through which the final goal of *oneness* can be achieved. Hatha yoga is a yogic

189 Ramacharaka, Yogi, *The Hindu-Yogi-Science of Breath,* London: L.N. Fowler & co., Ltd. P. 78 (1960); reported in Willis, op. cit., p. 233.
190 Bernard, Theos, *Hatha Yoga,* Arrow Books, London, (1950), p.19; re ported in Willis, op. cit., (1997), p.233.
191 Ramacharaka, *Yogi,* (nd), Raja Yoga, London: L.N. fowler & Co. Ltd., (1960), p. 10; reported in Willis, op. Cit., p. 233.

system in its own right, although in the West emphasis is generally placed on its exercises.[192]

Taking air in through the right nostril is said to be breathing in the *sun* energy. Breathing through the left nostril is said to be breathing in the *moon* energy. In the nostrils are believed to be two channels for carrying universal energy. These channels are called *ida* (left) and *pingala* (right) and are believed to start at the nostrils and go down to the lower end of the spinal column. They are said to be related to the activities of the lunar and solar forces in the body. The mystic moon of the body (microcosm) is said to be located in the head, pouring with its milky rays the elixir (amrita) which serves the channel *ida* on the left side of the body, etc. The antagonistic principle of devouring solar heat is supposed to be situated at the lower pelvis area of the body.[193]

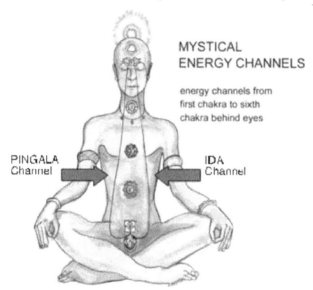

MYSTICAL
ENERGY CHANNELS

energy channels from
first chakra to sixth
chakra behind eyes

PINGALA
Channel

IDA
Channel

Figure 20. of man in yoga position with IDA AND PINGALA

Hatha Yoga, by definition, means *union of sun* (ha) *and moon* (tha). At a little higher level of yoga called *pranayama* the two channels in the nostrils become stimulated and union of the two breaths takes place at the "agya," the important chakra between the two eyes. One set of yoga exercises called *Surya*

192   Shealy, Norman M.D. Ph.D,, *The Complete Illustrated Encyclopedia of Alternative Healing Therapies,* Elelment Books Inc., Boston, MA, (1999), p. 52.

193   Jaggi, O.P.,M.D., PhD., Yogic and Tantric Medicine, Atm Ram and Sons, Dehli, India, (1973), p. 62.

Namatura, (Salutation to the Sun) is a set of easy movements and postures not held as long as most exercise postures. These exercises present a:

> Spiritual salutation to the rising Sun the source of all energy for life, and are found in many religious and pagan societies.[194]

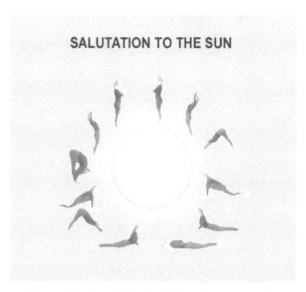

SALUTATION TO THE SUN

Figure 21. An artist's depiction of yoga exercises

Hinduism teaches that there is a great "latent" power within each person. Said to be located at the base of the spine, it is called *kundalini*, also referred to as the *serpent power*, as this is the definition of this Sanskrit word. To attain god-hood this *serpent power* must be awakened and moved up the body through the Hindu chakras to the highest one at the top of the head. The movement of this kundalini is believed to be accomplished by practicing meditation and yoga. Yoga asanas (postures) and exercises were designed to force flow of this serpent power up through the chakras and the body to the crown chakra on top of the head. The exercise positions are specifically designed to be snake-like in motion and are named after Hindu gods. One such position is called *the cobra.* Along with the positions of the exercises, great emphasis is placed on breathing. Remember *prana,* the *universal energy* of Hinduism, is believed to be in the air we breathe. In so-called Christian yoga (an oxymoron), there may be practiced what is called the breath prayer, a pagan practice given a Christian name, not unlike the centuries wherein paganism entered the church by simply giving Christian names to pagan customs.

---

194   Shealy, op. cit., p. 55.

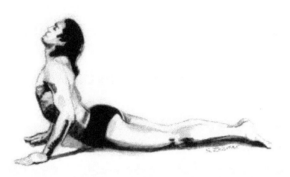

Figure 22. Cobra position

When the universal energy delivered to the body by breathing has traveled to the lower chakra, it will begin to ascend in an undulating manner, going through the chakras until it reaches the seventh crown chakra at the top of the head, whereupon one receives *immortality*. This may take many lifetimes to accomplish.[195] Yoga is a counterfeit of being yoked to Christ.

> Come unto me, all ye that labor and are heavy laden, and I will give you rest. Take my yoke upon you, and learn of me; for I am meek and lowly in heart: and ye shall find rest unto your souls. For my yoke is easy, and my burden is light. (Matthew 11:28-30).

Spreading across the world like a forest fire is the popular activity of yoga exercise and the breathing exercises that go with them. There may or may not be meditation involved, but most formal yoga sessions end with a few moments of meditation. This can easily lead to spiritualism experiences. Because the spiritual philosophy that is a part of Hinduism is not presented in a verbal manner with yoga exercises, or with meditation, people totally disassociate the Hindu religion and its "world view" of man's origin, from doing the yoga exercises. Yoga exercises are alleged to be purely physical with no mysticism involved. Yoga is yoga, and those various movements and stretching are designed to raise *kundalini* up through the chakras to join with the universal god of Hinduism. Partaking of these exercises places oneself on *Satan's ground.* He has used such activities for more than three thousand years and for his purposes only. Will we move his counterfeit system into our lives and into the church as paganism moved in during the fourth to fifth centuries, and call it *Christian?* An ex-Hindu Guru, now a Christian, has stated a very clear truth about the influences of participating in yoga. He said:

---

195   Jaggi, op. cit., p. 123.

There cannot be Hinduism without yoga and there can be no yoga without Hinduism.[196]

The highest goal of the Eastern religion is to realize *one's own divinity, to make contact with the spirit gods,* and *to escape the cycle of reincarnation* by joining the spirit world. These religions teach that this goal can be accomplished by our own works, not necessarily by good deeds, but by practicing meditation and yoga and its exercises. These practices were designed for these religions (by Satan's directions) to facilitate an alteration in one's state of consciousness wherein Satan can exert his power over them, and lead the person to believe he has attained godhood, and will at death join the spirit world.

To participate in these practices is to accept the foundation pillars of Hinduism. It is akin to dancing around the tree of knowledge of good and evil, and since it seems safe, eventually the urge to reach out and touch and eat of its fruit is too strong a temptation to resist.

MASSAGE

Ayurveda teaches that the body has special channels which not only carry nutrients throughout the body, but additionally conduct subtle energies which link mankind with the cosmos. Disease in Ayurveda medicine is said to be determined by knowing which of these channels is affected. Massage and yoga exercises are used to open these channels when they are blocked or are not flowing freely. The congestion of these channels is considered a source of disease.

In Ayurveda it is taught that there are one hundred and seven points on the body called "trigger points" (or *marma points*), and that by massaging these points we are able to facilitate the flow of energy that may be stagnant, blocked, or in some way congested. By massaging specific *marma points* with *essential oils,* then there is free flow of energy (prana). Different types of essential oils are used for different types of illnesses, and, in turn, these oils will be chosen for application to particular trigger points. The various trigger points are said to be associated with particular areas or organs of the body. None of the above comments is substantiated by science.

It is very important to understand that the *trigger points* in Ayurvedic medicine should not be confused with the expression *trigger point* as is used in today's conventional practice of medicine. A very frequent complaint encountered in family practice is a localized point of pain on a specific muscle. Examination will reveal a firm, tender nodule in the muscle. A twitch of the muscle group will occur when the tender nodule is touched or pressed on. The

---

196   Gods of the New Age: Video tape 1988 Jeremiah Films Inc., Hemet, CA.

cause of the nodule is most likely a section of muscle fibers in constant contraction. It can be very painful and can last days, weeks, or even months. There are various methods of treatment. Firm pressure held on the tender nodule for ten minutes may alleviate it. Injecting the nodule with a local anesthetic may also bring relief, and use of ultrasound over the nodule works well. I have personally treated hundreds of these tender nodules. They have no relationship to the *marma points* of Ayurvedic medicine.

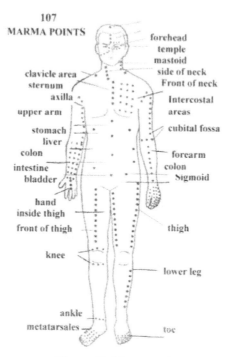

Figure 21 Marma points

Through memory of past emotional experiences, the Hindu believes we sometimes adopt postures and physical behaviors which create congestion of prana. Massage, above all else, involves the movement of energies, relieving congestion, thereby supposedly rejuvenating the mind-body.

Essential oils (oil of a plant) are extracted from plants having specific aromas, and are placed on specific marma points and massaged into the skin. Different marma points may require specific oils applied when massaged. These oils are used because they are believed to contain *spirit—universal energy* of high frequency.

In Ayurveda, food also imparts universal energy (prana) to the body. The diet philosophy is complex. There is a strong bent toward vegetarianism.

Another Eastern religion diet, the Zen Buddhist macrobiotic diet, consists of seven steps, with progressive restriction of diet choices. It is believed that food brings a type of energy (universal energy) apart from the energy obtained from the metabolism of food. It is also believed that foods of animal origin are stronger in rajas–tamas, yin–yang, and fruits and vegetables are more neutral in yin–yang and do not upset the energy balance, thus an additional reason for the choice of vegetarianism.

One may hear of *live enzymes,*" which can refer to the enzymes of plants unaltered by heat, or to the universal energy believed to be carried by the enzymes, and not a biochemical condition of the enzymes. Our bodies produce all of the appropriate enzymes we need and it is not necessary to assimilate *live enzymes* from plants for proper metabolism. The enzymes in plants are for facilitating the biochemical actions in the plant and do not function in our biochemical reactions. Previously stated in chapter five, also mentioned the choice of vegetarian diets due to the belief that eating plant food facilitated receiving energy from higher levels, or planes, which are then transferred to an individual's higher planes of energy.

HERBS & MINERALS

The use of herbs has been a fundamental practice in all ancient health and healing systems. Herbs are considered helpful in *bridging* the cosmic energies which are said to be internal and external to the body. In Ayurvedic practice, herbs are always to be used in conjunction with meditation, diet and other Ayurvedic approaches to health. According to these theories benefit from herbal therapy will depend upon it being added to other therapies; also, we must acknowledge the *consciousness* of the plant or it will be of no value or effect on us. Little to no benefit is to be expected when it is used alone.[197] A later chapter "Mystical Herbology" will enlarge on use of herbs in Ayurveda medicine.

Aromatherapy and the use of *essential oils* are very popular as a method of influencing universal energy within a person. The aroma is obtained by using oil concentrates of flowers and plant substances. It can be applied as oil or placed in vaporizers and diffused through the air. Many times plants are placed in water, and then placed in the sunshine for several hours. Sunlight is supposed to increase the *essence* of the plants. They are then processed by steam distillation of other methods of extraction into oils which are usually rubbed into the skin. This is one more way in which it is believed that the

---

197 Gerson, op. cit., p. 90.

universal energy (prana) is absorbed by the body. This subject will be dealt with in detail in a later chapter.

PANCHAKARMA: CLEANSING–PURIFICATION

Disease, by Ayurveda understanding, is the result of an abnormal accumulation of dosha (yin—yang) energies in the tissues of the body. One very interesting part of the Ayurvedic healing system belief is *panchakarma,* or purification treatment. It is believed that cells in the body contain residual impurities deposited in them as a result of improper digestion. The goal of purification is to rid the body of *ama* or impurities which imbalance doshas.

Ayurveda teaches that there is a *fire* in the body (called *agni*), which we call metabolism, that drives all of the vital chemical processes. It directs and supports digestion. If digestion is impaired by too little agni, or for any other reason, then impurities (ama) are produced. The ama is supposedly a *white sticky substance (*not recognized by scientific medicine) that is absorbed by channels (non-demonstrable by the anatomist), spreads to the tissue of the body, and if not cleaned out, often develops disease by causing imbalances of the dosha energies. The diseases might be called gallstones, cancer, heart disease, etc. Ayurveda recognizes two types of disease–outside disease and inside disease. Ama is said to be the root of all inside diseases.[198] The purification procedures are used both as preventative and restorative therapy.

The five cleansing therapies of Ayurveda are:

1. Nasal administration of substances that are believed to clear out the imbalanced doshas, or energies, from the head and neck area.
2. Emetics to induce vomiting, which clears the energies from the lungs and abdominal area.
3. Laxatives and strong purgatives to cleanse the blood, liver, spleen, small intestine, and sweat glands.
4. Medicated enemas to cleanse the colon, rectum, lumbar-sacral region, and bones of excess energies. "Ayurveda regards medicated enemas (Ayurveda lists over 100 different ones) as the most important purification method of all, because of the importance of the large intestine in health and disease." The loosened doshas (yin–yang, rojas–tamas) are believed to be washed out through the intestinal tract.
5. Bloodletting had long been a practice in Ayurveda until a change (140–150 years ago) when using herbs was substituted for taking blood. The concept behind drawing blood was that it eliminated toxins and excess energies from the blood, lymph, and deep tissues. The purpose

---

198   *Ibid.*, p. 49.

for bloodletting was to treat skin disorders, enlarged liver and spleen, gout, fevers, abdominal tumors, jaundice, etc. There are other cleansing practices such as the topical application of plasters and herbal pastes, etc. Bloodletting has nearly ceased and herbal use has been substituted in its place.

Ayurveda medicine is strongly connected to astrology, teaching that: ... For this reason, the zodiac was used in determining which area of the patient's body should be bled.

> The sun and moon have the strongest influence on health and healing and their movements indicate changes not only in the seasons but in human health and behavior.[199]

Another believed-in (supposed) cleanser is urine, applied topically, by drinking, by enema, and even by injection into the body.

> In traditional Ayurveda, alcoholism, poor appetite, nausea, indigestion, ascites (free fluid in abdominal cavity), and edema are treated with goat feces washed with urine; constipation is treated with a mixture of milk and urine; impotence is treated with 216 kinds of enemas (some including the testicles of peacocks, swans, and turtles); and epilepsy and insanity are treated with ass urine.[200]

These remedial substances were administered in enemas. Urine is the body's process of elimination of a multitude of waste chemicals. To drink or use urine waste in any way is simply putting back into the system a concentration of impurities. I have systematically presented the fundamental principles in Ayurvedic medicine because even today these practices are commonly promoted. It is common to hear of coffee or medicated enemas, or an electrical machine performing, continuous enemas, herbs, etc., to remove toxins caught in body tissues. Various cleansing practices of Ayurveda are accepted and used by many who have no idea of its origin.

In the practice of panchakarma (purification) in Ayurveda, the organs selected for stimulation to supposedly facilitate the removal of toxins from the system, are not all organs science recognizes as designed to eliminate impurities and toxic substances from the body. Ayurveda sometimes may apply irritating and/or toxic substances to the sinuses, stomach, lungs and intestines, which in turn causes them to secrete mucus and fluids, to vomit, or to have

199 Warrier, op., cit., pp. 170, 172.
200 Raso, op. cit., p. 89.

bowel movements. This is not a process of ridding the system of impurities; it is a method of adding impurities, which in turn causes the body to react.

The sciences of anatomy and physiology recognize the function of the lungs, kidneys, liver, and skin as the prime organs for processing and eliminating toxins from the body. The intestinal tract is not a prime detoxifying organ. However, it does carry out of the body the detoxified impurities discharged from the liver. Our bodies also need fresh air, water, and exercise to facilitate the elimination of toxins.

The following comment states:

> In health and in sickness, pure water is one of heaven's choicest blessings. Its proper use promotes health. It is the beverage which God provided to quench the thirst of animals and man. Drunk freely, it helps to supply the necessities of the system and assists nature to resist disease. The external application of water is one of the easiest and most satisfactory ways of regulating the circulation of the blood. A cold or cool bath is an excellent tonic. Warm baths open the pores and thus aid in the elimination of impurities. Both warm and neutral baths soothe the nerves and equalize the circulation.[201]

SENSIBLE CLEANSING DIETARY REGIMEN

A simple approach to cleansing follows: Eat a non-refined plant food diet; drink at least 5–6 glasses of water per day; breathe clean fresh air; exercise an hour per day, and bathe daily. Abstain from coffee, tea, alcohol and tobacco. In addition, it is prudent to be regular in habits of sleep, rest, and eating. Allow for five or more hours between meals, with nothing at all except water between meals. The fiber in a non-refined diet of plant foods will absorb many chemical by-products from the bowel and will promote elimination. There are several thousand types of phytochemicals in plants and some counteract various types of toxins. With this approach, the skin, lungs, kidneys, bowels, and liver are able to function at their best so as to eliminate impurities.

A fast for a day or even up to three days will allow the eliminating organs to neutralize and rid the body of substances we do not want in our systems. In the case of heavy metal poisoning such as lead, medical care is indicated. I recommend the reader read Appendix I an article about popular cleansing techniques.

I will share with you a clinical "gem" for promoting bowel function and avoiding constipation that I shared with patients in my medical practice. When first arising in the morning, drink two or three large glasses of quite warm to

---

201   White, E.G., *The Ministry of Healing*, Pacific Press Publishing Asso., Nampa, ID, (1905) p. 237.

near hot water. It must be drunk as a bolus and not in sips. Do not eat any food for at least fifteen minutes. This is most effective with a high fiber diet for bowel regularity. Do this daily for the rest of your life. I have had patients tell me that this solved their life-long problem with constipation.

COMPARISON OF HINDUISM'S AND THE BIBLE'S PLAN OF SALVATION

The path for the Hindu to reach nirvana, (spirit heaven), is by meditation—yoga, visualization (see next chapter), and with clearing the chakras by cleansing techniques such as nasal irrigation, cathartics, purgatives, and repeated colon irrigations. This is a self—works method, a counterfeit of the Bible's plan. The holy scriptures guide us to seek God through prayer and a mental process that is active and guided by the Holy Spirit; facilitated by the imagery of the Bible to point our minds to the great saving truths found in the scriptures. The Hindu looks to his various *cleansing* techniques to clear the spiritual impurities, so as to better move energy through his chakras which he believes will then carry him into the spirit world of nirvana. In sharp contrast, the Christian by faith trusts in the *merits of the shed blood of Jesus Christ* to cover (cleanse) his sin and be accepted into heavenly paradise by God the Father.

> And one of the elders answered, saying unto me, What are these which are arrayed in white robes? And whence came they? And I said unto him, Sir, thou knowest. And he said to me, "These are they which came out of great tribulation, and have washed their robes, and *made them white in the blood of the Lamb.* Therefore are they before the throne of God, and serve him day and night in his temple: and he that sitteth on the throne shall dwell among them." Rev. 7:13-15

> And I heard a loud voice saying in heaven, "Now is come salvation, and strength, and the kingdom of our God, and the power of His Christ: for the accuser of our brethren is cast down, which accused them before our God day and night. And they *overcame him by the blood of the Lamb*, and by the word of their testimony; and they loved not their lives unto the death. Therefore rejoice, [ye] heavens, and ye that dwell in them...." Rev. 12:10—12 (emphasis added)

CONVENTIONAL SCIENCE VS VIBRATIONAL MEDICINE

For the past three centuries the discipline of *science* was developed by experimenting, measuring, analyzing, and reproducibility. Conflict in beliefs occurred between the proponents of universal energy, vitalism, life force, etc., and modern science. The characteristics of the universal energy could not be measured, demonstrated, or explained by the known laws of physics. When electricity was discovered, and its laws of action understood, the proponents of universal energy felt that life force energy would now be demonstrated and explained to the non-believing skeptic scientists. It did not work out that way and there is still a gap in belief between the two.

In recent years, instruments for testing electricity and electro-magnetic energy fields have been greatly expanded and have become more sophisticated. Still, scientists cannot find common ground with those believing in, and teaching the universal energy hypothesis.

The scientist who believes in Eastern mysticism and energy hypothesis presents his work as proof. Points of *proof* proclaimed by universal energy adherents are:

A. Auras:

> All living things (people, plants, animals, etc.) are made up of a complex combination of atoms, molecules and energy cells. As these ingredients coexist, they generate a large magnetic energy field that can be sensed, felt and even seen around the physical body. This energy field is often called an Aura.[202]

Are there energy fields around the human body? Yes, sort of; but there are energy fields almost everywhere. The body's energy fields are commonly measured by medical devices such as electrocardiograph, electroencephalograph, or electromyography. To obtain a measurement with these devices, it is necessary to either insert needles into the skin to make electrical contact, or sandpaper the skin to prepare it for the application of an electrode that can pick up an impulse that reveals the electrical field. If either of these methods is not used, the machines will not be able to detect an electromagnetic field.

> Physics has some very advanced equipment. We can, for instance, measure one quantum of electromagnetic flux. That's more than a million times more sensitive than living tissue. After all, life as we know it is always warm and wet. Devices don't have that constraint. We can make devices out of poisonous metals. We can cool them to hundreds of degrees below zero, to make them superconductive. Even if the human nervous system turns out to be a thousand times better than I think, devices would still be hugely better at measuring energy fields.[203]

202 http://paganspath.com/
203 http://don-lindsay-archive.org/skeptic/ (Q—auras)

The human body has been measured with powerful machines that would detect an aura if such existed. The MRI machine is composed of extremely powerful magnets. When they are turned on, the hydrogen atoms in a person's body shift in position and when the magnets are turned off, the hydrogen atoms return to prior position. The movement of the hydrogen atom creates an electrical force that is measured by the instrument and the computer converts the information into a picture of the body's anatomy. No auras have been detected by MRI machines.

B. Kirlian photography.

In 1939, in Russia, Semyon Kirlian discovered by accident that if an object placed on a photographic plate was subjected to a high-voltage electric field, an image would be created on the plate. The image, though somewhat non-discreet and fuzzy, was accepted by believers in auras as proof of an *aura*.

This phenomenon has been shown to be the result of moisture, or gases around the test object reacting with the generated electrical field and therefore reacting on the photographic plate. When Kirlian photography is done in a vacuum where no moisture or gases can exist, the "aura" vanishes from the photographic plate. (Hines 2003). In spite of the scientific explanation, Kirlian photography is still referred to as *proof* that auras surround living and non-living objects.

C. Radiating energy fields are said to be projected from the hands:

James L. Oschman, in his book *Energy Medicine the Scientific Basis,* makes the comment that energy fields can be detected around the hands of "suitable trained therapists." Another author states that these same phenomena can be measured on "sensitives" but not on non-sensitives. As an illustration of energy radiating from hands, Oschman uses the story of Mesmer and his power of healing as done by magnets and then as he changed to using only his hands for healing. (See chapter on hypnosis.)

D. Claims that energy fields or auras can be felt:

Therapeutic Touch healing method is based upon this claim.

The spring issue of *Scientific Review of Alternative Medicine* reports a rare test of Therapeutic Touch designed by James Randi. The practitioner (of TT) was unable to detect the presence or absence of a human arm in a 'sleeve.' The test involved a patient flipping a coin. After each flip, they either did or didn't insert their arm into a sleeve. For the first twenty flips, the patient was in plain view, and the TT Practitioner was 100% successful (20 out of 20) in determining if the arm was or wasn't in the sleeve...The patient was then screened from the TT practitioner's view, and another twenty flips were done. The practitioners did no better than random (guessing) at telling if the arm was in the sleeve. They were asked if they would like to go on, and they refused.[204]

Emily Rosa, a nine year old girl, did a test of a similar type with the same results for a science project in school. Her project was written and appeared in three medical journals–*Lancet, The British Medical Journal*, and *The Journal of the American Medical Association.* Her experiment was also reported on nation-wide television.

E. Psychics and sensitives can see *auras*:

Ten thousand dollars was offered to any psychic who could accurately identify auras. A test was set up with twenty partitions on a large stage. The psychic, Berkeley Psychic Institute's best, was to identify which partitions had a person behind it. This was a live test on the Bill Bixby television show. The psychic agreed that the test was fair. Prior to placing the people behind the partitions, the psychic was asked if she could see the auras of the people. She said yes, and that they were from one to two feet above their heads. Six people were placed behind partitions, but fourteen did not go behind partitions and stayed out of sight. The psychic saw auras behind all twenty partitions. There is now a one million dollar offer for the psychic that can pass this same test.[205]

F. Magnetic therapy is used in conventional medicine:

Pulsating electromagnetic waves are used to facilitate bone healing, with ongoing research exploring its use in soft tissue injury. It is now recognized that with an injury to tissue there is an electromagnetic field *inside* the body surrounding the wound, but none on the outside. Pulsating electromagnetic forces can effect this energy field stimulating healing by attracting repair cells. Powerful magnetic pulses can be used in severe cases of depression; however, there may be significant memory loss. There is no evidence from double-blind studies that any benefit occurs from using stagnant magnets. It may be asked, why use terms such as electromagnetic frequencies, radio frequencies, etc.,

---

204   http://www.don-lindsay-archive.org/skeptic/ (Q---auras)
205   http://skeptic.com (Q---auras)

throughout this book relating to supposedly emanating energies from our bodies.

The reason is that there are no proper terms to use for an energy that does not really exist. I have used the terms that appear in writings of those supporting, believing in, and teaching the universal energy hypothesis. For example, from the book *The Way of Energy* by Lam Kan Chuen, we find:

> *You are a miniature field of the electromagnetic energy of the universe.*[206]

I must use the terms appearing in the literature so readers can relate the information in this text to that which they may read. A more accurate term might be *Satan's electric currents*. There are many highly trained scientists who are believers in Eastern mysticism. Several are superb authors. They are able to convincingly present the subject of the aura and hypothetical electromagnetic energy as radiating from our bodies and hands, which is said to be able to influence and correct the energy fields of others. I present two paragraphs from a book review which appeared in the *British Homoeopathic Journal* Vol. 87, July 1998, about one such author.

> Dr. Richard Gerber is a physician in Livonia, Michigan, USA described as 'the definitive authority for energetic medicine.' In his book he draws together a variety of complementary therapies, including acupuncture, homeopathy, flower essences, magnet therapy, hands on therapies and radionics, seeking to link their healing mechanisms together. He uses the term 'vibrational medicine' to cover these forms of energy medicine, a term that may not be instantly recognizable to all. In the introductory chapter there is an excellent section on the preconceptions of modern medicine, and how they evolved as a result of Newton's mechanical theory of physics. Energy medicine is more in tune with quantum physics. It was delightful to read a comprehensible explanation of such complex ideas, which would be clearly understood by those without a scientific background. Gerber shows his skill as a teacher in his ability to convey difficult concepts in an accurate manner. Gerber describes non-chemical information exchange between cells, which ultimately forms the basis of his theories on how these therapies may work. He creates a working hypothesis that embraces the ideas of chakras, meridians and energetic force fields. He expands on traditional Eastern philosophies of chi and prana, blending them together with fascinating results; there is a blending of scientific fact and esoteric philosophy that captures the imagination.[207]

---

206   Chuen, Lam Kam, The Way of Energy, Simon & Schuster Inc., (1991), p. 12.
207   http://www.minimum.com/reviews/vibrational-medicine.htm

Dr. Gerber presents in his book, *Vibrational Medicine (*and on DVDs), that universal energy frequencies above the first level or plane are faster than light frequencies. He refers to a William Tiller, a previous Physicist of Stanford University, for his authority on this subject. *This hypothesis is not entertained in conventional physics.*

I have listened to Dr. Gerber's explanation of vibrational energy medicine. He is highly trained in conventional science and medicine. He is so smooth and convincing that I began to wonder about my own beliefs. I have repeatedly experienced this same *self-questioning* after reading other well-trained scientists and skilled authors who are oriented in Eastern religion and metaphysics. I found that I had to back away from the immediate discourse and evaluate the overall picture that each of these doctors present. Where are they heading with this concept and their explanations of the physical workings of the universe?

As I continued to listen to Dr. Gerber, the subjects of astral travel, astrology, numerology, reincarnation, clairvoyance, channeling, psychic abilities, spiritual evolution, and divine-self were presented as wholesome objectives and realities. He teaches that we have a divine nature and are divine lights. There is the idea of chakras being the processors of energy which moves us onward in the spiritual climb toward the supreme self or godhood. Attaining perfection is a process of self-works which is obtained by the development of a higher energy level. Dr. Gerber is not the only scientist holding such beliefs.

I asked myself how it is possible that highly trained scientists, such as Drs. Gerber, Green, and Oschman arrive at conclusions so far from the accepted laws of conventional physics and chemistry? They at times speak of *intuition* as the source of their information. What is intuition? As I understand it, they are speaking of receiving intelligence from the universe that they are able to tap into. This is analogous to receiving *divine revelation.* The information received or arrived at by intuition, then is accepted as superseding conventional science.

Elizabeth Clare Prophet claims to have received seven dictated messages from Djwhal Kul, an "Ascended Master," (demonic spirit) which she placed in a book, these messages are:

> ...discussion of the chakras within the body as transmitters of light energy which is essential to the understanding of spiritual evolution.[208]

He, Djwhal Kul, (Djwhal Khul in some other writings), presents numerous meditations and techniques for "clearing the chakras" to facilitate their expansion and projection into the "macrocosmic-microcosmic interchange."

---

208   Prophet, Elizabeth Clare, *Intermediate Studies of the Human Aura*, Summit University Press, Colorado Springs, CO, (1974), p. 6.

These messages by Djwhal Kul are a guide for the pagan's pilgrimage and pathway to immortality and godhood.

We are told in Kul's messages that the aura is an extension of god "him–self" in us, and that the size of the aura is directly related to the mastery of god's energies within our chakras. The *god* spoken of in this book is not the God you and I think of. In reality, it is Satan. However, the description given in this esoteric book is that it is the highest plane (plane 7) of universal energy. It is believed to be the level of energy which imparts *immortality* and *Your Divine-Self.*

Why write about such blasphemy? What does it have to do with spiritualistic practices in health and healing? The alternative and complementary methods of treatment are about balancing body energy. They are not based on being in harmony with God's laws of health. If we choose to use these *energy* methods, we are accepting that they indeed may work in providing health and healing. At the same time we have accepted (perhaps not consciously) the energy hypothesis, which is the foundation and core of Hinduism and pagan religions.

DEEPAK CHOPRA M.D.

Deepak Chopra M.D. is a name you may have heard as a lecturer or in interviews on a T.V. show. He has authored 19 books promoting Ayurvedic medicine, produced many CDs teaching his style of Ayurveda, and established The American Association of Ayurvedic Medicine in 1991. In 1995 he opened The Chopra Center for Well Being in La Jolla, California, where he is Educational Director. His books are in twelve languages and sold around the world. The books have sold more than ten million English copies. He has produced TV and radio programs promoting his Ayurvedic teachings.

Chopra is a graduate of All India Institute of Medical Sciences; he took several years training in the U.S. at Lehey Clinic and University of Virginia Hospital, becoming certified in internal medicine and endocrinology. He taught at Tufts and Boston University Schools of Medicine, and was elected Chief of Staff at New England Memorial Hospital. He also established a private practice. Then his interests changed to Ayurvedic medicine. He no longer practices medicine, but applies his skills to the teaching and promotion of Ayurveda.

What does Chopra teach that catches so many people's interest? Central to his philosophy is that the human mind has latent potential and self-knowledge. To bring this potential to fruition he supports meditation, nutrition, yoga and exercise, herbal medicine, massage, sound, movement, and aromatherapy. He teaches detoxification and purification by fasting and enemas. His influence in this country and other nations has been vast. There are other medical doctors who also have taken up Ayurveda teachings and have great influence in this country, Drs. Weil and Coussens. They promote the association of Western scientific medicine with Eastern mysticisms which is called *integrative medicine.* See chapter "Those Who Do Magic Arts."

SUMMARY

Presented in this chapter are the basic principles of the Ayurveda system of health and healing. It is based on belief in astrology and the idea that man originated from the cosmic energy called the Creative Principle or Universal Energy. This is the *wisdom from the East* that so many consider superior to the knowledge gained through present-day science. It can be seen that many of the old practices of the West in past centuries were primarily the practice of Ayurveda without the spiritual names. There is a carry-over of many of the old practices that have been slow to disappear.

In the Bible we are told that God gave Solomon *wisdom*:

> Solomon's wisdom was greater than the wisdom of all the men of the East, and greater than all the wisdom of Egypt. ... Men of all nations came to listen to Solomon's wisdom, sent by all the kings of the world, who had heard of his wisdom. (I Kings 4:29–34, NIV)

God had blessed His people Israel, through the prophet Moses, with instructions for healthful living. Remember, Israel is the only nation in the history of the world to have a primary system of disease prevention. Today, we can give praise to God for the instructions in health and healing as given through the Bible and Ellen White, providing us with the most advanced knowledge in the world for healthful living. The end results have shown this to be true. Why would we even consider looking back to the wisdom of the East and of Egypt (paganism and sun worship), and reject God's directions for health and healing?

At this time of great advances in science, when this knowledge has been applied with great benefit, we see widespread belief in and the following after, these ancient methods that have no history of being effective for improving the health of man. There is no evidence that shows these practices have extended the life of man by even one day. The medical history in the areas of the world that practiced these methods has shown that health was dismal and never improved until the science that follows the physical laws of God, chemistry, physics, and hygiene were followed. How can we accept and use these pagan methods if we believe in a God who spoke and created by His power? We are sustained by His power and not by some power in us that can be turned off and on or stimulated by the practices presented in this book.

Why put so much effort into exposing the Ayurvedic system of health and healing? Because this system has had great influence on health and healing as practiced over the world for millennia. This system is being used as the right arm of the religious message of Hinduism and spiritualism. Ayurveda cannot be separated from Hinduism, and Hinduism cannot be separated from Ayurveda. Ayurveda has its basis in astrology. The sun is the all-powerful tenet of astrology, and to give homage to the sun is equivalent to Luciferic worship. To participate in these so-called healing methods is to partake of the *Tree of the Knowledge of Good and Evil.*

Addendum: Go to page 612 for additional information on yoga and yoga exercises relevant to the myth that they can be practiced without spiritual and physical influence.

CHAPTER 9

VISUALIZATION—GUIDED IMAGERY

I was a visitor at Christmas time in a large church filled to capacity. A young man home visiting his parents had been asked to offer prayer prior the sermon. When he came to the podium he asked the audience to join him in a special form of prayer. He explained that some years before while in a Christian college a teacher in the theology department had taught him a special way of praying. He asked us to follow him in our minds through imagination as he, by imagery, took a walk down a beautiful country path lined with trees, the leaves on the branches hanging low as we walked through them. We journeyed into a pleasant meadow with a stream running through, here we were asked to kneel and present our prayer. As we knelt, in this imaginative endeavor, we were advised that a beautiful little bird might fly to our shoulder singing a melodious song of praise. The young man then proceeded to pray a proper prayer for the occasion.

As he was leading the congregation in this imaginary walk prior his prayer, I wanted to stand up and shout "NO, NO, just get on your knees and ask forgiveness for what you are doing." It was an extremely strong impulse that came to me, being timid and a visitor I did not do what this impression was suggesting I do. "No one would understand," I reasoned and probably I was right, but I was concerned about what he was doing even if he was not. He had received direction by his college professor in "guided imagery." Well so what! He had made a beautiful prayer and presentation so why all the fuss in my mind?

Within the past year I received an e-mail message from an alarmed mother of a college student telling me of her daughter's recent experience in a nearby Christian college. A guest speaker was featured at the usual Friday evening vespers, who, during his sermon asked the students to get out of their chairs and walk to some location within or just outside the auditorium in which they were meeting. At their selected location they were to put away all outside thoughts and begin to visualize—in their minds placing them selves' on some distant planet. In this imagery they were to find a bench or place where two could sit. Continuing, they were to conjure up Jesus Christ, then invite him to sit and join in conversation.

The following story was shared with me by a participant in a Church sponsored seminar. In 2010 a special seminar was conducted at a church

Conference's convention center. In one of the classes, at the later part of the seminar, the subject of handling stress and burnout was presented. The participants were asked to get comfortable, put feet flat on the floor, close their eyes, and relax. Music began to play that was without melody, and played continuously in the back ground. A man's monotone voice, friendly and welcoming, was heard coming through the music asking that each one go deep down inside themselves to find any negative energy. Again to go deep, deeper down, pushing out through the arms, legs, hands, feet, fingers and toes the bad energy.

Once the bad energies were pushed out then in imagination they were to conjure up in their mind a forest scene with a path lined with golden stones. The invitation came to wander down this path observing the birds and listening to the noise of the nearby stream. When coming to a small clearing the invitation came from the voice to choose a *spirit guide* to assist in the rest of the journey. This guide could be anything of our choosing, bird, dog, an angel, whatever. Next on the path a fountain of water was observed and the voice suggested taking a cup and to drink in positive energy from the water. Then the voice said "let us take time now and thank the spirit of the earth." To close, the voice suggested that positive energies could be sent out from each one to others who might need it.

The participant, who shared this story with me, said that when it was all over (22 minutes) he expressed his concerns to the instructor and the class about the practice, and mentioned that the only time he could remember a creature guiding in a decision, led to the fall of our first parents. Then came the accusations from some of the class— "narrow minded."

Recently I was reading a book, written by a Christian psychiatrist, who had gained my attention and admiration in a very convincing way. I believed God had impressed this author with wisdom from on high. Suddenly I came up short in my reading as I looked at the next sentence in the book. The doctor was commenting on the value and benefits of a technique referred to as "guided imagery." I had a feeling of concern as to how he might be using guided imagery; does he use it in a way that points to power of the Creator God or to a power that is supposed to be immanently within *self*, the counterfeit of the power of God? What is it with me that trigger these responses to words and phrases naming certain techniques which others may consider proper and even valuable? Allow me to share with you why I have these feelings when encountering the word and the expressions "visualization" and "guided imagery." You will need to make your own decision concerning the appropriate use of such nomenclature and the techniques in their use after you read the explanation of why I am affected so, as I choose not to make the conclusion for you.

In the past thirty years I spent thousands of hours reading and studying the topic of this book, looking for answers to questions I had, as well as questions of others concerning many popular healing techniques that are herein presented. While reading about many different techniques of alternative style healing, I frequently encountered the word "visualization" and the expression "guided imagery." It was obvious that I needed a better understanding of the origin, history, use of, and the meaning of these terms. Let me share a little of what I learned.

First, the following is what I understand these expressions to mean as I have seen them used. The two terms *visualization* and *guided imagery* are used synonymously. I have found them to be used that way in many writings. A definition of, *visualize, guided imagery* follows: by imagination in one's mind forming a picture, an action, a change of something, etc. As one repeatedly forms and thinks upon the imaginary mind picture, a happening, etc., there is the belief that doing such will actually cause it come about or to form. Is it analogous to being a creator, by the power of your mind?

A definition, from another source, of *visualization* and *guided imagery* is given:

> Creative visualization is the technique of using one's imagination to visualize specific behaviors or events occurring in one's life.[209] Advocates suggest creating a detailed schema of what one desires and then visualizing it over and over again with all of the senses (i.e., what do you see: what do you feel? what do you hear? What does it smell like?).[210]...

What is its origin? Michael Harner, the leading shaman of today claims it is ancient with the shamans. He points out that holistic medicine of today is trying to re-invent many of the old techniques of shamanism. He cites, *visualization*, altered states of consciousness, aspects of psychoanalysis, hypnotherapy, meditation, positive attitude, mental and emotional expression, etc.,[211] as some of these techniques.

We know that Hinduism was formed more than 3500 years ago and that visualization or imagery is a fundamental doctrine. The goal in Hinduism is to bring the latent *divinity of man* into full godhood, then to leave this world of reincarnation and join the spirit world, nirvana. This is done by raising the

---

209 Fink, Ronald A., *Creative Imagery: Discoveries and Inventions in Visualization,* Routledge Publishing, (1990), ISBN 0805807721 reported in Wikipedia/visualization.

210 Roeckelin, Jon E., *Imagery in Psychology:* A Reference Guide, Greenwood Publishing Group, (2004), ISBN 0313321973 reported in Wikipedia/visualization; Fezler, William, *Creative Imagery: How to Visualize in All Five Senses,* Published by Simon and Schuster, (1989), ISBN 0671682385.

211 Harner, Michael, The Way Out, Harper Collins Publishers, New York, NY, (1990), p. 136.

latent *kundalini* (Mother serpent god power) in the chakra at the base of the spine, up through the other six chakras to meet the male serpent god *Shiva* at the crown chakra (top of head) where they (male and female) meet in sexual embrace, and thus immortality and full godhood are achieved. *Meditation, visualization, and chakra clearing (or cleansing) are necessary to achieve such.*[212] This information comes from a book that was dictated by a spirit calling itself *The Tibetan Master* or *Djwhal Kul* the same name given by the spirit that channeled through Alice Bailey the information in the books that are the "Bible" for the New Age Movement. The thought comes to me perhaps this channeling spirit is Satan himself?

From the book *Milarepa: Tibet's Great Yogi* we have the following comment in regards to entering the state of *Tranquil Rest.*

> In realizing the non-existence of the personal Ego, the mind must be kept in quiescence. On being enabled, by various methods, to put the mind in that state as a result of a variety of causes, all thoughts, ideas, and cognition cease, and the mind passeth from consciousness into a state of perfect tranquility, so that days, months, and years may pass without the person himself perceiving it; thus the passing of time hath to be marked for him by others. This state is called Shi-ney (Tranquil Rest) ...Thus, by *thought –process* and <u>*visualization*</u> one treadeth the path.[213] (Emphasis added)

John Ankerberg and John Weldon in their booklet *The Facts on Holistic Health and the New Age Medicine* present additional insight to the subject of visualization:

> ...the practice of visualization is ancient and claims to work in a variety of ways. For example, by using the mind to contact an alleged inner divinity or "higher self," practitioners claim they can manipulate their personal reality to secure desired goals such as optimum health and the acquisition of wealth.... visualization is often used as a means to or in conjunction with altered states of consciousness and it is often accompanied by occultic meditation. It has long been associated with pagan religion and practice such as shamanism and shamanistic medicine. It is frequently used to develop psychic abilities and in *channeling* to contact "inner advisers" or spirit guides.[214]...

Dave Hunt and T. A. McMahon stir the muddy water with their following statement:

212 Prophet, Eliazbeth Clare, *DJwal Kul Intermediate studies of the Human Aura,* The Summit Lighthouse, Inc. Colorado springs, Colorado, (1974) p. 78, 114, 121.
213 *Milarepa, Tibet's Great Yogi:* Oxford University Press, (1971), p. 141.
214 Ankerberg, John, Weldon, John, *The Facts on Holistic Health and the New Medicine,* Harvest house Publishers, Eugene, Oregon, (1992), pp. 45, 46.

Paul Yonggi Cho declares: 'Through *visualization* and dreaming you can incubate your future and hatch the results.'[215] Such teaching has confused sincere Christians into imagining that "faith is a force that makes things happen because they *believe*." Thus faith is not placed in God but is a *power directed at God*, which forces Him to do for us what we have believed He will do. When Jesus said on several occasions, "Your faith has saved (healed) you," He did not mean that there is some magic power triggered by believing, but that faith had opened the door *for Him to heal* them. If a person is healed *merely because he believes* he will be healed, then the power is in his mind and God is merely a placebo to activate his belief. If everything works according to the "laws of success," then God is irrelevant and grace obsolete.[216]...

As stated previously, *visualization* and *imagery* are fundamental, core concepts of Hinduism, and have spread into many holistic healing techniques such as crystal healing, biofeedback, and most self-healing methods. Elmer Green in his book *Beyond Biofeedback,* states that visualization seems to be the quickest way to program the body. He feels that the body will follow "*command visualization*" and the whole body will respond to this directive given by thought and imagery. He explains:

> ...Instead, we visualize what we want to have happen globally and body converts the command visualization into the individual neural process for execution. The body seems to know what to do if the person knows what is desired.[217]...

Green further explains his use of visualization in therapy relating to biofeedback (self-hypnosis, see chapter on biofeedback).

> *In attempting to make a physiologic change through the focus of attention, it is important to realize that it is not accomplished by force or active will. It is done by <u>imaging</u> and <u>visualizing</u> the intended change while in a relaxed state.* (Mind in passive or neutral state) *We call this* passive volition (passive will). *Relaxation is important because* it is easiest then to have the casual, detached, and yet expectant attitude that is useful in bringing about the desired change. (Underline by author)

> "It has been found helpful to try to visualize clearly the part of the body that is to be influenced while using the autogenic phrases (which means "self-regulating

215   Cho, Paul Yonggi, *The Fourth dimension* (Logos, 1979) p. 44; Reported in Hunt, Dave, Weldon, John, *The Seduction of Christianity Spiritual Discernment in the Last Days,* Harvest house Publishers, Eugene, Oregon, (1992), p. 24.
216   Ankerberg, John, Weldon, John, *The Facts on Holistic Health and the New Medicine,* Harvest house Publishers, Eugene, Oregon, (1992), pp. 24, 25.
217   Green, Elmer & Alyce, *Beyond Biofeedback,* Knoll Publishing Co., Inc., (1989), p. 168.

phrases"—mantras) that I will give you. In this way a contact appears to be set up with that particular body part." This seems to be important in starting the chain of psychological events that eventuate in physiological changes." [218]

Elmer Green is telling us it takes a *mind in an altered state of consciousness* to effectively respond to visualization. *Stilling* the mind is done by meditation. And then, by using visualization, healing that is said to come from *within* is "tapped" into.

Visualization has gained great popularity and is presently used as a way to bring about success in many endeavors and enterprises, business, sports, education, psychology, religion, military, and even health and healing. This world-wide popularity can to a great extent be credited to the efforts and writings of Shakti Gawain. In 1978 she wrote *Creative Visualization* and by 2002 six million copies had been sold, and the book translated into thirty-five languages. It truly has had a world- wide impact. Other authors had written on visualization prior, but without the popularity and extensive circulation that Shakti 's writings have gained.[219]

In the following paragraphs a short summary of the information contained in Shakti's *Creative Visualization* will be presented. The principles she presents as to the source of power of visualization, methods of utilizing such, and application to life experiences are shared by other authors. Ophiel wrote the text *The Art and Practice of Getting Material Things through Creative Visualization* in 1967; Ronald Shone wrote the book *Creative Visualization* in 1988, and there have been many others with the same basic concepts. The purpose and goal of visualization is to create what one desires or feels need of. To make use of visualization in our own life, Shakti tells us, *it is not necessary to* "have Faith" in any power outside of our own selves, we need only utilize the *principles* that govern the working of the universe.

> Creative visualization is Magic in the truest and highest meaning of the word. It involves understanding and aligning yourself with the natural principles that govern the workings of our universe, and learning to use these principles in the most conscious and creative way.[220]

Let us review the principles that writers, who give support to creative visualization, tell us are the forces that govern the universe. The concept of universal energy, life force, chi, etc., is foundational. Every material thing is

---

218   Green, Ibid., p. 33.
219   Gawain, Shakti, *Creative Visualization,* Nataraj Publishing a division of New World Library, Novato, California, (2002) p. xi.
220   *Ibid.,* p. 6.

energy turned into solid matter. Energy is said to vibrate at various frequencies having different qualities, from lighter to denser. *Thought* is considered a light form of energy and is easily changed and transformed into something else. Creative visualization is the act of *thought* being transformed into what we have imagined or image in our minds; it is proclaimed to be a simple act of rearranging the form of energy by the power believed to be within our mind, that is *Self*. In reality it is the attempt to mimic the creative power of God.

To effectively perform visualization one has to experience a mind altering status, by bringing the brain wave pattern from beta to alpha rhythm. This is done using the same procedures and acts as is done in meditation. Actually it is a form meditation.[221] The mind comes to the attitude of "letting go of attachment" which is really *passivity of the mind* allowing the opening of channels to the soul and causing creative energy to flow.[222] Shakti tells us that only good can be produced from creative visualization; how is it that if there is power to transform energy by the power within man's mind it can only form that which is good? Behind this concept is the belief that man is inherently good, that there is no sin, and that man will judge himself.

Another point presented in how to be successful in visualization is to have a feeling of being connected to "your inner spiritual source." What is this inner spiritual source? We are told it comes from the infinite supply of love, wisdom, and energy that roams the universe. In her book, Gawain gives several names by which she feels one may identify his or her source, such as, "God, Goddess, universal intelligence, the Great Spirit, the higher power, or your true essence, the higher self, the wisdom that dwells within, etc. This power is identified by those writing on this subject as coming *innately* from within SELF. Simply stated, it is the *pagan's god*. Shakti expresses it in the following comment.

> Almost any form of meditation will eventually take you to an experience of your spiritual source, or your higher self. If you are not sure of what this experience feels like, don't worry about it. Just continue to practice your relaxation, visualization, and affirmations. Eventually you will start experiencing certain moments during your meditation when there is a sort of "click" in your consciousness and you feel like things are really working; you may even experience a lot of energy flowing through you or a warm, radiant glow in your body. These are signs that you are beginning to channel the energy of your higher self.[223]

---

221   *Ibid.*, p. 43.
222   *Ibid.*, p. 37.
223   *Ibid.*, p. 53.

We can agree with comments made in Gawain's book concerning the positive effect of our thoughts relevant to our health, that of entertaining thoughts that are positive, happy, of gratitude, appreciative, etc., instead of negative, constrictive, accusative, and other similar moods. Our expressions of appreciation and gratitude are to be directed to the Creator God, Jesus Christ the Son of God as the source of our strength and wellbeing, not some power that is lying latent within one's self which is said to be a part of the universal mind and just waiting to be found and put into service. We also are aware that as we express thoughts of praise and gratitude to others it can in turn be positive in their lives. This truth is counterfeited by the adversary of God in the following way.

The teaching in the Eastern and pagan dogma is that the universal energy throughout the cosmos of which our mind is a part, is interconnected to everything in the universe and also to other people's minds. By creative visualization one is able not only to influence one's self toward healing, but by visualization one is able to affect someone else's health, even if at a far distance by the visualization act. This is said to bring "instant cure" many times even without the other person being aware of your act on their part. This healing by visualization and at a distance, unknown to another, is believed to occur by having universal energy flow through that person doing the visualization and on to the person chosen to receive this energy. Ones *higher energy is* connected to another's *higher energy.*[224]

Remember in the chapter on Ayurveda we learned that the goal of the Hindu is to move the flow of universal energy through the chakra system so efficiently that the connection with the energy of the universe is so strongly connected as to cause one to be "one with all," "as above so below," "one is all and all is one," and that this status brings a person into "nirvana," connected with the "spirit world" of bliss. Visualization combined with meditation is taught to be a necessary and an integral part of this ascension to godhood by opening the energy centers, the chakras.

The beginning of this chapter presented the story of a young man asking the church congregation to join him in a visualization experience during his prayer. He had received guidance in this style of prayer from his religion teacher in a Seventh-day Adventist university; he had been guided to create a sanctuary in his imagination. The *sanctuary* was the meadow through which a small stream flowed and a bird singing its song of praise flew and lit on his shoulder. This sanctuary is promoted (falsely) to be a place of retreat, a place of rest and relaxation, of safety, that one can go to when weary and tired.

---

224 *Ibid.*, p. 83.

Shakti Gawain, as well as other teachers of visualization present the way to meet our *"inner guide"* after we have created the *"sanctuary"* in our imagination. The inner guide has many names, such as counselor, spirit guide, imaginary friend, master, etc. To meet this guide, place yourself in meditation and by visualization walk down the path to your personal sanctuary. As you come down the path into the sanctuary your guide will come from the opposite direction to meet you. This guide may be a bird, squirrel, rabbit or any type of animal as well as a human being. You then begin a conversation with this guide and show it around the sanctuary. You ask the guide what advice it has for you, express your appreciation for its presence and assistance. Invite this entity back; thereafter the guide is there for you to call on anytime you have need of counsel, wisdom, knowledge, support, love, or guidance of any type.[225]

Ronald Shone is Senior Lecturer at Sterling University in the United Kingdom and author of *Autohypnosis*, *Advanced Autohypnosis*, *First Steps to Freedom*, and *Creative Visualization, Using Imagery and Imagination for Self-Transformation.* While Sakti Gawain has gained vast popularity with her book and lectures over many years, Shone presents a more intellectual expose' of his understanding and belief in imagery and visualization. Although Shone is in agreement with Gawain on this subject of visualization he does add to her explanations in several areas. These additional points will be presented in the following paragraphs.

A most fundamental precept to visualization is to be in a *relaxed state. T*his, he tells us, is best achieved by the use of autohypnosis; he actually refers to it as a *hypnotic state*. One needs to arrive at a condition wherein the eyes are closed, breathing is slow and regular, and muscles totally relaxed, words or phrases are verbally being repeated. This state can be accomplished either in a lying position or sitting. To arrive at this situation practice is necessary, and eventually it will happen almost suddenly as one chooses to place themselves in this deeply relaxation or hypnotic state. To illustrate to the reader the depth of "relaxation" of which Shone is writing. I will take a quote from page 139 of his book *Creative Visualization, Using Imagery and Imagination for Self-Transformation.*

> One final observation: before you **awaken,** you should picture yourself totally free from pain and doing all the things you want to do. (Emphasis added)

Shone teaches that this act of visualization is carried out in the brain; it is a "right brain" function. What does he mean by the expression "right brain"? He teaches that the left side of the brain has to do with logic, reason, mathematics, reading, writing, language, and analysis while the other, right,

---

225 *Ibid.*, pp. 94-97.

side functions for such acts as recognition, rhythm, visual imagery, creativity, synthesis, dreams, symbols, and emotions. Why is it important to form an image in one's mind? Shone tells it this way:

> Why are visual images in the mind so important? The most important things about visual images are that they can influence the body....A strongly formed image will lead to an emotional response or some other bodily response. *It does not matter whether the image is about reality or something totally imaginary.* Both will create changes in the body that are consistent with the image....
>
> But it is not only the body that is influenced by images. Behavior, too, is influenced by them. Again the result is similar. *A strong image leads to behavior consistent with the image being formed in the mind's eye.* It does not matter whether the image is one of reality or unreality. What matters is whether the image is *strong* and whether you have *belief* in the image.[226]

He makes reference to the *power of the will.* He refers to such as a force which belongs to the *inner self,* and which gives direction and purpose to our actions. There is no outward manifestation of this entity; it simply directs, or makes the choice of our actions. It is a force which in our use will command, stimulate, regulate, and direct all activities.

Elmer and Alyce Green in their book *Beyond Biofeedback* frequently refer to the use of visualization with biofeedback therapy. In the preface of their book they comment that the principles of psycho-physiologic self-regulation has been known for 2500 years but primarily used by shaman (witch doctors). They have attempted to translate the writings of a shaman into modern language as follows:

> ...(1) we can more easily understand how involuntary process of body and mind, the major part of the "internal cosmos," are continuously influenced and controlled by VISUALIZATION, and (2) we begin to understand that the "external cosmos," outside our skins, also responds to visualization—though only shamans and occultist seem to have known much about the latter.... From our view point, the development of full human potential starts most easily with mastery of *body* energies through internal control of images, emotions, and volition (the will), and the process can be extended to energies which influence the outside world. It is striking that in yogic theory ten pranas (ten kinds of energy), which can be self-regulated, control the World inside the skin — and the *corresponding* prana affect the outside world. "As below — so above!"...[227]

---

226 Shone, Ronald, *Creative Visualization, Using Imagery and Imagination For Self-Transformation,* Destiny Books, Rochester, Vermont, (1988), p. 6.

227 Green, op. cit., p. xix.

I wish to add a comment made by E.G. White concerning the power of the will.

> Through the right exercise of the will an entire change may be made in the life. By yielding up the will to Christ, we ally ourselves with divine power. We receive strength from above to hold us steadfast. A pure and noble life, a life of victory over appetite and lust, is possible to everyone who will unite his weak, wavering human will to the omnipotent, unwavering will of God.[228]

That which is critical to the use of the will is to whom do we yield it? Christ or Belial? As I understand the use of visualization as outlined in the books I have read I believe that to participate in imagery and visualization as taught, I would be yielding my will to Satan. Later in this chapter I will write about the proper use of imagery and visualization wherein we give our will to Christ, not to Satan, for his direction and guidance in our lives.

The subject of "Self" is frequently written about in most disciplines in alternative healing techniques. Ronald Shone expands beyond the usual explanations of the beliefs behind the term "Self." It is important to have an understanding of this term to better comprehend the subject of "inner guides" which are, in truth, fallen angels, workers for Satan—*demons*.

To help in understanding this teaching let us use the following illustration. Envision a core circle somewhat like a *nucleolus* of a cell, which *Eastern thought and Western occultism* refer to as the "true self"; encircling this first small circle in this illustration is another circle, the *nucleus*, referred to as the "conscious self." Enclosing both of these small circles would be the cell, a much larger circle containing the entire contents of the cell and is referred to as the "unconscious self." At one end of this cell visualize a small area separate from the rest of the insides of the cell; this area would represent the "Super conscious self." We have one more term to list in our pursuit of understanding the terms used in this subject. "Collective unconscious" which is the area outside the cell we have envisioned, representing a large area of influence which acts upon and, in turn, influences the components of the interior of the cell. Think of it as the universal energy concept. Now let us define them:

The Conscious Self: This is the part of our consciousness of which we are directly aware and function within.

The Unconscious Self: A complex term referring to all thought, feelings, sensations, etc., that goes on *below* our level of consciousness but influences our behavior. The unconscious self is said to be influenced by imagination, dreams, and symbols and everything that enters our mind. It is actually thought

228   White, E.G., *Counsels on Health;* Pacific Press Pub. Assn., Nampa, ID, (1923), p. 440.

of as higher level than just the accumulation of influences, it is believed to contain latent wisdom of the universe.

The True Self: Think of it as a screen to show pictures on. Many different pictures can be shown on it, but it remains the simple plain white screen without change from the pictures. It is also considered to be the "divine within".

The Super Conscious: Area of highest thought, hopes, goals, aspirations, love, etc. Level of consciousness that connects with the "collective unconsciousness", in Eastern teachings this is where the person's consciousness and unconsciousness connects with the Universal mind or Creative Spirit (man joins and is a part of the godhood).

The Collective Unconscious: The above conscious and unconscious divisions constitute the cell in symbolism; a cell belongs to a group of cells or an organism. The organism exists within a sphere of influence is called the collective unconscious, equivalent to the Eastern thought of universal energy, vital force, life force, prana, chi, etc.

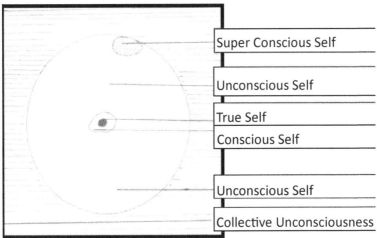

Figure 24. consciousness/unconsciousness

The author Shone now presents to us the idea that each of the above unconscious entities has an "inner guide" that we can call upon to assist us in life and gain wisdom and advice from. Within Eastern thought and Western occultism concepts, the unconscious levels of the mind have available, latently, the entire wisdom of the universe. To access this wisdom "inner guides," are contacted, discussion ensues and the information or understanding which we wish to know is obtained.

The technique of contacting an inner guide necessitates a deep state of relaxation, a quieted mind, (*hypnotism*), or the attempt will not be successful. Notice the following quotation.

In this section I wish to discuss how you can use creative visualization to call on your own inner guides. The technique itself is straightforward, but it does require a little practice. First, get yourself into the deepest relaxed state that you can, ...For this particular use it is important to get as deep as possible because your inner guides reside in those layers of consciousness not so easily accessible while conscious thoughts "cloud" the mind. Only when the mind is quietened can you even begin to approach an inner guide, or earlier attempts will be wasted.[229]

Shone goes on to explain that we not only have a guide for each of the unconscious selves but a male and a female guide as well. We are said to have the privilege to contact whichever guide we wish to speak to, and be able to talk and ask questions. The guides are to help us reach "our other selves." We are to invite the guides to return and thank them for their service. In this way they are available whenever we desire their presence and service. It is also important to express to the guides that we desire to be able to contact them in the future. Using visualization in health and healing is a common practice.

The basic principle is that your body and mind are inseparable. The whole person must be treated—mind and body. In holistic medicine prevention is also important. First and foremost one must obtain a deep relaxed state, a *hypnotic state*, to be able to use visualization in healing. In an infection one will image white blood cells attacking the germs and destroying them. In a broken bone imagine repair cells laying down bone, restoring intact bone, etc. An additional practice for which some may use visualization is the diagnosing and detecting of a disorder in the system. It is done in the following way.

An Inner Body Search: Start with very deep relaxation, then the body must be changed into a very small entity, then enter yourself through the blood stream, through the nose, through the throat, through a sweat gland, etc. Once inside you may make your way around the body inspecting all regions. You find a tumor in the brain, you clear it away with a laser, and then you leave via the tear duct.[230] There seems to be no level to which visualization cannot function. If you think the above-mentioned beliefs and practices are a bit out of the ordinary then consider the next proclamation that author OPHIEL makes as to our origin.

OPHIEL has written several books which by the titles alone a person can gain an appreciation as to the belief system he supports. Titles:

Art and Practice of Astral Projection; Art and Practice of the Occult; Art and Practice of Clairvoyance; Art and Practice of Cabala Magic; etc. and also *The*

---

229 Shone, op. cit. p. 28
230 *Ibid.*, pp. 147, 148.

Art and Practice of Getting Material Things Through Creative Visualization. I present his answer as to where we came from:

> WE CREATED OURSELVES, FOR OURSELVES, AND BY OURSELVES, BY OUR OWN MENTAL POWERS!
>
> Naturally we did this creating ignorantly but we did it nevertheless. As I said before the time can come that you can take, and will take, your own Personal Divine Powers into your own hands and direct the Right Use of the power. AND THEN ONLY WILL YOU BEGIN TO USE YOUR DIVINE POWERS AS THEY SHOULD BE USED AND AS YOU SHOULD USE THEM— IN THE RIGHT WAY AND FOR YOUR OWN BENEFIT!!![231] (Emphasis from original text)

And the Buddhist says: "We have created our own bodies."[232] Think back to the incident I spoke of in the opening paragraph, the prayer imagery. After walking down a path covered with foliage, a bird appeared as you kneeled to pray. I read of such a scenario occurring after repetition of the imagery, the bird, squirrel, rabbit or whatever creature appears in this guided imagery appears quickly and may even dialogue with you. It may become your "guide," appearing even without imagery initiation.

I wish to share with the reader comments and information relevant to guided imagery and visualization presented by Richard Gerber M.D. in the book he authored, *Vibrational Medicine.* He is considered one of the outstanding scientists and writers in New Age scientific writing. He is an internal medicine specialist, yet governed in his thoughts by his deep belief in the pantheistic Eastern belief system. In his book he states that he and his wife are "clairvoyant," and that much of the information in the book has come *from channeling,* I quote:

> I would like to point out to the readers of *Vibrational Medicine* that I believe this book is the result of cooperation between healers and researchers on the physical plane and beings who exist on the higher spiritual planes. This cooperation has made possible the transmission of a wealth of information that is much needed on the planet at this time. Many of the sections of this book are actually "*messages from spirit*" that I have accumulated over the years, *channeled* through various sources.[233]

231　*OPHIEL, The Art and Practice of Getting Material Things through Creative Visualization,* Samuel Weiser, Inc., York Beach, Maine, (1967) p. 12.

232　Govinda, *Foundations of Tibetan Mysticism,* Samuel Weiser, NY, (1969), p. 159.

233　Gerber, Richard, Vibrational Medicine, *The #1 Handbook of Subtle—Energy Therapies,* Bear and Company, Rochester, VT, (2001), p. 37.

In a discussion of the value and use of a type of meditation which Dr. Gerber labels "active meditation" which involves use of visualization combined with imagery, he gives an illustration as to how they can be used to obtain advanced knowledge. A person will imagine himself enrolling in a school of higher education, one that grants advanced degrees. Continue by imagining yourself attending classes in a school of higher learning:

> ...Often times the *advanced meditator*, when visualizing him or her attending classes in a school of higher learning, may actually be working with *inner teachers* (spirits) and learning on an *astral* level.[234]

Gerber adds another illustration of visualization and guided imagery. The individual *stills* the mind and body by various *relaxation techniques* then turns their consciousness to their *"Higher Selves"* (innate inner knowledge) concerning aspects of the past, present, and the future. The person then listens for meaningful information which may come in the form of *words, images, or feelings*. An additional illustration gives us added depth in the use of imagery in a spiritistic manner.

This example has to do with *dialogue* with "Higher Self" (a spirit) while being dedicated to higher learning. This dialogue will be combined with various types of visual *imagery exercises* which involve cleansing the *auric field* and the *chakras*, as well as creating a greater alignment of the *physical* and *subtle bodies*. An example of an imagery exercise is as follows. Take a crystal in each hand, hold your hands in front of the third eye center (forehead) and visualize subtle energy in the form of colored and white light entering into the body through the crystals. The energy taken into the body causes a rising of the vibrational rate of the body and raises the consciousness to a higher frequency level. The person can see one's self shrinking and entering into the crystal. You can then decide to enter a hall of knowledge within the structure of the crystal:

> This hall of knowledge can be set up like a library. Only this unique library allows one access to information about oneself in present and past lives, as well as allowing one to obtain general information about any number of historical subjects. The visual metaphor of the library allows one to use imagination to tap into higher levels of cognitive processing. The technique of visualization itself, when used in conjunction with the meditational process, allows human beings to not only reprogram their own biocomputers (as in biofeedback and autonomic control) but also to access levels of inner potential not ordinarily

---

234   *Ibid.*, p. 397.

available to waking consciousness. Visualization and imagery holds the key to unlocking the hidden reserves of human thoughtpower.[235]

...Behind imagination lie the doors to higher levels of reality. The ability to use symbolic imagery also holds the key to tapping into vast inner sources of creativity and insight.[236]

The deception of imagery and visualization has entered the church like a "Trojan Horse" according to Hunt and McMahon, in *The Seduction of Christianity*. How did it get there? Let's follow the trail as authors Hunt and McMahon unfold the story.

To understand our present society and our world, it is important to understand the influence that secular psychology has had on its formation. The great expansion of this influence took place following World War II. In 1946 U.S. Congress passed a National Mental Health Act, establishing a federally funded program to expand the study of psychology in universities, including seminaries, throughout the nation. This was new to seminaries. Hunt & McMahon tell us that by 1950 nearly 80% of these seminaries were offering advanced studies in psychology. Paul Vitz, in the 1980's a professor of psychology at New York University wrote the following:

Psychology as *religion* exists...in great strength throughout the United States.... (It) is deeply anti -Christian... (Yet) is extensively supported by schools, universities, and social programs financed by taxes collected from Christians.... But for the first time the destructive logic of this secular religion is beginning to be understood....[237] (Italics by author)

In 1951 Carl Rogers, one of the foremost proponents of secular psychology spoke of *"professional interest in psychotherapy,"* as being the most rapidly growing subject in social sciences of that time. Hunt and McMahon comment that by the mid 1980's psychology had attained the status of a "guru" and "who's who": "Scientific standards of behavior" are relieving consciences of obedience to God's moral laws. In this way, as well as through introduction of sorcery as science, psychology is the major change agent in transforming society.

---

235 *Ibid.*
236 *Ibid.*, pp. 397, 398.
237 Vitz, Paul Clayton, *Psychology As Religion: The Cult of Self-worship*, Erdmans, (1997), p. 10 : Reported in Hunt and McMahon, op. cit., p. 29.

...Humanistic and transpersonal psychologies have now embraced the entire spectrum of sorcery. For example, the 22nd annual Meeting of the Association for Humanistic Psychology held in Boston August 21-26, 1984 was heavily flavored with Hindu/ Buddhist Occultism. The official daily schedule included "early morning; Yoga, Tai chi, Meditation." About half of the "Pre-Conference/ Post-conference Institutes" involved blatant sorcery, with such subjects as Visualization and Healing...Trance States and Healing...operation of alchemy... guided imagery... Shamanic (witchcraft) Ecstasy and Transformation...Being the Wizard We Are.[238]

Dr. Beverly Galyean, consultant to the Los Angeles school system, wrote in an article in *The Journal of Humanistic Psychology* the following:

...Human potential is inexhaustible and is realized through new modes of exploration (i.e., meditation, guided imagery, dream work, yoga, body movement, sensory awareness, energy transfer (healing), reincarnation therapy, and esoteric studies.)...

Meditation and guided imagery activities are the core of the (confluent/holistic education) curriculum.[239]

Is it any wonder that *visualization* and/or *guided imagery* have entered the Church? Few religious or science leaders have perceived that this sorcery is not neutral and is in fact anti-Christian. To partake of the use of visualization is to partake of the world view out of which it has its origin, pantheistic concepts, and the belief that within ourselves divinity exists which can be articulated to actually *create*. At the root of modern and humanistic psychology is "SELF," while the Bible teaches us to die to self.

I am crucified with Christ: nevertheless I live; yet not I, but Christ liveth in me: and the life which I now live in the flesh I live by the faith of the Son of God, who loved me, and gave himself for me. (Galatians 2:20)

I can of mine own self do nothing: as I hear, I judge: and my judgment is just; because I seek not mine own will, but the will of the Father which hath sent me. (John 5:30)

What about visualization, imagination, imagery, which I do in my mind and that I use to plan my future, to do work for today, to invent, to solve

---

238   Hunt and McMahon, op. cit., p. 30.
239   Galyean, Beverly-Colleene, Guided Imagery in Education,, *Journal of Humanistic Psychology,* Fall (1981), Vo.. 21, No. 4,; Reported in Hunt and McMahon, op. cit., p. 30.

problems? Has the author of this book lost his judgment, his common sense by incriminating any imagination or originality? What may seem like an unbalanced attack on visualization and guided imagery, by careful analysis will reveal a distinct difference between Satan's counterfeit and God's true gift of imagination and use of imagery. God in creating man gave him a mind that has attributes making it capable of reflecting upon the mind and character of God; he was given the ability to reason, to imagine, and to use imagery to grow in mind and wisdom. These activities are to be guided by God and under His influence.

When we allow the influence of Satan to be our guide, accepting his concept that we have divinity within ourselves, and by using the techniques of visualization and guided imagery, we are led to believe that we are able to use that divinity to achieve certain accomplishments. Remember from previous paragraphs we learned that those activities are part of the Hindu's trek to reach the Supreme Self—Godhood.

We must ask a question: the author E.G. White, writes a great deal about our imagination, which can be used to gain health or to destroy it, or to learn great truths from the Bible. That is true, so what is the difference between the imagery written about in the previous pages and this *imagination and imagery* White speaks of? Answer: One method seeks to transform thought into action or change, from a power believed to be within *self,* while the positive value of the imagination from E.G. White's point of view is that the power in imagination and imagery does not come from within but from *above.*

> And whatsoever ye shall ask in my name, that will I do, that the Father may be glorified in the Son. If ye shall ask any thing in my name, I will do (it). (John 14: 13, 14)

Let's take a look at some of those statements on imagination and imagery.

> All who profess to be followers of Jesus should feel that a duty rests upon them to preserve their bodies in the best condition of health, that their minds may be clear to comprehend heavenly things. The mind needs to be controlled; for it has a most powerful influence upon the health. The imagination often misleads, and when indulged, brings severe forms of disease upon the afflicted. Many die of diseases which are mostly imaginary[240]....

> Thousands are sick and dying around us who might get well and live if they would; but their imagination holds them. They fear that they will be made worse if they labor to exercise, when this is just the change they need to make them

---

240 White, E.G., *Counsels on Health,* Pacific Press Publishing Association (now in Nampa Idaho), Mountain View, California, (1951), p. 95.2.

well. Without this, they never can improve. They should exercise the power of the will, rise above their aches and debility, and engage in useful employment, and forget that they have aching backs, sides, lungs, and heads.[241]

Even imagery is described as being of value.

The minister who makes the word of God his constant companion will continually bring forth truth of new beauty. The Spirit of Christ will come upon him, and God will work through him to help others. The Holy Spirit will fill his mind and heart with hope and courage and *Bible imagery,* and all this will be communicated to those under his instruction.[242]

If the Bible were studied as it should be, men would become strong in intellect. The subjects treated upon in the Word of God, the dignified simplicity of its utterance, the noble themes which it presents to the mind; develop faculties in man which cannot otherwise be developed. In the Bible a boundless field is opened for the *imagination.* The student will come from a contemplation of its grand themes, from association with its lofty *imagery* more pure and elevated in thought and feeling than if he had spent the time in reading any work of mere human origin, to say nothing of those of a trifling character.[243] (Emphasis added)

The Bible contains imagery throughout the Old Testament and the New. The sacrificial system pointing to the future death of the Son of God as a substitute for sinful man was initiated by God Himself. This ceremony was to help man realize that sin resulted in death of the sinner, but through accepting by faith the merits of the shed blood and death of Christ the Divine Son of God, as man's substitute, man could regain paradise and eternal life. The entire Tabernacle service was imagery and teaching God's plan of salvation for man. The parables Jesus told used imagination and imagery to teach saving truths. They were written to stimulate the mind of man to seek for eternal truths stored in the Bible. The prophecies of Daniel and Revelation are filled with imagery.

To close this chapter the following quote has been chosen to emphasize that imagery has a place in our thoughts and minds but it is imperative that we have chosen the Holy Spirit to guide our imagination and not the power of Satan.

---

241 White, E.G., *Testimonies for the Church* Vol. 3, Pacific Press Publishing Association, Mountain View, California, (1948), p. 76.
242 White, E.G., *Gospel Workers,* (1915), p. 253.
243 White, E.G., Vol. *1. Mind, Character, and Personality,* Southern Publishing Association, Nashville, Tennessee, (1977), p. 92, 93.

When the teacher will rely upon God in prayer, the Spirit of Christ will come upon him, and God will work through him by the Holy Spirit upon the minds of others. The Spirit fills the mind and heart with sweet hope and courage and Bible imagery, and all this will be communicated to the youth under his instructions.[244]

---

244 White, E.G., *Christ's Object Lessons,* Pacific Press Publishing Association, Nampa, ID, (1900), pp. 131,132.

CHAPTER 10

ACUPUNCTURE AND CHINESE TRADITIONAL MEDICINE

Chinese traditional medicine practices were little heard of in the West until the early 1970's. I became involved in medical education in 1954, and not until the 1970's did I hear of acupuncture or other traditional Chinese healing methods. The march toward scientific medicine in the first years of the 20th century had been almost complete.

The medical disciplines of eclectic medicine, homeopathy, osteopathy, and naturopathy had either converted toward scientific medicine or had slowly faded and/or ceased to exist. Medical students were told about some past medical treatments, such as the use of heavy metals, emetics, blistering compounds, purgatives, and bloodletting, but I heard no mention of Ayurvedic or traditional Chinese medicine, such as acupuncture or moxibustion.

Since the late 1970's, there has been widespread acceptance of the oriental healing methods. Most of the older physicians rejected them, but a large number of younger doctors did not, and amazingly some of the alternative therapies have gone "Main Street." For some practitioners, it has been mainly a financial interest; but for others, it has been a belief in these alternative methods. Now, we see in many medical training institutions and at the National Institutes of Health research being done on alternative treatment methods, acupuncture being one of the more common.

Segments of the Ayurvedic system have been used more widely than has Chinese traditional medicine. However, the Chinese methods are often used along with Ayurveda. Let us examine the roots of the traditional Chinese system of healing. You are probably very familiar with the symbol of two fish swimming in a circle with eight trigrams of all possible combinations of the two, which in Chinese is called *pa kua* and referred to in English as *circle of harmony.* Emperor Fu His, in 2900 B.C., is credited with its origination. It is a symbol representing all the conditions of interior—exterior, hot—cold, deficiencies—excesses, yin—yang. This Emperor's works are the most ancient upon which traditional Chinese medicine is based.[245]

---

245 Lyons, Albert S. , Petrucelli, R. Joseph II; *Medicine An Illustrated History,*Harry N. Abrams, Inc. Publishers, NY, (1978), p. 125.

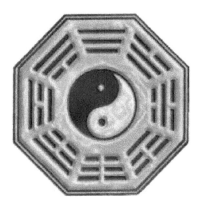

Figure 25. picture of pa kua (circle of harmony)

Another Emperor, Shen Nung, in 2800 B.C., compiled a text *"pentsao"* which was the first medical text for the use of herbs. It contained three hundred and sixty-five drugs, which he had tested on himself.[246]

The most celebrated ancient medical text in China is called the "Nei Ching." It was written in 2600 B.C. by the Yellow Emperor, Hwang Ti. From this text is garnered information that gives us insight into the early approach to Chinese medicine and its orientation.[247]

January 1, 1912, Sun Yat Sen, a Western trained physician, was inaugurated President of China following the revolution and over-throw in 1911 of the Imperial dynasty. Shortly following, he initiated improvements in hygiene practices in China such as having garbage cleared from the streets and installing running water in major urban centers. A bureau to combat epidemics was established and Western style medical schools were developed by a few Western-trained Chinese physicians. The old practice of traditional Chinese medicine was discouraged and in 1929 outlawed. This caused a great furor from the traditional Chinese medicine doctors who banned together to fight the new restrictions. The masses of China were on the side of traditional medicine, and the attempt to eradicate the old style practice failed primarily because of the belief of mostly uneducated Chinese masses in Taoism and the philosophy of *chi* with its *yin—yang* divisions. That attempt to modernize China failed.

The changes initiated by Sun Yat Sen were almost insignificant compared to the size and degenerate condition of the country. From 1916 until 1949 China suffered great political turmoil and instability, with minimal progress made in hygiene and health of the nation. Following Mao's rise to power under Communism in 1949, public hygiene was made a priority. Eradicating the

---

246   *Ibid.*, p. 124.
247   *Ibid.*, p. 124.

vectors of parasitic diseases, closure of open sewers, immunization programs, and clean water were measures taken to combat a deplorable health status, as documented by Paul Bailey in his book *A History of Chinese Medicine*. He tells us of epidemics continuously of cholera, plague, black fever (500,000 afflicted in 1949), and 10,000,000 were infected by a parasite called bilhariza, 1,000,000 died each year from tuberculosis, epidemics of scarlet fever, and typhoid; untold millions were infected with malaria. The average life span was 35 years. This health status was a result of the mind-set of Taoism and the other Eastern religious concepts. The medical approach to illness was based on such beliefs, which allowed these conditions to exist. Traditional Chinese medicine is based on Taoism ("The Way"). The basic beliefs of Taoism are:

1. The Creative Principle (or universal energy) is called *chi* and is composed of two parts–*yin* and *yang (*dualism);
2. *Five basic elements* are involved in transformation in creation: *metal, air, earth, fire, water*. (synonyms for five planets, Saturn, Venous, Jupiter, Mars, Mercury, believed to be source of creation)
3. Man is the *microcosm* of the universe—*macrocosm*

In contrast the Biblical account of creation tells us how God created:

> For He spake and it was done and He commanded and it stood fast. (Psalms. 33:9.}

Man was created by God forming the dust of the ground into man's form; God breathed into it "the breath of life" and man became a living *soul*. Early on in the history of the world Satan's counterfeit changed this story in such a way that left out the Creator, Jesus Christ the Son of God. This formed the myth of a great power, energy, voice, breath that existed throughout space which was of two parts, good and evil and when it became properly balanced creation occurred. The Greeks called this cosmic spirit that they believed pervades and enlivens all things, and produces change, *pneuma*, this equates with the Hindus' prana, those of the South Seas mana, and the Chinese chi.

The Chinese explanation for origins is that with the proper balance of yin and yang (which are divisions of *chi)*, transformation occurred which brought the cosmos, earth, and man into existence. Fundamental to traditional Chinese medicine is the astrological concept of the planets being closely associated with earth and man, with the sun and moon having the strongest influence. They had a belief in a "cosmological correspondence" between the houses of the Chinese zodiac and "chinglo channels" (now called meridians) that are said to be in man. Sheila McNamara, in her book, *Traditional Chinese Medicine*, makes the following statement:

> To the Chinese, the human body is the cosmos in miniature. The universe is an organism and man is a microcosm of the universe...Yang is masculine: sun.... Yin is feminine: moon, ...[248]

This belief gives expression in the saying "as above, so below." This concept was prevalent throughout the ancient world but often expressed in different terms. A statement made by Gregor Reisch (c. 1467-1525) in *Margarita Philosophica,* published in 1503:

> The pagans believed that the zodiac formed the body of the Grand Man of the Universe. This body, which they called the Macrocosm (The Great World), was divided into twelve major parts, one of which was under the control of the celestial powers reposing in each of the zodiacal constellations. Believing that the entire universal system was epitomized in man's body, which they called the Microcosm (the Little World), they evolved that now familiar figure of "the cut—up man in the almanac" by allotting a sign of the zodiac to each of twelve major parts of the human body.

These beliefs led to *astrological medicine* which was dominant in Europe up until the seventeenth century. The physicians of that time used special *tables,* called *ephemerides* or *Alfonsine tables,* to make predictions based on astrological conjunctions, alignments, and the angle between planets. These predictions were then used to perform various healing acts, such as drawing off blood from the body (venesection), cupping, (causing great blisters to form), cauterization, surgery, and to choose herbs for medicines with special astral powers. Disease, they believed came from an interruption of the free flow of pneuma or prana, as well as an imbalance of four body fluids called *humors.* Each humor was believed to be connected to a planet by correspondence.

To correct a supposed imbalance of humors, bloodletting (bleeding) was instigated and used by European and early American practitioners, and is still done by some Muslims today.

> ...The practice of lancing, bloodletting and cupping, (*hijama*) to affect specific organs or to mitigate specific diseases based on a postulated relationship between the internal organs and points on the surface of the skin is still prevalent amongst the Muslims worldwide and nowadays video instructions for it are available, even on YouTube. It is plausible that the same principle is at the origin of acupuncture channels in China because the distribution of the regions of astrological influences and the related venesection points portrayed

---

248   McNamara, Sheila, *Traditional Chinese Medicine*, Basic Books, (Perseus Books) New York, NY, (1996), p. 26.

in medieval Islamic and European manuscripts significantly resembles the allocation of master, command influential, and other key points.[249]...

The Chinese followed a similar concept and saw disease as being a result of disharmony in the balance of yin and yang. This imbalance can occur for many reasons, such as lifestyle. It is believed that some physical disorders are caused by *winds*. Foods are considered yin or yang and the balance of such will influence so as to maintain health, or imbalance to allow illness. The beliefs of what causes imbalance in the yin and yang of the body are complex. I will not go into the causes of imbalance, but rather will direct our attention to the practices that are said to be capable of restoring balance.

In Ayurveda, *prana,* universal energy is said to be centered in whirling vortexes of energy referred to as chakras. The flow of energy through the body is said to be facilitated by meditation, yoga exercises, diet, herbs, aromatherapy, and cleansing therapies. In *traditional Chinese medicine* (TCM) the energy is described as flowing through the body in "meridians" which are (imaginary) channels perpendicular to the body. Many smaller channels branch from the meridians and distribute the energy throughout the body. Here too, meditation, exercises, food—drink, moxibustion, acupressure, acupuncture, and other *sympathetic remedies* are used to facilitate the flow and balance of chi.

All creation depended upon *correspondence, association*, and *sympathy* between the various phases outlined above and yin—yang balance of chi. All disease of animal and man is considered to be an imbalance of yin—yang. Correcting the imbalance is believed to restore health, therefore methods to balance chi and treat disease were developed over millennia of time.

Diseases are classified according to four different states of disharmony and make up eight syndromes, which include all varieties of disease. These previously mentioned conditions are: imbalance of yin/ yang; interior/exterior; hot/cold; and deficiencies/excesses.

The customary way to diagnose an imbalance of energy in traditional Chinese medicine was to observe the tongue and feel the pulse. The tongue was felt to demonstrate changes in chi energy distribution throughout the body. Taking the pulse was done not to check the rate and rhythm of the heart, but to find where an imbalance of chi existed. One ancient author of Chinese traditional medicine wrote ten large volumes on *pulse diagnosis*. From the pulse and observation of the tongue, those physicians determined the imbalance of chi (qi), where it existed, and then prescribed to balance it.

249   Kavoussi, Ben MS, MSOM, Lac, *Science-Based Medicine,* Astrology with Needles, Posted (9-4-09), pp.5,6; http://www.sciencebasedmedicine. org/?p=583.

DISEASE TREATMENT METHODS

In this chapter is presented those methods of treatment most commonly known and accepted by Western society. These include the use of herbs, martial arts, and acupuncture. The Chinese practice disease prevention, with special emphasis on exercise and diet. Disease prevention is directed toward maintaining a balance of body energies.

In traditional Chinese medicine, herbs and foods are considered to have a *signature* and *like cures like*. For instance, walnuts resemble the brain therefore walnuts are especially nourishing to the brain. For a child to eat the pig's tail, is to assure a straight strong spine as he or she grows (in China pigs have straight tails). If an herb looks like an organ of the body, then it is considered to have special healing powers for that part of the body.[250]

Ginseng root can resemble the body and its limbs and is therefore considered good for all bodily ailments. The horn of an animal represents a phallic symbol and so is used as an aphrodisiac. Consumption of animal parts, such as a tiger's heart, will give courage. This type of belief has resulted in a large number of herbs being used because of their appearance rather than from their biochemical properties. Many animal parts are likewise used in this way. I visited a very large Chinese pharmacy in Vancouver, British Columbia, Canada, and was amazed to see dried parts of animals, fish, and many other products I could not identify. The store had a thousand or more different substances, some in bottles and some in open boxes.

The idea of *like cures like* is an *association–sympathy* concept and not at all due to the biochemical action of our systems. The Chinese found many herbs and substances that really do have significant biochemical action which are used world-wide. Herbal books will often label herbs as either hot–cold and/or yin–yang. The herbs may then be chosen for medicinal use accordingly, so as to influence a sick person's balance of yin-yang and or hot and cold.

MARTIAL ARTS—QI GONG

> Qi gong is the forerunner of traditional Chinese medicine, since *qi*/chi, the subtle breath or life energy, is at the heart of everything.[251]

Qi gong or (Chi Kung) means manipulation of vital energy (psychic energy), and is also the precursor of martial arts that have been practiced in China for thousands of years. Qi is comprised of yin and yang, each

---

250   McNamara, op. cit., p.117.
251   *Ibid.*, p. 130.

contributing to health when in proper balance. Gong refers to achieving the ultimate balance of the two parts. Qi gong is a variety of physical exercises and actions practiced to facilitate the harmony of yin and yang. If one is able to superbly balance these parts of qi, he will be able to accomplish extraordinary feats with his powers and will be a *master* of qi gong.

Qi gong is a system of body/mind discipline of traditional Chinese medicine and is the foundation of martial arts, which are practiced under various names, such as ninjutsu, tai chi chuan, ikido, tae kwon do, judo, kenpo, karate, etc.

> Fundamentally, qi gong is a method of meditation exercise aimed at the cultivation of physical and spiritual perfection.[252]

Meditational forms involve stillness, standing, sitting, or lying motionless. More physically active forms will involve breathing exercises in order to inhale the *"vital essence of life."* Physical activity is frequently a slow, smooth, and rounded movement. Concentrating on breath and emptying the mind are very important. These activities are *"always with a spiritual element".*[253]

(See page 614 for addendum on "origin" of martial arts.)

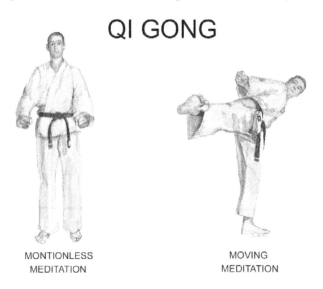

QI GONG

MONTIONLESS
MEDITATION

MOVING
MEDITATION

Figure 26. Martial Arts

---

252   *Ibid.,* pp. 127–128.
253   *Ibid.,* p. 128.

The exercises can be performed alone, or by a qi gong Master for another person, which involves exercising around the other person's body, without making any physical contact. This is supposed to activate the qi within another's body so that the person can be brought into the qi gong state. Balancing the qi is the objective, for too little qi is equivalent to illness. When people do their own exercises, or when masters do the exercises for them, qi, it is said, can be directed towards different areas within the body.

> One of its main precepts concerns finding the center of the body, to attain perfect balance as a prerequisite to health. Students will be taught to visualize the soles of their feet reaching hundreds of yards deep down into the earth, or a rod passing down their spine via entering of their head and penetrating deep into the ground. Once they achieve perfect balance, no one will be able to knock them off-balance. It proves that the qi is perfectly centered, neither too weak in one part of the body nor too strong in another.[254]

I once presented this information to an assembly and a gentleman came to me afterward. He spoke of taking *karate,* one of the disciplines of qi gong, and how he and two other students tried to push their instructor off-balance, and were unable to do so. The question to ask is what power held him to the ground?

A delegation of Chinese physicians traveled to the United States to present to American doctors this particular aspect of traditional Chinese medicine. They desired to convince the American doctors of the scientific basis of this therapy for which they made great claims. They described studies showing that the power associated with this life force showed up as making changes in electrical brain wave potential; in the molecular rotation of liquid crystal molecules; and in cancer cells, bacteria, and viruses. The following was reported in *The Medical Tribune*:

> After the Chinese Qi Gong scientists described their research, Dr. Li Xiao Ming, a Qi Gong master at the Qi Gong Research Institute at the Beijing College of Traditional Chinese Medicine, demonstrated his art on Dr. Alfonso Di Mino. As Dr. Li did his exercise around Dr. Di Mino, Dr. Di Mino shouted for Dr. Li to lower his hands as he said that he felt as if he "were ready to fly." Later he said that it felt as if he had an "electric magnetic power inside his body" "My mind was not aware of my body."
>
> Dr. Di Mino, a biophysicist, described this "life force" as "the medicine of the future."[255]

---

254 *Ibid.*, p. 128.
255 *Medical Tribune,* Feb. 5, (1986) by Elizabeth Mechcatie (medical newspaper)

Robert Leeds, the vice chairman of the Sino-U.S. Qi Gong Center, then told the audience that Dr. Li was able to:

> ...manipulate energies we allegedly are not sensitive to or do not understand." He added that for four thousand years, the Chinese have been able to map out this energy field and manipulate it to such an extent that it can heal.[256]

(See appendix L p. 584 for additional information on Martial arts.)

All across China in the early morning, people can be seen outside practicing various exercises of qi gong. All qi gong methods are supposed to produce equal flow of energy through the body and thereby promote health. Remember, there is a *spiritual aspect* connected to qi gong exercises.[257]

Tai chi is one of the popular styles of qi gong. It is felt to be totally free of any spiritual association by most people practicing it. Sheila McNamara in her book, *Traditional Chinese Medicine,* says of the different qi gong exercises:

> ...but they all spring from the same ancient root, and all are based on the meridians which interconnect the internal organs and viscera with the exterior of the body, through which the qi flows.[258]

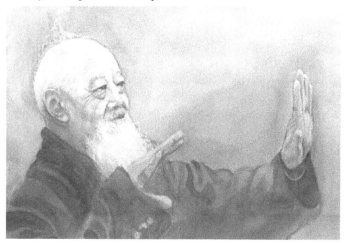

Figure 27. Chinese doing tai chi

In *U.S. News and World Report*, Feb. 22, 1999, there was an article by Bay Fang, entitled *An Opiate of the Masses*? This article referred to an advanced type of qi gong exercise. Grand Master Li Hongzhi leads sixty million Chinese

---

256 *Ibid.*
257 McNamara, op. cit., p. 128.
258 *Ibid.*, p. 128.

in the practice of Falun Gong "Rotating the Law Wheel." Tape recordings of the voice of the Master were played as thousands gather to do exercises. With eyes closed the people raised their arms together, and in perfect unison their hands swept slowly in a circle and came to rest in a prayer position.

> Adherents in China say the Falun Gong Master can cure cancer, heal the blind, and make white hair turn black. ...Throughout history, Qi Gong masters have captivated the public with their miracle cures, soothsaying and other tricks ranging from levitating objects to communicating with aliens and changing the odor of cigarettes.[259]

We have seen how energy manipulation has progressed from the use of hands and needles, to exercises, and finally to energy manipulation without touching, just by using the mind to bring about *miraculous* changes. This type of progression, in whatever art being practiced, proves that the method used is not the real power, but is, instead, the *mental connection* with hidden powers of the occult.

ACUPUNCTURE AND CHINESE PHYSIOLOGY

Chinese physiology has astrology as its foundation. All qi gong exercises are based on the Chinese concept of physiology which teaches that there are fourteen meridians. Qi is believed to circulate through these meridians–the invisible lines of energy channels which are said to travel through the system, six on each side, plus one in the middle of the front, and one in the middle of the back. They run perpendicular on the body and have multiple small channels which are said to connect to various organs of the body. Acupuncture is performed by needling these meridians at specific points in order to balance the distribution of energy (qi) to organs. Those who are proficient in qi gong can bring about this same balance simply by mind power and without needles.

The Chinese describe the distribution of *chi* (life energy) in a manner different from the Ayurvedic system. It is believed that the energy comes close to the skin in various places and can be influenced in those areas to alter its flow.

Stephen Basser M.D. did a very extensive review of studies evaluating acupuncture. His report *"Acupuncture: A History,"* appeared in the Spring/Summer issue of *The Scientific Review of Alternative Medicine, 1999.* He learned from his research that in the early 1970's, manuscripts dating from 168 B.C., describing medicine as it existed in the third and second centuries B.C., were discovered in China at the Ma-wang-tui graves. From these manuscripts, descriptions of all procedures used in Chinese medicine during that period of

---

259   U.S. News and World Report, Opiate of the Masses, by Bay Fang, Feb. 22, (1999), p. 45.

time were obtained. Acupuncture was not mentioned. It first showed up in the Shi-chi text in 90 B.C.; however, there are descriptions of sharp stones being used to drain blood from veins prior this date.[260]

> The Ma-wang-tui texts describe eleven 'mo', or vessels, that were believed to contain in addition to blood a life force known as chi or pneuma.[261]

It was not appreciated at that time that blood circulates in a closed system. The most important text of the end of the first century B.C was the Huang-ti nei-ching. It describes twelve vessels (mo) instead of eleven, and gives different courses for the vessels from those given in the earlier descriptions. The vessels are called "conduits" (ching) or "conduit vessels" (ching-mo); by this time it was understood that blood flows through a system where the vessels interconnect. The text also tells of a large number of holes located over the body of these vessels. At the time of this text, there was no distinction made between vessels on the basis of content, and no explanation as to how the blood and chi circulated in the vessels. The texts reveal that the belief later developed that chi flowed through a separate system of vessels (today called *meridians*) which did not contain blood.[262]

Early in the history of Chinese medicine disease was attributed to imbalances of chi, and was caused by demons (hsieh-kuei); and that demons were carried by winds, and that winds dwelt in caves or tunnels. The demons (evil spirits) were believed to lodge within the vessels carrying chi and disturbing the flow. To dislodge the demon which was clogging the flow of chi, needles were inserted in the holes (tunnels) over the vessels allowing escape of chi and relieving the congestion.[263]

> The vessels, and not the openings, were the central feature of 'ancient' acupuncture, whereas in modern practice the points appear to be of prime importance. The vessels have, over time, lost their association with the vascular system and in the West are now viewed primarily as functional pathways lining the openings. The term 'meridian' rather than 'vessels' merely serves to aid in clouding the issue.[264]

---

260 Basser, Stephen M.D. , Acupuncture: A History, *Acupuncture Watch;* http://acuwatch.org/hx/fdac1973.shtml Feb. 22, (2005).
261 Epler, Jr DC. , *Bloodletting in early Chinese medicine and its relation to the origin of acupuncture.* (1980), Basser, op.cit. p. 1.
262 Bassar, op. cit., p. 2.
263 Epler, Jr DC. *Bloodletting in early Chinese medicine and its relation to the origin of acupuncture.* Bull Hist Med. 1980l54L357-367; Reported in Basser, *Ibid.*, p. 2.
264 Unschuld PU. *Medicine in China: a History of Ideas,* Berkeley, CA: University of California Press; (1985), Reported in *Acupuncture Watch;* Basser, *Ibid.*, p. 2.

Pulse diagnosis was developed during the time that chi was believed to flow through blood. It was believed that the location of blockage of chi could be determined by feeling the pulse.

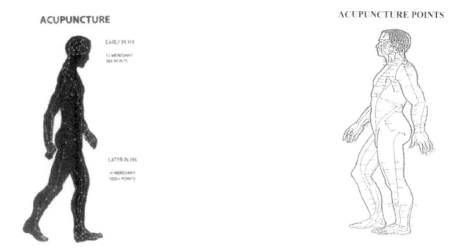

Figure 28. acupuncture points

> Over time the connection between needling and chi, which formed the basis of acupuncture, was described in the context of an emerging cosmological view of the world, not evident in the earlier descriptions of medical bleeding. Organic medicine was subsumed under this emerging system of *cosmological correspondences*.[265]

Early in the history of acupuncture, there were twelve meridians and 365 points, one point for each day of the year. This has changed and now many more points and fourteen meridians are said to exist. The body is supposed to have twelve organs. The Chinese day is considered to be twelve hours which covers the 24 hours we have in a day. One hour of Chinese physiology time equals two hours of our time. The chi is claimed to flow around through the twelve organs, on schedule, where one organ will have the dominance of chi for one Chinese hour (two hours), then another organ, so covering all organs in twelve divisions of the day. This is analogous to the zodiac and the planets, and reflects the belief that man is a small cosmos.

Acupuncture at specific points is believed to cause a change of the energy (chi) flow running through that specific point to bring a desired balance of the

---

265   Unschuld PU. Nan-ching: *The Classic of Difficult Issues.* Berkeley, CA: University of California Press, (1986), p. 5; Reported in Basser, op. cit., p. 2.

yin and yang. This method is used for all types of illnesses, even for overcoming habits such as smoking. Some people claim to have experienced great relief from pain. Others have stopped smoking. What are the believed causes of the presumed imbalance of energy which results in disease? Lifestyle, different foods, and many other things are believed to influence the balance of energy. Winds are also believed to be a source of over 100 different diseases.

Treatment entails balancing the energy (chi), or using *Like Cures Like* therapy. Prevention involves meditation, and/or meditation in exercise (no motion, stillness of position), exercise, and balancing foods. It is also important to have balance in the home, such as the proper placement of furniture.

As mentioned previously, energy balancing techniques of Chinese traditional medicine are as follows: meditation, meditation in exercise, breathing exercises, qi gong, tai chi and martial arts of all types, diet, drugs, minerals, herbs, moxibustion, acupressure, and acupuncture. Acupuncture is by far the most popular healing methods of traditional Chinese methods in the West. Today the proponents of acupuncture commonly use the term "energy" in referring to chi, however this is misleading as:

> The core concept of chi bears no resemblance to the western concept of energy (regardless of whether the latter is borrowed from the physical sciences or from colloquial use).[266]

This is true in Ayurveda (prana) as well as traditional Chinese medicine.

The Christian believes in a God of Creation who, by the power of His spoken word created the heavens and the earth. The universe and man are sustained by His power, and in healing. And salvation of man is obtained through faith in the sinless life of Jesus Christ, in the merits of His shed blood in His death at Calvary, and His resurrection.

The pagan denies the living God (Trinity), yet he recognizes there is a power that created and sustains the universe. We learned in chapter 4 of his explanation for creation, of the vital force believed to sustain us, and of the balancing of the supposed force's two (yin—yang) divisions to heal. This power was considered a *spiritual* force; therefore a system was devised whereby man believed he could manipulate and influence this power to sustain well-being, to heal, as well as to obtain eternal life.

The creative power of God is not measurable or demonstrable by mechanical measuring instruments, and is not under the control of man. The power, which paganism separated from God, had many names, such as vital force, prana, chi, qi, and more recently, universal energy. The term *energy medicine* is commonly used to refer to the various techniques used in holistic

---

266   Unschuld PU. Nan-ching op. cit., p. 5; Reported in Basser, op. cit., p. 2.

health therapies. Scientists who are believers in these theories desire to show that this power (chi) is truly in the field of modern science and attempt to measure and demonstrate such. It is most likely that the common use of the term *energy* in reference to the *vital force* power has come from this desire. To the established believer in Hinduism or Taoism, the term energy may be an insult to his beliefs. The words prana, chi or qi, mana, etc., are not true synonyms of the word energy.

DOES ACUPUNCTURE WORK?

Acupuncture seems to do something for some people but nothing for others. Could it be a placebo effect? Why have we not had studies that really determine if it works by the placebo effect or not? Part of the confusion and lack of solid *yes* or *no* answers rises out of the difficulty of doing quality scientific studies on this procedure. It is difficult to do a mock acupressure or acupuncture procedure. However, hundreds of studies have been done to test the effectiveness of the procedure over the past 35 years.

In 1981, the Academy of Sciences of the German Democratic Republic produced a statement regarding the effectiveness of acupuncture. Their summary, written by Rudolph Baumann, and published in *Zeitschrift fur Experimentelle Chirurgie* 14:66-67, 1981, concluded the following:

1. Points of acupuncture are unknown to science and are not demonstrable, and different schools of acupuncture have charts that do not match for specific points.
2. All procedures attempting to prove their presence have failed.
3. Equal effects are obtainable in acupuncture when no attention is paid to specific points on the body.
4. There is no benefit to be expected to organic disease.
5. Infectious diseases have no response to acupuncture.
6. Acupuncture does not give better results than hypnosis, suggestion, or autosuggestion.
7. There was not enough evidence of effect to recommend research or to teach the subject to medical students or physicians.

Dr. Basser reported in 1999, that:

Carefully designed and conducted scientific studies have so far failed to demonstrate that the Chinese acupuncture is associated with more effective pain relief than either placebo or counterirritant stimulation such as TENS (transcutaneous electrical nerve stimulation).[267]

---

267 *Ibid.*, p. 6.

TENS has been used for many years for mild to moderate chronic musculoskeletal pain. Basser has concluded that from a scientific viewpoint it can now be said with confidence:

1. The concept of chi has no basis in human physiology.
2. The vessels, or meridians, along which the needling points are supposedly located, have not been shown to exist and do not relate to our current knowledge of human anatomy.
3. Specific acupuncture points have not been shown to exist—as noted earlier, different acupuncture charts give different numbers and locations of points.[268]

For the past forty years science has not been able to explain the physiologic actions from acupuncture or to detect any true lasting value from the use of acupuncture. Many proponents of this technique will rise up in alarm by this statement, but this is what I have found.

In November 1997, The National Institute of Drug Abuse held a Consensus Conference on acupuncture. The meeting was arranged by a Dr. Trachetenber, who is reported to be a strong advocate of acupuncture. Wallace Sampson M.D. FACP, presents a critique of the conference, in *Acupuncture Watch*.[25] He mentions that the first question that arose was, why investigators who had previously made studies on acupuncture, which showed no measurable effect from acupuncture, were not a part of the presenting scientists? There seemed to be present only proponents of acupuncture. Prior analyses of research of acupuncture (1986, 1988, 1990) had revealed that the best quality of research showed negative effects, and the low quality studies were mostly positive.

Dr. Sampson makes the following comment:

> The lack of critical, scientific thinking was apparent in the panel's report, which was sixteen pages long. It obviously was composed before the conference and changed somewhat after the presentations. Despite the uneven literature and the lack of firm evidence to support the conclusions, the consensus statement panel recommended acupuncture for musculoskeletal pain, some headaches, and nausea. It recommended use for nausea due to chemotherapy, based on only three papers.[269]

---

268 Basser, op. cit., p. 8.
269 Sampson, Wallace I. M.D. , *Acupuncture Watch*, Critique of the NIH Consensus Conference on Acupuncture, March (2005), http://acuwatch.org/

Dr. Sampson continues:

That the consensus Conference was engaged in pseudoscientific reasoning is further illustrated by the rejection of the most obvious and probable reason for perceived effects. Those are natural history of the disease, regression to the mean, suggestion, counter-irritation, distraction, expectation, consensus, the Stockholm effect (identifying with and aiding the desires of a dominant figure), fatigue, habituation, ritual, reinforcement, and other well-known psychological mechanisms. With such an array of obvious alternative explanations and such fertile areas for productive research, strong bias would be needed to agree to the conference conclusions.[270]

Why would physicians make a consensus statement labeling acupuncture as being scientific if there is really no hard data confirming it? There could be several reasons, among which is the desire to place it in an acceptable light with patients and the scientific community. Those physicians who believe in Eastern mysticism and practice its techniques, do not enjoy being considered as on the fringe of scientific medicine; so when an organization such as the National Institute of Health puts out a consensus opinion that acupuncture is science-based, this elevates its status. Also, if there is a consensus from an influential medical body that a particular procedure is science-based, it is easier to persuade insurance companies to pay for its use. Acupuncture is cheap to perform, the risks are low, it is popular, and the financial returns are very good. Never underestimate the financial interest.

Reports of studies testing acupuncture, some with positive results as to benefit over and above more conventional methods, continue to appear. Most of these studies are dealing with discomforts and disorders that have strong subjective type complaints. These include headaches, a variety of aches and pains, etc. To do true double blind studies with acupuncture is almost impossible. There have been some sham acupuncture studies where the patients cannot detect if the needle is inserted or not, and other studies that place needles anywhere but on the acupuncture points. The results of the sham and wrongly placed needles compared to the correct acupuncture procedures are almost the same. Do they work? Yes, many times, as do the fake procedures. I have never seen a study done using acupuncture for pneumonia, diabetes, coronary heart disease, meningitis, or other serious disease. We have had studies going on for forty years and still the results are questionable. If it is so good should it not be easy to show a difference, a large difference, using acupuncture versus not using it?

---

270 *Ibid., p. 2.*

A positive report appeared about fifteen studies made by Duke University Medical Center in North Carolina, of the use of acupuncture for post-surgical pain, and which was reported on the Internet by Reuters Health Service on October 17, 2007. Acupuncture was done before and after surgery. There was less pain on those receiving the acupuncture than the controls, but not freedom from pain. There was less nausea, dizziness, and also of urinary retention. Urinary retention often occurs with abdominal surgery due to reflex from pain.

Remember, surgery has been done on people using acupuncture as the anesthetic, so too was surgery done without pain in years past in India by use of hypnotism.

In the report by Reuters Health a comment is made that doctors at the National Institutes of Health do not understand how acupuncture works. Many proponents of acupuncture will claim that the case is settled, and may give you answers as to how they believe it works. In the following paragraphs I will share with you information as to that which is known about possible physiologic actions of acupuncture. This information comes from the New England Journal of Medicine, July 17, 2010/363:454-61

I obtained a report of a study done in 2008 and reported in *Science Daily*, January 21, 2009. I will share with you the report:

Headache sufferers can benefit from acupuncture, even though how and where acupuncture needles are inserted may not be important. Two separate systematic reviews by Cochrane Researchers show that acupuncture is an effective treatment for prevention of headaches and migraines. But the results also suggest that faked procedures, in which needles are incorrectly inserted, can be just as effective.

In each study, the researchers tried to establish whether acupuncture could reduce the occurrence of headaches. One study focused on mild to moderate but frequent 'tension-type' headaches, whilst the other focused on more severe but less frequent headaches usually termed migraines. Together the two studies included 33 trials, involving a total of 6,736 patients.

Overall, following a course of at least eight weeks, patients treated with acupuncture suffered fewer headaches compared to those who were given only pain killers, in the migraine study, acupuncture was superior to proven prophylactic drug treatments, but faked treatments were no less effective. In the tension headache study, true acupuncture was actually slightly more effective than faked treatments.[271]

Why are we so hung up on using something that is so difficult to prove as to whether it has true benefit? If this procedure is what I understand it to be, then if I choose to use it, I have subjected myself to the influence of Satan's counterfeit healing system, with little chance of true lasting benefit above that of a fake procedure. We know that it has been used as an anesthetic wherein people undergo surgery and are wide awake and even can eat during a surgical procedure. Is there power in acupuncture? Yes, but whose power? The results of applying acupuncture may well be as dependent upon the connection of the therapists to the powers of the occult as the Theosophy Society states that radiesthesia is in radionics. (See Divination, chapter 16). Studies on acupuncture never consider this factor.

In 1893 and 1958, the British Medical Society and the American Medical Society, respectively, made a consensus statement on hypnosis as being based in science even though there were no explanations as to how it worked. That it worked no one disputed, yet the Christian may recognize the source of its power as of the occult. (See chapter on hypnosis). I have observed reports on acupuncture for more than forty years, waiting for the definitive evidence that this technique works in the hands of anyone (not just sensitives); that it works consistently on all people; and that it convincingly produces lasting benefits. I am still waiting. I recognize that there has been an occasional person who had severe pain of the back or in some other location and experienced dramatic relief, or someone stopped smoking easily, etc. Such testimonies can be persuasive, but in no way add up to conclusive evidence.

When we choose to receive medical treatment from an acupuncturist, a serious concern is that of placing oneself in the hands of a person who has poor or no understanding as to proper diagnosis and treatment, thus allowing serious disease to continue without identification and proper care. Many diseases are difficult to recognize even by highly trained and experienced physicians.

Steven Barrett M.D. illustrates the above comment with this story:

A study published in 2001 illustrates the absurdity of TCM (*traditional Chinese medicine*) practices. A 40-year old woman with chronic back pain who visited 7 acupuncturists during a 2 week period was diagnosed with "Qi stagnation" by 6 of them, "blood stagnation" by 5, "kidney Qi deficiency" by 2, "yin deficiency"

271 Linde K, Allais G, Brinkhaus B, Manheimer E, Vickers A, White AR. *Acupuncture for tension-type headache.* Cochrane Database of Systematic Reviews, (2010), Issue 1. Art. No.:C D007587 DOI: 10.1002/14651858. CDOO7587 Linde K, Allais G, Brinkhaus B, Manheimer E, Vickers A, White AR. Acupuncture for tension-type headache. Cochrane Database of Systematic Reviews, Issue 1. Ar. No.:CD001218 DOI.

by 1, and "liver Qi deficiency" by 1. The proposed treatments varied even more. Among the 6 who recorded their recommendations, the practitioners planned to use between 7 and 26 needles inserted into 4 to 16 specific "acupuncture points" in the back, leg, hand, and foot. Of 28 acupuncture points elected, only 4 (14%) were prescribed by 2 or more acupuncturists.[272]

One would think, that with the lack of studies reporting positive effects of acupuncture, interest in its use would subside; but just the opposite has happened. More young physicians who have embraced the Eastern philosophy have matured into experienced physicians and by their numbers alone have considerable influence. Many of them have been promoted to positions of leadership in medical institutions and schools. Public pressure to try these "wonderful methods" has caused many hospitals to offer some type of alternative therapies. Scientific investigational studies on acupuncture and its potential for being physiologically therapeutic to certain disorders continue.

A physician is faced daily with common ailments that are difficult to treat, such as fibromyalgia, migraine headaches, and osteoarthritis of back, hips, knees, and fingers. The medications used in an attempt to control the ever present pain are of themselves fraught with problems and danger. So physician and patient alike are always looking for an effective and safe way to bring relief. The physical risks of using acupuncture are low and many feel that if it is not helpful, what have they lost? When pain is unrelenting, a person is driven to try anything suggested, and this is why "testimonials" as to the great benefit received by some type of therapy have ready followers. I will present three short summaries of studies, using acupuncture as therapy, done recently on fibromyalgia, migraine headaches, and osteoarthritis.

In the *Annals of Internal medicine*, July 2005, Dr. Dedra Buchwald of the University of Washington in Seattle, reported a study on fibromyalgia using acupuncture. Acupuncture was administered twice a week for twelve weeks. The final report was that people with fibromyalgia were no more likely to report decrease of pain than people who received acupuncture designed for a different condition, wherein needles were inserted into random locations rather than specific acupuncture points, or they received simulated acupuncture but without needles.[273]

Reuters Health Information 2006-03-02, reported on a German study using acupuncture for migraine headaches. Nine hundred patients were randomly

272 Barrett, Stephen, M.D., *Quackwatch Hone Page*, Be Wary of Acupuncture, Qi Gong, and Chinese Medicine, p. 7 Jan. (2004). http://quackwatch.org/

273 *Reuters Health Information*, (2005-07-05) Acupuncture may do little for fibromyalgia,http://www.reutershealth.com/archive/2005/07/05/elinelinks/2005070elin003.html (available to Reuter's subscribers only).

selected to receive Chinese traditional acupuncture, sham acupuncture, or drugs, all showed equal effectiveness. Drug therapy for migraine is far from satisfactory so this comparison does not reflect as much benefit for acupuncture as it may seem.[274]

The British medical journal, *Lancet,* July 9, 2005, carried an article by Dr. Claudia Witt, from Charite University Medical Centre in Berlin, in reference to a study she and her colleagues conducted on osteoarthritis. This study involved 294 patients, age's fifty to seventy-five years of age with osteoarthritis of the knee. The average pain intensity of the group was 40 (the higher the score the greater the pain). The final analysis reported 149 patients were assigned to acupuncture, 75 to minimal acupuncture (inserting needles in distant non-acupuncture points), and 70 to a waiting *control* group. The treatment groups received twelve treatments over eight weeks. At that point, average scores on a standard osteoarthritis scale were 26.9 point nine for the acupuncture group, 35.8 for the minimal acupuncture group and 49.6 for the controls. At 26 weeks and 52 weeks there were no differences between groups.

> The editorialists, both from The Churchill in Oxford, UK conclude: 'We are still some way short of having conclusive evidence that acupuncture is beneficial in arthritis or in any other condition, other than in a statistical or artificial way.[275]

Some might say, "But there was benefit for the migraine sufferer and drugs were not needed." Allow me to speak of another factor not considered in any of these studies, that of the power of Satan. If a practitioner of acupuncture is a believer in the Eastern thought or Western occultism and the patient has allowed him or herself to participate in this technique that comes from Eastern mysticism, is it not possible that the power of Satan can cause apparent benefits?

I wish to share another more recent study on acupuncture done in Hong Kong and reported on the Internet from Reuters Health on November 13, 2008. The study was to test the power of acupuncture in promoting in-vitro fertilization among 370 women, half receiving true acupuncture and the other half sham acupuncture. The sham procedure was done in a way that the women could not detect which type acupuncture they were getting and they would not know that they were in a testing group. Acupuncture points were the same for both groups.

274 *Reuters Health Information,* 2006-03-02: Acupuncture shown to relieve migraines: study, http://www.reutershealth.com/archive/2006/03/02/eline/links/20060302eline006.html (*available to Reuter's subscribers only*)

275 *Reuters Health Information,* (2005-07-08): acupuncture may ease knee arthritis, for a while, http://reutershealth.com/archive/2005/07/08 /eline/ links/20050708eline019.html

The acupuncture was given 25 minutes before the ovum implants were placed and 25 minutes after. The acupuncture group had 43. % take (pregnancy) from the implant and the sham acupuncture group had 55%. A weakness in the study was that there was no group that received neither sham nor real acupuncture.

Have there been studies showing a benefit from acupuncture? Yes, there have been. It seems that almost all of the studies I read have been on conditions that involve pain, nausea, or various types of discomfort. For these symptoms the studies will often show a positive benefit, however, those benefits are usually only mildly better than sham or no acupuncture. After a few weeks to three months the difference between those tested and the controls usually have returned to being equal.

Let us consider a study where acupuncture was used for control of nausea and vomiting caused by receiving chemotherapy, also a study of patients receiving radiation for cancer treatment of the throat and neck area, and receiving acupressure therapy for the resulting xerostomia (dry mouth) reported in *CA: A Cancer Journal for Clinicians* volume 59/#9/ September/ October 2009. The studies used acupressure bands which caused pressure to be applied to a specific acupressure point on the wrist. Previous studies have shown acupressure bands to be beneficial for control of nausea. Peter Johnstone M.D. and William A. Mitchell Professor and chair of Radiation Oncology at the Indiana University School of Medicine report the study for chemotherapy nausea.

The study was divided so that there were controls not receiving therapy with acupressure bands as well as those wearing the bands. Rigid record taking was instituted of the time of nausea symptoms, the amount of medications taken to control nausea, and the number of times vomiting occurred for those receiving therapy as well as the control group.

At the conclusion of the study those receiving acupressure therapy had a reduction of nausea and associated symptoms of 28% and the controls a reduction of 5%. However when the records of how much anti-nausea medication was taken and the number of times vomiting occurred there was no difference between those taking the acupressure treatment and the controls.

Investigators at University of Texas M.D. Anderson Cancer Center in Houston tested acupressure on patients having received radiation to the neck area that resulted in xerostomia (dry mouth). They had patients record the degree of dry mouth and the amount of time it caused distress. They also tested the amount of increase of saliva in the mouth that occurred from the acupressure treatment.

The conclusion of the study was that there was very significant difference in relief of symptoms of those taking the acupressure treatment versus those not taking. However there was no difference in the amount of saliva produced between the two groups.

In the final evaluation of the two groups it was clear that those receiving acupressure therapy reported beneficial (subjective) results, yet the measurements in each of the two studies did not reveal a difference in physiological changes between therapy and no therapy (objective results). Dr. Johnstone states the following: "we have evidence now *proving that a disconnect* often exists between a patient's reported symptoms and objective evidence of those symptoms." (Emphasis added)

In June 2010 The Center for Inquiry Office of Public Policy located in Washington D.C. presented a paper entitled ***ACUPUNCTURE: A SCIENCE-BASED ASSESSMENT***, a position paper from this center and authored by Robert Slack, Jr. This report brings an up to date assessment of the scientific status of acupuncture as revealed by improved testing techniques in the past several years. The optimistic conclusions about the effects reported by use of acupuncture in past research during the 1970-1990's was due to the placebo effect, but was not recognized due to not having a *placebo* in testing. This new and changed understanding is a result of the development of "sham" acupuncture technique which has caused a *"complete unraveling of nearly all acupuncture claims."* The 1997 National Institutes of Health report on acupuncture as being effective for nausea, headache, and dental pain now carries the following disclaimer.

> This statement is more than five years old and is provided solely for historical purposes. Due to the cumulative nature of medical research, new knowledge has inevitably accumulated in this subject area (...) thus some of the material is likely to be out of date, and *at worst simply wrong.*[276] (Emphasis added)

The **Cochrane Collaboration**, one of the world's most trusted evaluator of medical literature, undertook a recent systematic review of the research concerning acupuncture. The results of this analysis were included in an article presenting recent acupuncture research by Edzard Ernst in *The American Journal of Medicine.* He states:

> During the past ten years, however, researchers have begun to take a more rigorous look at acupuncture, designing studies that are properly randomized and adequately controlled for placebo effect. Though research is ongoing, an increasingly robust body of literature has accumulated showing that acupuncture has no intrinsic clinical value.

276 http://ww.csicop.org/uploads/files/Acupunctue_Paper.pdf) p. 11.

> After discarding reviews that are based on only three or fewer primary studies, only 2 evidence-based indications emerge: nausea/vomiting and headache. Even this evidence has to be interpreted with caution; recent trials using [...] placebos suggest that acupuncture has no specific effects in either of these conditions. (Ernst, 2008, 10-27)[277]

In *Acupuncture: A Science Based Assessment*, Robert Slack, Jr. pointed out that there are many articles to be found that do conclude that there has been "encouraging effectiveness" from the use of acupuncture. For individuals that are not acquainted with scientific testing it seems that these types of articles present solid evidence of benefits of acupuncture. Truth in science is better demonstrated by studies that test by use of a double blind, randomly selected, and having 1) test group; 2) placebo group; 3) control group; and with a large number (hundreds) in each group. The evaluation of results will also be double blind, that is, the individual doing the acupuncture treatments will not be the person to do the evaluation. The person evaluating will not know which test group of individuals he is evaluating. This helps reduce bias and comes closer to revealing truth.

Slack further states that with this development of an effective sham— placebo technique of acupuncture, there has been much better evaluation, with the results indicating: 1) that real acupuncture is not more effective that when a placebo procedure is done; 2) for many conditions there is no benefit for either acupuncture or sham procedure.

In this same review by Robert Slack Jr. he mentions that there have been leading proponents of acupuncture and other alternative therapies, such as Andrew Weil M.D. , that emphasize that these therapies have far less potential to cause harm than many conventional treatments. Therefore they should be judged by a "sliding scale" as to their value of effectiveness. The less the risk of side effects of therapy the less strict should be the criteria for effectiveness. This is not science; it is bias of the highest order. One cannot use two standards to evaluate therapeutic effectiveness decided upon the degree of potential side effects. It does, however, often enter into the decision as to whether to use a therapy or not.[278]

A study (638 patients) of the use of acupuncture and its effectiveness for chronic low back pain was reported in May 2009. This research study was conducted by Daniel Cherkin Ph.D. senior researcher with the Group Health Research Institute in Seattle Washington. Patients were divided into four

277 http://www.csicop.org/specialarticles/show/acupuncture_a_science-based_assessmentp.2 (www.csicop.org/uploads/files/Acupuncture_Paper.pdf) p. 2

278 Slack, Robert Jr. , Acupuncture: A Science-Based Assessment, *A Position Paper From the Center For Inquiry Office of Public Policy,* June, (2010). p. 15.

groups: 1) standard acupuncture; 2) individualized acupuncture; 3) placebo acupuncture using tooth picks to touch the skin; 4) standard medical treatment without acupuncture.

The patients treated with any of the three styles of acupuncture were reported to fare better than no acupuncture. Dr. Cherkin concluded that acupuncture was beneficial in treatment of low back pain and that the study had stimulated the question as to how acupuncture works. Other scientists reviewing the study conclude that this study does not prove that acupuncture works, but that it shows the results are equal to use of a placebo; hence the obvious is that acupuncture of itself does not work. However, the lay press and proponents of acupuncture accept and voice the opinion that the study proved acupuncture is effective and does work.[279]

The New England Journal of Medicine, July 29, 2010; 363:454- 61 contained an article that reviewed recent research on acupuncture. In this scientific article the studies mentioned in the above paragraphs were included in its evaluation of acupuncture. This article in the NEJM originates from the Center for Integrative Medicine, University of Maryland School of Medicine, and the University of Maryland Dental School; also from Department of Neurology, and the Program in Integrative Health, University of Vermont College of Medicine, Burlington; and the Institute for Social Medicine, Epidemiology, and Health Economics, Charite' University Medical Center, Berlin.

Integrative health programs seek to bring together therapies of Western scientific medicine and alternative (non science based therapies such as Ayurveda and traditional Chinese medicine) therapy. Thousands of offices and clinics across America and several medical schools have combined these methods. As seen by the names of the organizations behind this particular article one recognizes the potential bias to be expected, however, I found the article to be quite scientific with an obvious attempt to avoid bias.

In this article a short explanation is presented of the Chinese theory of chi and yin—yang, meridians, and Chinese traditional medicine's concept of physiology that was presented earlier in this chapter. Then this statement is made on page 3:

...Efforts have been made to characterize the effects of acupuncture in terms of the established principles of medical physiology on which Western medicine is based. These efforts remain inconclusive, for several reasons....[280]

279 Acupuncture for Chronic Low Back Pain, *The New England Journal of Medicine,* Boston, MA July 29, (2010); 363:454-61.
280 *Ibid.*

These reasons are given in the following summary of findings from studies testing for physiologic changes from acupuncture performed mostly in animals;

1. Acupuncture will activate peripheral-nerve fibers of all size.
2. Acupuncture experience is dominated by a strong psychosocial context, including expectation, beliefs, and therapeutic milieu.
3. Injecting the skin at the spot of presumed acupuncture point with a local anesthesia will block the analgesic effects of acupuncture.
4. Endorphins are released by the brain-stem, sub-cortical and limbic parts of the brain.
5. In rats electrical acupuncture has shown release of hydrocortisone from pituitary (adrenal) gland which, in turn, results in anti-inflammatory responses.
6. MRI studies have revealed changes in the limbic and basal forebrain areas when prolonged acupunctures stimulation is done.
7. Positron-emission tomography has shown that acupuncture increases u-opioid-binding for several days in the same brain areas as stated above.
8. Acupuncture has mechanical stimulation effects on connective tissue.
9. Adenosine is released at the site of needle stimulation.
10. There is increase blood flow at the local site of acupuncture

In spite of what may look like to some as powerful positive proof of the physiological action of acupuncture; the article in the New England Journal of Medicine, July, 29, 2010 states the following:

> However, the various observations that have been made are not sufficient to permit a unified theory regarding the effect of acupuncture on mechanism of chronic pain.[281]

The article tells us of a meta-analysis study (information of many studies placed into one study and analyzed) in 2008 which included 6359 patients with low back pain. *The real acupuncture treatment was no more effective than sham treatment.* However, with real or sham treatment there was *subjective* improvement over conventional treatment without acupuncture. This same finding was reported in the previously described *Cochrane Collaboration Study.* This information is to be found in the Supplementary Appendix available with the original article in the *New England Journal of Medicine,* July 29, 2010.

---

281   *Ibid.*

Two additional studies are referred to in this article in *NEJM* July 29, 2010, they come from German investigators. One study with 1162 patients over eight years compared real acupuncture versus sham procedure for chronic low back pain. There was little difference between the groups and at six months they were identical yet somewhat better than the control group that did not receive acupuncture. The other German study involved 3093 patients over seven years and this study on low back pain was measured by use of a *questionnaire* concerning reduced back function. Two groups were tested, one with conventional therapy and one with acupuncture. The acupuncture group had significant improvement above the non-acupuncture group as revealed by *questionnaire*. The results are taken from subjective responses of the patient.

Your attention is now directed to the setting in which acupuncture is delivered. In the traditional practice the insertion of the needle may be accompanied by a variety of other procedures, such as palpation of the radial artery in the wrist, as well as pulses in other locations. The tongue may be inspected in detail, recommendations as to use of herbs etc. All of these actions are based on the application of the principles of traditional Chinese medicine in contrast to Western scientific physiological medical concepts.

To the credit of the authors of this article we are not left at this point with the conclusion that acupuncture functions on a physiologic basis, actually they suggest its function may well be explained from a *psychological* standpoint and more research is needed in that direction. See quote below:

> There is continuing debate in the medical community regarding the role of the placebo effect in acupuncture. As noted above, the most recent well powered clinical trials of acupuncture for chronic low back pain showed that sham acupuncture was as effective as real acupuncture. The simplest explanation of such findings is that the specific therapeutic effects of acupuncture, if present, are small, whereas it's clinically relevant benefits are mostly attributable to contextual and *psychosocial* factors, such as patients' beliefs and expectation, attention from the acupuncturist, and highly focused, spatially directed attention on the part of the patient. These studies also seem to indicate that needles do not need to stimulate the traditionally identified acupuncture points or actually penetrate the skin to produce the anticipated effect...

In the closing part of this extensive article recommendation is given for additional studies to further evaluate the efficacy of sham (placebo) acupuncture without skin penetration, since it *may be possible to achieve the same benefits by not doing invasive needle punctures*. The master of Qi Gong tells us he can accomplish feats and healing equal to using needles in acupuncture simply by performing Qi Gong about a person. Light beams shined on the skin are said to work as well as needles, on and on it goes.

Wow, this reminds me of the experience of Mesmer, first he used magnets to effect healing, and then he learned he did not need magnets as he could accomplish the same simply by his hands. From there he moved on to the use of only the mind in bringing apparent healing; Mesmerism— hypnotism. In this chapter on traditional Chinese medicine I have not had the motive or desire to prove that the therapies are simply—fake. I believe at times quite remarkable changes may occur and apparent healing takes place, yet I ask the question *BY WHAT OR WHOSE POWER DOES IT WORK?* That is the concern.

For the past three thousand plus years the power of Eastern healing has been accepted and referred to as *spiritual power*. It is only in the last seventy-five to one hundred years has there been an attempt to describe its action in terms of modern physics. There are only two sources of spiritual power, that from Satan and that from God, there is no other.

Why do I warn against using therapies of traditional Chinese medicine if one does not believe in the astrological concepts upon which acupuncture is based, but only want to take of the *good* of the method? I believe that as a person understands traditional Chinese medicine's origin and theory of man being the *microcosm* of the *macrocosm* (universe) and that a balance of a two sided universal energy referred to as chi when rightly balanced created the universe and man, and when out of balance creates illness and malfunction; it would be impossible to participate in these so called healing methods without acceptance of that power. Is it a treatment method that will cure infectious or chronic diseases or increased life span? Thus far no evidence has been presented to support such.

In China, for at least 3000 years, traditional Chinese medicine was part of medical care (acupuncture for 2000). What was the health status under this system? It was dismal. Neither public nor personal hygiene was practiced. Chairman Mao attacked these conditions head-on in the 1950's and a national movement to improve hygiene personally and publicly was instituted. By the end of the 1950's, great progress had been made in reducing infectious diseases. This was done by making changes that were scientific, not by practices based on astrological concepts. Clean water, closed sewer systems, cleanliness of body and homes, controlling vectors of infectious disease and parasites, and immunization brought improvement.[282] Life span doubled in fifty years, it was one of the most remarkable medical feats of the twentieth century.

---

282   Dominique and Marie-Joseph Hoizey, *A History of Chinese Medicine,* UBC Press University of British Columbia, Vancouver, B.C, Canada (1993), pp.173–174.

As the infectious diseases came under control and living habits along with diet changed to include use of more animal products, the degenerative diseases of the West began to replace infectious disease. Today, the #1 cause of death in China is vascular disease, followed by cancer.

Chinese cuisine is planned according to five phases or food divisions: metal, water, wood, fire, earth. Proper planning and use of foods from the five divisions is said to assure the flow of chi energy from food to the body.

Traditional Chinese medicine uses many herbs, which are often classified as hot/cold, yin/yang. The Chinese pharmacy contains a great variety of medicinals, which are not necessarily there because of their biochemical properties. The early chemists, (Alchemists) believed they could find a potion that would prolong life and bring immortality. In this search they experimented with numerous plants, minerals, and different animal parts.

This has been a very brief glimpse of the most commonly used healing methods of traditional Chinese medicine, which have been practiced in China for at least 2000 or more years. The end result has been abysmal, and it took the introduction of scientific medicine to improve health and increase life span in China, doubling in fifty years. None of this can be attributed to traditional Chinese medicine.

What is so attractive about a system that has no proven track record of improving health? What causes us to flock to it as if it was something new and wonderful? Could it be we have accepted its *spiritual philosophy* and have chosen to partake of the "tree of knowledge of good and evil?"

The following quotations from E.G. White should help give a proper perspective of traditional medicine practices.

> The apostles of nearly all forms of spiritism claim to have power to heal. They attribute this power to electricity, magnetism, the so-called sympathetic remedies, or to latent forces within the mind of man. And there are not a few, even in this Christian age, who go to these healers instead of trusting in the power of the living God and the skill of well qualified physicians.

> The mother, watching by the sickbed of her child, exclaims, 'I can do no more. Is there no physician who has power to restore my child?' She is told of the wonderful cures performed by some clairvoyant or magnetic healer, and she trusts her dear one to his charge, placing it as verily in the hand of Satan as if he were standing by her side. In many instances the future life of the child is controlled by a satanic power which it seems impossible to break.[283]

---

283   White, E.G., *Mind, Character, and Personality* Vol. 2, Southern Pub. Assn., Nashville, TN, (1977), p. 701.1.

Those who give themselves up to the sorcery of Satan may boast of great benefit received; but does this prove their course to be wise or safe? What if life should be prolonged? What if temporal gain should be secured? Will it pay in the end to have disregarded the will of God? All such apparent gain will prove at last an irrecoverable loss. We cannot with impunity break down a single barrier which God has erected to guard His people from Satan's power.[284]

In the next chapter, we will look at the emergence from the West of other energy balancing therapies.

284　White, E.G., *Conflict and Courage,* Pacific Press Pub. Assn., Mountain View, CA, (1970), p. 219.6.

CHAPTER 11

REFLEXOLOGY AND OTHER ENERGY-BALANCING THERAPIES

At the heart of alternative medicine therapies is the doctrine of correspondence, or sympathy, between the cosmos, earth, and man. This concept is central to the term *life force energy. T*his energy in theory is emanating from the cosmos, from which all things are said to be made, and within which all are *one* (pantheism*).[285]* Let us look at some popular therapies for health disorders developed from this theory.

Early in the development of the astrological system in Europe, the 12 houses of the zodiac were assigned to various parts of the body starting at the head with Aries, the ram, and ending at the feet with Pisces, the fish. The organs of the body were then assigned to the remaining individual houses.[286] The Chinese divided the body in a vertical manner believing that a special universal cosmic energy they (referred to as *chi*) ran through the body following 12 vertical divisions called meridians. These meridians had side channels to distribute the energy to the various organs of the body. In contrast, the Hindus described the distribution of vital energy as being concentrated in seven centers in the body called chakras. The chakras utilized nadis (small channels) to distribute energy to the tissues surrounding each chakra. When the energies of the chakras were combined; an aura was believed to surround the individual.

As previously explained the cosmos was considered the macrocosm and man the microcosm. Man was then divided into micro-microcosms. Specific locations on the body were believed to have developed association in such a way as to represent the entire body. It was believed that cosmic energy influenced man by correspondence, association, and/or sympathy.[287]

One of the first body locations considered to reveal this sympathy, or correspondence, was the hand. It probably began in the Sumerian civilization.

285   Levington, Richard, East-–West *Journal of Natural Health and Living,* The Holographic Body, Aug. (1988), Kushi foundation, Brookline, MA, p. 46.
286   Bessy, Maurice, *Magic and the Supernatural,* Spring Books, NY, (1970), p.73.
287   Levington, op cit., pp. 36–47.

Birth omens were obtained by inspecting a newborn infant for any sign which would predict the child's future. Palmistry likely had its origin in this manner.[288]

Palmistry, or Chiromancy, had roots in the ancient Vedas of India 4500 years ago.[289]

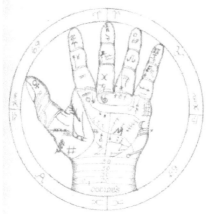

Figure 29. Palmistry and Zodiac

Additional areas of the body that were believed to have correspondence with all other areas of the body were added over time. Now, a total of 18 areas on the body are considered to be *holograms* of the whole.[290] The most common locations are ear, hand, foot, the web between thumb and forefinger, tongue, etc. Apart from the hologram locations, the musculature and fascia (membranes, tendons, ligaments) of the body are also believed to have many points that may impede the flow of universal energy so as to influence the function of body, mind, and spirit. Pressure, or some type of physical stimulation to those points, is said to affect—correct the flow of universal energy.

Why so many types of therapies if the treatments are effective? Because none of them are based on physical science but on the paranormal or psychic; the actual physical method used matters little in medical treatment. It depends on the mental attitude and acceptance of the theory of *universal energy* or *cosmic intelligence*.

Zone therapy—now called reflexology, Rolfing and similar massage, Shiatsu, Reike, craino-sacral therapy, polarity, and applied kinesiology, are techniques used by various holistic healers. These methods are collectively

---

288 Garrison, Fielding H. A.B., M.D.; *History of Medicine,* W.B. Saunders and Co. Philadelphia, PA. (1929), p. 63.
289 Levington, op. cit., p. 38.
290 Levington, op. cit., p. 43.

referred to as *body therapy* or *soma therapy*. Martial arts, tai chi, and qi gong are body or soma exercise-type treatments also providing *Life Force Medicine*.

Since it is believed that physical disease is a condition of unbalanced life force, universal energy, or chi, within the body due to congestion or blockage of flow, then correction of the imbalance would be achieved by manipulating points of correspondence. This is the foundation of acupuncture, acupressure, reflexology, and several other techniques collectively labeled *soma* (body) therapies.

REFLEXOLOGY

In 1913, an American doctor, William H. Fitzgerald M.D. , initiated a method of applying pressure to localized areas on the body to affect anesthesia for performing ear, nose, throat, surgery. By 1923 it had been expanded to treat most all medical disorders and was very popular with self-appointed healers.

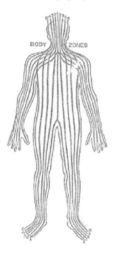

Figure 30. Zone Therapy

Doctor Fitzgerald was an admirer of, and influenced by Swedenborg, the famous Swedish spiritualists of the 1700's. Fitzgerald believed in *universal energy,* or as it was called in those times *vitalism*. He was not the absolute originator of using pressure to areas on the body to effect healing; rather he borrowed this concept from the Chinese and Egyptians. An issue of *EAST WEST* Journal (March 1990), relates that a form of reflexology was in use in China during the earliest period of China's history. In addition a hieroglyph depicting reflexology was found in a physician's tomb in ancient Egypt. Fitzgerald "determined" from his own reasoning, that the body was divided into ten specific zones, five on each side (not substantiated by science), believing that each zone carried its own bioelectric energy which made direct connection to the brain. He applied pressure to specific points on the body, and then proceeded with operative procedures to the ear, nose, or throat area without the patient experiencing pain. Fitzgerald further theorized that such pressure would treat disorders of body organs that he had allocated to correlate with the ten zones.

Eunice D. Ingham, an American, took up this therapeutic approach (zone therapy) in the 1930's, and carried it further, making it popular. She mapped out specific points on the feet and hands that she determined were sympathetic to specific organs. By rubbing those points on the hands or feet, beneficial effects or cures seemed to be accomplished. A lady in England, Doreen Baylay, called Fitzgerald's and Ingham's zone therapy, *reflexology,* and it is now very popular and practiced around the world.

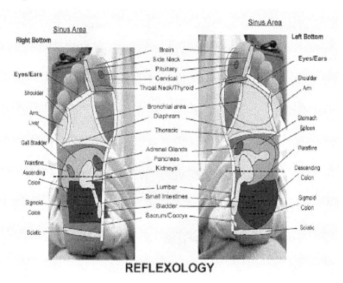

REFLEXOLOGY

Figure 31. Reflexology chart of foot.

Reflexology is the discipline of massaging the hand, foot, or ear to diagnose, predict future disease, and effect healing of present disease. It is founded upon belief in universal energy, vitalism, prana, chi, etc. Reflexology is also a variant of acupressure and/or Shiatzu, which are based on body correspondences and the meridian concept of Chinese Traditional Medicine. Reflexology has a similar philosophical background.[291]

However the theoretical Western explanation of reflexology contends that there are nerve connections directly from the feet or hands to the brain

291   Levington, op. cit., pp. 36-47.

connecting to various organs of the body. By rubbing a very specific point on a hand or foot, the nerve impulse is said to travel to the brain and is transferred on to a particular organ, thus correcting any abnormality of that organ.[292] Reflexologists may or may not teach that there are *crystals* of calcium or uric acid and/or other substances on the nerve endings in the hands or feet. These crystals are supposed to have caused congestion of universal energy flow about and through nerves which are purported to connect directly with organs of the body. Massage is said to break up the crystals, which will relieve nerve or energy blockage, the nerve can then impart health to the area of affliction.[293] No one has ever found these crystals by anatomical dissection or by any other method.

Reflexology purports the ability to diagnose, as well as to treat, by massaging either the hand, foot, or ear. Foot therapy in reflexology is the most common area for performing therapy, but hand treatment is supposed to be just as effective. Reflexologists proclaim that there are 7200 nerve endings on the bottom of a foot. I have never seen an anatomy or neurology book that said such, and even if it did, that does not mean the proclaimed point has specific connections to the various organs. There is no evidence that rubbing nerve endings would correct abnormal function of tissues elsewhere in the body.

If a person looks on the Internet for information relevant to *re-flexology* there will be found 6.5 million web sites. It is a worldwide phenomenon. What disorders are claimed to be improved by use of reflexology? Some reflexologists speak only about relief from stress while others make no limits as to types of problems that can be treated and will be benefitted. Have there been any studies of scientific quality? There can be found on some web sites studies that claim to show benefit to many various medical disorders. Quality studies are another thing. It is very difficult to design a study for testing reflexology that uses randomly selected, double blind, placebo, and a control group.

William T. Jarvis, Ph.D. a prior professor at Loma Linda University taught research methods to aspiring scientists. He often challenges a new group of students to devise a study design to test reflexology. I will share with you some of the studies done using designs created from his classes.

Using questionnaires, 70 subjects were asked to record any health problems they had encountered on any of 43 anatomical locations in the past two years. A reflexologists then examined each of the individuals in a blinded manner. The feet were exposed but a sheet covered the individual and no voice contact was allowed. From this test the results of determining a diagnosis by reflexology were no better than guessing.

---

292   Bergson, Anika; Tuchak, Vladimir, *Zone Therapy,* Pinnacle Books, Inc., New York, NY, (1974), p. 2.; Levington, op. cit., pp. 36-47.
293   Levington, op. cit., pp. 40–41.

In another study, three practicing reflexologists examined 18 individuals that had at least one to six different conditions identified by physicians. The end results were that there was no correlation between the reflexologists' findings and those identified by a physician.

A third study dealt with 35 women with premenstrual syndrome (PMS) which were randomly selected and assigned to either ear, hand, or foot reflexology, or a placebo group which had sham reflex points massaged. The women selected their personal symptoms from a list of 38 symptoms which are commonly associated with this syndrome. They then received reflex therapy. The results were that the treatment group had a modest reduction in symptoms compared to the placebo group. The placebo group complained that their treatment was rough and with discomfort. The group with improvement had thirty minutes of pleasurable relaxing treatment. This study suggested there may be some reduction of symptoms from PMS. There was no proof of a connection between reflex points and body organs.

A fourth study was done on patients with asthma, a disorder that is frequently claimed by many web sites to be benefitted by reflexology. Ten weeks of therapy was given to a treatment group and to a control placebo group. Lung function studies were conducted on both groups which did not change on either group. The conclusion was that no evidence of improvement beyond placebo was shown.[294]

Dr. Jarvis, in an article found on the Internet, shares with us his experience over several years as he did studies on reflexology. In the classes he conducted for post graduate studies in methods of research at Loma Linda University, he would bring a registered reflexologist to the class and have this individual present the theory and demonstrate the practice of reflexology. As previously mentioned he would challenge the students to design a method of testing the theory presented by the reflexologist. Eventually the reflexologist confided in Dr. Jarvis that even as he believed in reflexology he would like to see a study testing it.

Since reflexology claims to be able to prevent and to predict future disease, how do you test for that status? You cannot. Dr. Jarvis decided to test whether reflexologist could detect a present disorder of an individual and if the reflexologist failed that test then there would be no reason to try to design a test that determines whether or not future disease can be detected. The study that was done in response to the reflexologist's request is the one reported above on the 70 people. At the conclusion of the study the reflexologists agreed that it was not possible to diagnose present problems by reflexology, thereby

294   http://www.quackwatch.com posted Sept. 16, 1997. (Reflexology: A Close Look by Steven Barrett M.D.) accessed 3-30-11

accepting the conclusion that reflexology would not be able to predict future disease or even to be therapeutic.

> From that time on his practice would involve simple foot massages for people who wanted them with no diagnostic or therapeutic claims.[295]

A good foot rub is relaxing and without ill effects and no one should avoid such if they enjoy it. Just do not expect it to be diagnostic or correct health problems. Do not get caught up in such thinking, for if we do, we are then venturing into a system that is founded upon the doctrine of universal energy which leads us away from God's system of health. The danger of accepting this type of therapy is that if people feel they have gained help in their personal discomforts from such a therapy, they begin to believe the philosophy by which the benefits are explained. This allows acceptance of the *vital energy* concepts and leads in to accepting Satan's counterfeit health system, the "right arm" of his false message of salvation.

In a subset of reflexology, the ear is believed to represent the entire body by reflex. When the ear is used in therapy it is termed "auricular therapy." In the *East–West Journal of Natural Health and Living*, Aug. 1988, p. 43, the claim is made that there are at least 18 known locations on the body, labeled holograms, wherein a specific point is claimed to influence a specific organ. The hand, the thumb, a tooth, the tongue, and many other areas are said to be micro-microcosms of man and of the cosmos.

An abstract from the Med J Aust. Sept 7, 2009: *Is reflexology an effective intervention? A systematic review of randomized controlled trials.*

> OBJECTIVE: To evaluate the evidence for and against the effectiveness of reflexology for treating any medical condition.
>
> DATA SOURCES: six electronic data bases were searched from their inception to February 2009 to identify all relevant randomized controlled trials (RCTs). No language restrictions were applied.
>
> STUDY SELECTION AND DATA:
>
> Extraction: RCTs of reflexology delivered by trained reflexologists to patients with specific medical condition. Condition studied, study design and controls, primary outcome measures, follow-up, and main results were extracted.

---

295   http://www.ncahf.org/articles/o-r/reflexology.html

DATA SYNTHESIS: 18 RCTs met all the inclusion criteria. The studies examined a range of conditions: anovulation, asthma, back pain, dementia, diabetes, cancer, foot oedema in pregnancy, headache, irritable bowel syndrome, menopause, multiple sclerosis, the postoperative state of premenstrual syndrome. There were 1 study for asthma, the postoperative state, cancer palliation and multiple sclerosis. Five RCTs yielded positive results. Methodological quality was evaluated using the Jadad scale. The methodological quality was often poor, and sample sizes were generally low. Most higher-quality trials did not generate positive finding.

CONCLUSION: The best evidence available to date does not demonstrate convincingly that reflexology is an effective treatment for any medical condition.[296]

Reflexology is practiced around the world. It is a sympathetic remedy based on the concept that man is the microcosm of the macrocosm (the cosmos). Again, reflexology can be considered a variant of acupressure or Shiatzu.

MASSAGE

The early health centers of the SDA church utilized *Swedish massage* as a treatment for their patients. Massage combined with hydrotherapy will result in an increase in circulation of blood and body fluid. The delightful sensation of a good massage to the muscles is beneficial for anxiety, mood and happiness. Massage for a bed-ridden patient is refreshing and restful.

Perfect health depends upon perfect circulation.[297]

Patients attending these live-in health centers were taught to look to God, not only as the Source of healing, but also as the Sustainer of life. In short they were taught a new lifestyle and way of living, giving their Creator God respect, loyalty, and worship.

Today, there are several forms of massage being used by New Age healers, using different names, but based on the same basic dogma, that is, a physical disorder is the result of an imbalance of cosmic energy forces. Their form of massage is directed at correcting the flow of these supposed cosmic forces within an individual. Massage treatment itself is appropriate but often it is *hi-jacked* and used by the devil to insert his doctrines through medical therapeutics into the mind of man. His methods are *spiritually* based and are not dependent upon the physical laws of God.

---

296   http://www.ncbi.nlm.nih.gov/pubmed/19740047
297   White, E.G., 2 *Testimonies For the Church*, Pacific Press, Nampa, Idaho, p. 531.

Let us review several of these modified massage methods, whose therapeutic effects are explained by "balancing of energies," or relationships to earth's forces.

ROLFING

In the MID 1940's, Ida Pauline Rolf initiated a form of massage therapy to correct a physical disorder that she postulated existed, that of an imbalance of structure and movement of the entire body. Rolf presented a theory that "bound up" fascia (connective tissue) often restricts opposing muscles from functioning in concert with one another. Her special massage method was aimed at separating her hypothesized bound up fascia, by deeply separating the fibers manually to loosen them and allow effective movement patterns.

She called her method *Postural Release* and later *Structural Integration of the Human Body*, and presently the *Rolfing Method of Structural Integration*. The *Rolf Institute of Structural Integration* states that Rolfing:

> ...is a form of bodywork that reorganizes the connective tissues, called fascia, that permeate the entire body.[298]

Such a physical condition has not been recognized by science and there is no literature to support value in use of Rolfing in a disease group.[299]

Rolfing therapists believe that their techniques facilitate flow of *universal energy*. The pagan world view of astrology, is that of association, of correspondence and sympathy of man with the cosmos as a base doctrine. They look to a counterfeit creation power, apart from a living Being/God and teach this as they apply and explain therapeutic measures. Even as some therapy might have beneficial aspects in and of itself, this world view may be presented as the source of healing. This in turn initiates a change in the recipient's world view as a result of the treatment. It is not just the therapeutic modality that can influence us, but the very concepts of the therapist and the explanation given, crediting the movement of universal energy for healing. By partaking of these therapies applied by *healers* with this pagan world view we place ourselves on Satan's ground.

It is also taught that this type of treatment brings a higher level of *consciousness* through mind/body rejuvenation.

---

298 http://www.rolf.org
299 Jones, T.A., "Rolfing", *Physical Medicine & Rehabilitation Clinics of North America,* (2004), 15 (4): - 799–809. Doi:

Rolfing is based upon Wilhelm Reich's theory of 'Character armor'—that the 'consciousness' can be found in the body as well as the brain, and that energy blockages cause lots of problems. 'Because mind and body are inter-connected, the results of past traumatic experiences show themselves in a person's posture....' Through deep muscle massage—which may be painful, even torturous, these blocks can be broken down and a harmonious mind body system achieved. (The physical massage causes emotional release hence it is an emotional as well as physical treatment).[300]

In 2007 Dr. Mehmet Oz while on the Opra Winfrey T.V show endorsed Rolfing and likened it as someone doing yoga for you, Christian beware.

SHIATZU

Shiatzu finger pressure is another form of mind/body energy balancing therapy in the massage group. It is considered diagnostic as well as therapeutic. Skilled fingers are said to be able to detect energy imbalances and in turn, correct such. It claims to be able to stimulate the immune system, thereby benefiting the whole body.

A large variety of Shiatzu therapy disciplines exists in Japan and throughout the world. It has similar basis in the meridian concept as acupressure and acupuncture. This massage is gentle and is done close to the diseased organ.[301] It, too, is a treatment based on the correspondence or sympathies of the body to the cosmos—man as the microcosm of the macrocosm. It has its origin from Japan.[302]

Shiatzu claims to be able to treat the following without needles:

Ankle sprains, appetite, asthma, bedwetting, blood pressure, chills, constipation, diarrhea, eyestrain, fevers, hangovers, headaches, heart pain, hemorrhoids, hiccups, indigestion, insomnia, knee pains, leg cramps, nervousness, neuralgia, nosebleed, numbness, menopause, menstrual cramps, morning sickness, nausea, motion sickness, nasal congestion, common cold, neck cramps, nervousness, neuralgia, rheumatism, sciatica, sexual problems, sinusitis, swelling, toothache, whiplash, and much more.[303]

Acupuncture uses needles, zone therapy (reflexology) concentrates principally on applying pressure to the hands and feet, and Shiatzu employs its own type

---

300   Eldon, John, Wilson, Clifford, *Occult Shock and Psychic Forces,* Master Books, San Diego, California, (1980), pp. 229, 230.
301   Bergson, Anika, Tuchak, Vladimir, *Shiatzu*, Pinnacle books, (1976), p. 13.
302   *Ibid.*
303   *Ibid.,* face cover back side.

of pressure. It does not matter much that the key points might be called by different names— reflexes, acupuncture points, or Shiatzu points. The seed of thought, basic to all, is the same. The history of Shiatzu then goes back to this deeper understanding of its essential nature. Thus we owe our thanks not only to Namikoshi but to the ancient Chinese and to the American pioneers of zone therapy as well.[304]

The difference among the various treatments seems to lie in the kind of pressure treatment recommended by each method; yet, in all methods, results are obtained. To this day, no one quite knows why....[305]

POLARITY THERAPY

Polarity therapy is a combination of ancient Eastern and Western holistic health care ideas, adhering to the energy field hypothesis, and formed by Randolph Stone in the 1940's. Universal energy is described as becoming unbalanced when unequal distribution occurs to the poles of the body's energy field, divided into the body's right and left side. The right side is charged with *positive sun heat energy*, and the left with *cooling moon receptive energy*. Balancing techniques used are 1) touch (massage or acupuncture), 2) stretching and exercise, 3) diet, and 4) mental-emotional process. They correct the disturbance of balance of the *etheric electric*.

There is no scientific basis for this belief, nor any reproducible measurements of this system. Stone referred to the unproven energy as Breath of life, ki, chi, prana, and or life force.

REIKI

Reiki is a popular "body-mind-spirit" therapy imported from Japan. It is a soma therapy, and which the next chapter will deal with at length.

CRANIOSACRAL THERAPY

Craniosacral therapy is another body—mind—spirit therapy quite like Reiki in its application, with a very soft touch to the head and neck area. It could be considered a continuation of phrenology with therapy directed more to the body than to the mind. This therapy, too, will be presented in depth in the next chapter.

---

304   *Ibid.*, p.2.
305   *Ibid.*

APPLIED KINESIOLOGY

Kinesiology is a true science of muscles and body movement and is not to be confused with *Applied Kinesiology.* Applied Kinesiology is another method of energy manipulation, diagnosis by divination, and treatment that has become popular with some chiropractors, naturopaths, an occasional dentist and physician, and with many in the public sector. (originated by George Goodhart D.C., by   psychic means 1964, *Can you Trust Your Doctor* p. 157) The practitioners of this technique say they are more interested in prevention of illness than with treatment. It is their claim that they can evaluate five body systems—nervous, lymphatic, vascular, cerebrospinal, and meridian (no such system has been demonstrated to exist). They do not separate the systems in testing. It is a test of a specific muscle for strength and is done by pushing and/or pulling against a muscle group, with the patient resisting. The test is supposed to reveal the chi, or universal energy flow, through specific areas of the body.

> Applied Kinesiology claims to induce proper structural and chemical -nutritional organization in the body, as well as 'left and right brain' hemisphere balance. It claims to evaluate and correct problems of the nervous, circulatory, lymphatic, skeletal-musculature, and 'meridian' systems, thereby maintaining health. Its practices are believed to permit the even flow of *cosmic energy* throughout the body, thus nurturing individual organs and systems with the proper supply of chi energy.[306]

This same technique is claimed to detect vitamin and/or mineral deficiency. There are supposedly specific points at various places on the body which will correlate with these deficiencies. If a finger is held on one of these points, that is said to correlate with a specific vitamin or mineral, testing of the correlating muscle group is believed to reveal a deficiency or normal level. If a person wishes to test for allergies to a substance or food, then this substance can be held in one hand or in the mouth and again the muscles are tested. If a weak response occurs as judged by the examiner, the diagnosis of an allergy is made. This is a form of *divination*.

---

306 Ankerberg, John; Weldon, John, *Can You Trust Your Doctor?,* Wolgemuth and Hyatt, Brentwood, TN, (1991), p. 154.

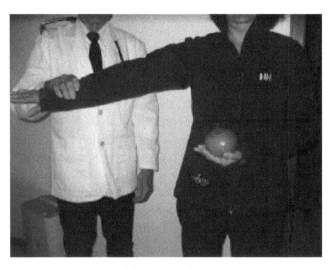

figure 32. Applied kinesiology

BI-DIGITAL-O-RING TEST

A method quite similar to *applied Kinesiology* but not so well known is the *Bi-Digital-O-Ring test* (BDORT). This test has its origin from Yoshiaki Omura, M.D., Sc.D. of the USA. Dr. Omura's web site opens with the statement seen below:

> Through the methods and materials presented here you may witness a revolution in medicine, dentistry, and technology, because Dr. Yoshiaki Omura has discovered a way to test which materials (pharmaceutical or "natural" medicines, drugs, hormones, vitamins, minerals, supplements of any type, anesthetics, herbs, dental restorative materials, food, clothing, cell phones, chemicals, etc.) are potentially health-giving and life-promoting for a person, and those which are potentially harmful.

> Yoshiaki Omura, M.D., Sc.D. is an early non-invasive diagnostic test for intractable medical problems with their safe and effective treatment. Such diagnosis is often achieved within an hour. It can involve the detection and treatment of early stages of cardiovascular disease, Alzheimer's disease, Autism, and cancer (often long before any known laboratory test can detect any abnormality or malignancy). It may be the *ultimate in preventive medicine* available today. BDORT evaluation can not only diagnose many medical problems, but can also help manage conditions such as malignant tumors,

chronic severe pain, cardiovascular diseases, Alzheimer's disease, Autism and neuromuscular diseases.[307]

What is the test that this article says is the ultimate? It involves the testing person holding his thumb and forefinger of one hand together to form a *O-ring* and then he places a finger from his other hand on the patient, or he may use a wand to touch the patient at acupuncture points or over an organ, etc. Another person will attempt to pull apart his thumb and finger. If the finger and thumb circle is weak at any time when the probe or finger is placed at a location on the body it signifies disorder in this area. The wand—probe can be placed anywhere on the body or on any medication, herb, etc., and the test tells the practitioner the diagnosis, chooses the therapy, etc. It is essentially the same as *applied kinesiology*. It is simply another form of *divination* performed by "hands on."

TOUCH FOR HEALTH

Touch for Health is another variant therapy and is explained on the same concept as for acupuncture, *i.e.*, the flow of chi through *meridians*. Instead of using needles or massage, this form of therapy involves determining approximately which meridian is involved, then running the hands up and down the meridian, to correct the energy imbalance. Gentle massage is applied by the practitioner's finger to the same energy centers as pierced by the tiny acupuncture needle. This finger massage is known as acupressure.

THERAPEUTIC TOUCH

Another practice in the West which is similar to qi gong, or Falun gong of Chinese traditional medicine, is *Therapeutic Touch*. It is not an exercise, but a technique of (supposed) energy transfer which does not involve touching the patient. It is done by placing the hands a few centimeters above the body and traversing the body to determine the balance of *life force energy*. This technique has swept through the nursing profession in the UK and America. The *British Medical Journal* (April 4, 1998, p. 1042) reported that over 100,000 people have been trained in this modality, with 43,000 being professionals. How many today?

---

307   http://bdort.org

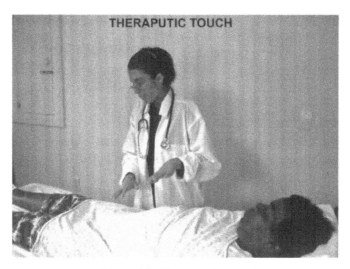

Figure 33. Therapeutic touch

I have read that in Russia this treatment method has been standard training in medical schools for years.[308] It has gained great popularity because it claims to get results without adverse side effects. It has gained acceptance in the highest academic centers for training nurses. Many hospitals have had teams of nurses who administer this *touch*. The practitioners of therapeutic touch say that they can improve a wide variety of medical conditions, such as decubiti ulcers (pressure sores), Alzheimer's disease, and thyroid disorders, etc., by correcting the energy-field disturbances, which they are able to feel and *re-pattern:*

by passing their hands over a patient's body at a distance of 5–10 cm.[309]

The originator of this type of energy medicine is Dora Kunz, a past president of the Theosophical Society.

Dora Kunz is herself a 'spiritualist' who looks to 'invisible intelligences," 'angels' and theosophy's "ascended Masters' for inspiration and guidance."[310]

308   Swain, Bruce, *East-West Journal of Natural Health and Living,* Shushi Foundation, Brookline, MA, May (1989), p. 30.
309   McCarthy, Michael, Therapeutic Touch Fails Child's Test, *The Lancet,* April 4, (1998), (A British Medical Journal).
310   Kunz, Dora, *The American Theosophist,* Dec. (1978), Viewpoint, reported in Ankerberg, Can You Trust Your Doctor? op. cit., p. 393.

Delores Krieger R.N. credits Dora Kunz for her knowledge of this practice. Krieger also had additional training in occult healing techniques. She studied yoga, Ayurvedic medicine (Hindu occultism applied to medicine), occultic Tibetan medicine, and Chinese traditional medicine.[311] Delores Krieger has been a leading promoter of therapeutic touch in the nursing profession. Therapeutic touch is an example of the Hindu concept of *prana* (vital energy, chi), under a new guise. Krieger stated that the Hindu version of universal energy is the basis for healing energy that is said to be transferred. She comments that the practitioner of this so-called art is the *conduit* not the generator, of the energy believed to be present.

> …prana may be transferred from one individual to another and may not be so readily apparent to us unless we have gotten into the practice of and literature of hatha yoga, tantric yoga, or the martial arts of the orient.[312]

The therapeutic touch technique is based on four steps:
a.   Centering type meditation by therapist prior to applying treatment.
b.   Assessment–scanning the patient's energy fields with the hands, feeling for energy imbalances.
c.   Unrufling the field–checking for stagnant energy and sweeping this energy away with the hands.
d.   Transfer of energy–moving energy via the hands to the patient so as to correct energy imbalance.

> Whatever their initial appeal, energy therapies inevitably beckon the budding healer into more hard core 'New Consciousness' thinking since these systems are in essence profoundly mystical.[313]

In April 1998, three medical journals, *Journal of the American Medical Association, British Medical Journal* and *Lancet* (also a British medical journal), reported a study done by Emily Rose, a nine- year-old girl testing the ability of practitioners of therapeutic touch. In her test, the therapeutic touch practitioners put their hands through a small hole in a shield that prevented them from knowing if anyone was on the other side or not. Then a person's hand would be put very close to the therapist's hand and the therapist was asked to tell when a hand was near his or her hand. The results were no better than guessing. This was done as a school project and the quality of the experiment

311   Ankerberg, op. cit., p. 393.
312   Krieger, Delores, *The Therapeutic Touch,* p. 13; Reported in Reisser, Paul C. M.D. , Reisser, Teri K., Weldon, John, New Age Medicine, Global Publishers, Chattanooga, TN, (1088), p. 45.
313   Reisser, op. cit., pp. 47–48.

was such that when written up by adults it was accepted and placed into three prestigious medical journals. The conclusion of the journals editors were:

> Twenty-one experienced Therapeutic Touch practitioners were unable to detect the investigator's *energy field*. Their failure to substantiate Therapeutic Touch's, *most fundamental claim,* is unrefuted evidence that the claims of Therapeutic Touch are groundless and that further professional use is unjustified.[314]

As we close this section concerning various massage methods a little should be said concerning various mechanical apparatuses that are sold to effect massage. Swedish type massage by hand or by machine can and may be a desirable experience and should not be considered as "spiritualistic." It is when the therapist may describe or explain benefits and actions of the massage as being a method of unclogging, diffusing, or imparting *energy* we know we have a therapist that is connected to the power of Satan. Therapy from this person then becomes of concern.

MASSAGE MACHINES:

There are many machines, chairs, and/or beds sold to effect massage. I see no concern here. However if in purchasing for my own use or going to a place to receive treatment from such an instrument, and its benefits are explained as coming from a manipulation of universal energy to impart health and I accept that concept, then I believe one is on Satan's ground.

I am often asked about a particular machine as to whether it is a part of the above described occultic pseudoscientific electronic gadgetry. One such machine is the "Chi Machine." There are several close copy duplicate machines with changed names and selling for a lesser price. I opened the web site for the Original Chi Machine" and found that the site makes comments about the *me-too* machines and how one will not receive the real therapy from these copy-cats.

The Chi Machine was imported into the U.S. from Japan where its originator received a Japanese patent. It is a device that moves the legs in a figure eight motion. One lies down, with legs together and outstretched with ankles on a holder, the holder then moves the ankles and legs side to side in a smooth figure of eight motion 140 times a minute. The motion is not more than four inches in width. It does cause some motion of the pelvis and extension into the spine, similar to the motion of a fish swimming.

---

314   Linder, Rosa, BSN, Rosa, Emily, Sarnor, Larry, Barret, Stephen M.D., The Journal of American Medical Assn. April 4, (1998), pp. 1005-1010.

The Federal Drug Administration has given it a class III status. It has been shown to lessen swelling in the legs when edema is present. Therefore, there is some physiologic action, but very minimal. It was not compared with the benefits for reduced swelling in legs by lying down with legs elevated.

But what about questions as to its spiritualistic influence? I read through the website of the Original Chi Machine and there seemed to be nothing I could find that gave a hint that spiritistic ideas were incorporated into its use. After a long list of attributes of the proclaimed physiological benefits of using the apparatus, I found what I suspected from the beginning—that it was a machine developed to promote the movement of the Eastern dogma of chi—universal energy. See the paragraph below taken from the energywellnessproducts.com website.

> **Exercising Internal Organs and Building "Chi."** "Chi is a Chinese word referring to the life force or life energy. Chi increases the feeling of aliveness and wellbeing. Ch'in is the permeating energy within the universe and creates vitality: Western medical science is beginning to consider ancient Eastern traditions. These Eastern traditions emphasize healing and good health based on a *life force energy*, which flows in channels through all living forms. The Ch'in Machine aids in unblocking the "Ch'in" pathways and ensures a maximum flow of healing source throughout your body and organs.

This is another example of a pagan healing method presenting itself under the banner of science and proclaiming all sorts of non-proven benefits from a scientific standpoint, when in reality the whole objective is to introduce the Eastern pagan dogma. Early in the chapter on *Mystical Herbology*, I write about a book on aromatherapy which made the statement that twenty years earlier the introduction of aromatherapy was done through strict promotion as if its value was only physiological benefits. But now the acceptance of the spiritual nature of aromatherapy is so accepted there can be direct comments on its spiritual power.

What about receiving therapy from a person who has definitely accepted the universal energy— spiritualistic doctrine but gives me regular physical therapy as the doctor prescribed? Should I look elsewhere for a therapists that is not tied into such beliefs? I will leave that to you, I cannot answer for you, and it is between you and God. However let me draw your attention to the following quote:

> **Danger in Consulting Cultist Physicians.**--There is danger in departing in the least from the Lord's instruction. When we deviate from the plain path of duty, a train of circumstances will arise that seem irresistibly to draw us farther and farther from the right. Needless intimacies with those who have no respect for

God will seduce us, ere we are aware. Fear to offend worldly friends will deter us from expressing our gratitude to God or acknowledging our dependence upon Him. . . .

Angels of God will preserve His people while they walk in the path of duty; but there is no assurance of such protection for those who deliberately venture upon Satan's ground. An agent of the great deceiver will say and do anything to gain his object. It matters little whether he calls himself a spiritualist, an "electric physician," or a "magnetic healer...."[315]

I wish to share with the reader concerning a particular massage table that is sold around the world coming from a foreign country and marketed in many countries that does give some concern. There are a number of web sites on the Internet advertising this massage table under the name *Nuga Best*. It is widely promoted and very popular throughout the countries Ukraine and Russia. In my investigation of this table I once went to a treatment center in Ukraine that had several tables and where the therapist was treating up to forty patients each day. Due to lack of an interpreter at the time of the visit I was not able to hear what a new patient would be told about the machine and its benefits. The price for a treatment was expensive. While visiting the therapy center I did read the machine's manual from the manufacture. There were no comments made anywhere as to the effectiveness or improvement of disorders that one could expect from therapy. It totally avoided any comments as to its use. This is a customary pattern for machines that are not shown to be of true therapeutic value. The manufacture avoids any legal conflict. However the agents who sell machines and those directing treatment may have a story to tell which may not be bound to reality or truth.

I am going to share with you what information I obtained on a web site promoting the *Nuga Best Therapeutic Thermal Massage Table*. I opened this web site one day, and on the following day I could not pull up this article. There was a web site for the clinic that the article had originated from but not this article. Fortunately I had printed out the four page article about the Nuga Best massage table and its description. The article had been withdrawn, why? (Now 3-28-11, replaced) The other articles advertised by this chiropractic clinic in Montana, USA were still on the web site, strange? First, the opening paragraph:

The special genius of Nuga Best, the result of extensive research and development, lies in the *marriage of the ancient Eastern healing arts of acupressure, massage, and moxibution (heat therapy) with modern chiropractic*

---

315   White, E.G., Education, Pacific Press, Nampa Idaho, (1903), 607.

theory, far-infrared light therapy, and modern technology. Thus, through our products and services, we contribute to society and to the health of the human race. (Emphasis added)

The web site contains four pages of written comments, it intermingles the pantheistic Eastern thought and healing traditions with the comments on the value and benefits of the machine. This intermingling is careful however to never really say directly that the machine influences the power that those Eastern healing traditions proclaim. It lets the reader assume so, but has protected the author from being accused of teaching that the machine accomplishes such. This technique I have frequently run into in the subject of alternative healing. The article talks about chi, life force, power, the universal life energy that is said to run through everything. It is written so as to appear that the machine will aid the movement of this imagined energy. See the quote below:

> Nuga Best automatically massages the muscles and tendons around the spine, relaxing hardened nerve roots, relieving tension, and improving the flow of chi, lie back relax and enjoy![316] (Emphasis added)

As one lies on the massage table the "highly therapeutic" heated jade rollers emit far-infrared light beams as they roll up and down the spine. A comment is made about a massage phase and an acupressure phase. Massage from the table is said to stimulate major acupuncture meridians along the spine causing powerful bioelectric impulses to course throughout the nervous system. Massage from the machine is said to increase circulation of the blood and of vital force energy—chi.

We are told that Nuga Best massage does the same as acupuncture yet without the needles or the focused pressure of acupressure. The physiological benefits are widely known so says the article: relaxed muscles and tendons, reduced anxiety, less insomnia, increased circulation and over all improved flow of chi. Let the Christian beware. (Article on nuga best not now on this web site)

Magnets

A long-time patient of mine, a retired nurse and institutional church worker, sat on the exam table in my office. He complained of pain in the feet. I removed a shoe and found magnets inserted in various locations in his shoe. This nurse and his wife informed me that, that very day they were to have delivered to their home, a mattress and pillows filled with magnets. Earlier

---

316   http://bigskywellnesscenter.com (info about Nuga Best now removed from web site

that week they had attended a special retreat for retired church workers. A demonstration of the supposed health benefits of magnets had been made at the retired workers retreat by a member of the church who was in the business of selling magnets. I shared with these friends my concern and gave them some references to study and urged them to re-think their choice. The mattress and pillows were sent back.

The use of magnets has become popular in the treatment of pains and aches and a variety of other distresses. It is a billion dollar industry. Magnets are being used in sports; housewives have also been convinced of its value. Magnets are applied to various places on the body and left for hours or days. They are placed in shoes, in pillows, in mattresses. This practice is supposed to make one stronger, increase circulation, and generally restore health. There is not a shred of scientific evidence to support these claims, but that does not seem to matter as long as someone testifies as to how much it helped them. There seems to be no concern that the magnet might create some abnormal function. The belief is that it can only benefit.

What seems silly and harmless, except for the money transferred into someone else's hands, is really a technique quite like the others we have been studying. There may be no talk of balancing energy, yet it is implied that the application of magnets at various places on the body corrects unbalanced polarity. There may be claims made that the influence of the earth's magnetic field has been altered in some way and by use of magnets this imbalance will be corrected. Consider this statement from a magnetic healer:

> Magnet therapy focuses on electromagnetic energy surrounding and infusing the body and works with this energy in much the same as subtle energy practices work with subtle energy.[317]

A study was done on the use of magnets in treating plantar fasciitis of the heel by Mark Winemiller MD at the Mayo Clinic. 96 people with heel pain participated in the study. Fifty percent received magnets in their shoes and fifty percent were given fake magnets. At the end of three months there was no difference between the two groups. There was improvement in both groups but no difference one from the other.[318]

In September 25, 2007 the Canadian Medical Association Journal carried an abstract reporting a meta-analysis study done on the use of static magnet therapy by Max Pittler M.D. and colleagues at the Peninsula Medical School

---

317   *New Age Encyclopedia,* Gale Research, Detroit MI, (1990), p. 28.
318   Reuters Health Information (2005-09-21): *Magnetized insoles don't appear to relieve foot pain,* http://www.reutershealth.com/archive/2005/09/21/ eline/links/20050921 eline003. html (archived).

of the University of Exeter and Plymouth. This meta- analysis contained 29 studies and found "no convincing evidence to suggest that static magnets might be effective for pain relief." The studies looked at foot pain, fibromyalgia, lower back pain, carpal tunnel syndrome, diabetic peripheral neuropathy or delayed onset muscle soreness. Results were mixed for osteoarthritis so no conclusions were made for this disorder.

History tells us of the use of magnetism millennia ago. Probably the first electrified substance (static electricity, by rubbing) used in treatment was amber, then lodestone—ferrous oxide was found in Magnesia (Western Turkey) as a natural magnet. Magnetic substances were carved in the shape of body organs and placed over the organ as therapy. At various times in the past, magnetic therapy became popular and then faded. In the 16th century, a historically famous physician, Paracelsus, used magnetism in his treatments. Magnetism was believed to be the same power as in hypnosis.

Franz Anton Mesmer (1733–1815), is known as the father of modern hypnotism. He graduated and received his degree in medicine from the University of Vienna in 1766. In his book, *On the Influence of the Planets*, he proposed:

> That stroking diseased bodies with magnets might be curative.[319]

He affected his first cure by passing magnets over the body.

> ...Like Paracelsus, Mesmer believed that the microcosm of the human body reflects the macrocosm of the universe; he also believed that the corresponding parts are tied together by a universal magnetic fluid....

> ...In 1776, Mesmer met Gassner and became convinced that all of Gassner's cures (passing hands across a body without magnets) could be explained by his own theory of animal magnetism. Before this meeting, Mesmer had achieved cures by (passing magnets over the patient's body), but the fact that Gassner achieved the same results with his bare hands led Mesmer to wonder whether the healing power might reside in the human body itself, rather than in the magnets; dispensing with the magnets, he too began to pass his hands alone over patient's bodies.[320]

When these practices eventually progressed on to hypnotic trances and psychic experiences, magnets were discarded.

---

319 *New Age Encyclopedia,* Gale Research, Detroit MI, (1990), p. 29.
320 *Ibid.*

The above comments are not to be confused with the use of magnetism such as the MRI diagnostic machine, and the use of pulsating electromagnetic field about a fractured bone to promote healing. These methods work on known laws of science. It is interesting to note that no one has ever heard of a person being healed of a disorder by being placed for an hour in an MRI diagnostic machine, though it is one the most powerful magnets on earth. Powerful magnets that are electrically pulsated are used occasionally to treat the most severe forms of depression. There can be benefit from this treatment. It is not to be confused with the popular use of magnets in shoes, pillows, mattresses, etc.

This comment bears repeating:

> Not a few in this Christian age and Christian nation resort to evil spirits, rather than trust to the power of the living God. The mother watching by the sickbed of her child, exclaims, 'I can do no more. Is there no physician who has power to restore my child?' She is told of the wonderful cures performed by some clairvoyant or magnetic healer, and she trusts her dear one to his charge, placing it as verily in the hands of Satan as if he were standing by her side. In many instances the future life of the child is controlled by a satanic power which it seems impossible to break.[321]

> An agent of the great deceiver will say and do anything to gain his object. It matters little whether he calls himself a spiritualist, an 'electric physician,' or a 'magnetic healer.' By specious pretenses he wins the confidence of the unwary. He pretends to read the life history and to understand all the difficulties and afflictions of those who resort to him.[322]

IRIDOLOGY

An alternative method of making a medical diagnosis for the present, and predicting disorders in the future, is *iridology*. This is a divination method which involves examining the iris of the eye, and inspecting the color, texture, and location of various pigment flecks in the iris. The practitioners say they can detect *imbalances* in the body's system which in turn can be treated with vitamins, minerals, herbs, and in other ways. Iridology is practiced around the world. However, the technique is rarely accepted by a conventional medical doctor. Some chiropractors and naturopaths utilize it, and there are many non-medical people who present themselves as iridologists.

---

321 White, E.G., *Counsels on Health,* Pacific Press Pub. Assn., Mountain View, CA, (1951), p. 454

322 White, E.G., *II Mind, Character, Personality,* Southern Pub. Assn., (1977), p. 700.

Modern iridology had its start from Ignatz von Peczely, a Hungarian physician, who, in his youth, had broken a leg of an owl and noticed a black stripe in the lower part of the owl's eye. He theorized that the broken leg caused the black stripe. However, this does not happen.

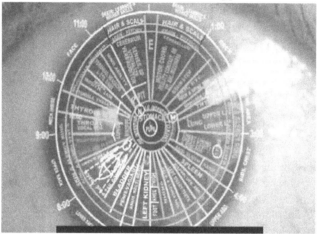

Figure 34. iris chart

The right side of the body is said to be represented by the right iris and the left side by the left iris. The iris is divided into ninety sections with each section supposedly representing relationship to a specific part of the body. Disease or disturbances in those areas of the body are said to present changes in the iris which can be seen by the skilled examiner. Jessica Maxwell, in her book *The Eye–Body Connection,* claims that:

> The basis for iridology is the neuro-optic reflex, an intimate marriage of the estimated half million filaments of the iris with the cervical ganglia of the sympathetic nervous system. The neuro-optic reflex turns the iris into an 'organic etch-a- sketch' that monitors impressions from all over the body as they come in.[323]

Ophthalmologists have not found the above statement to be true. Only a rare optometrist will accept it. The technique has been scientifically tested a number of times and each time it has failed to support the claims of its adherents. The iridologist might make claims as to the accuracy and scientific basis for iridology, such as that it is based upon a neuro-optic reflex, a connection between the optic nerve and the iris and the rest of the body. The

---

323   Maxwell, Jessica, What Your Eyes Tell You About Your Health, Esquire, January (1978). Reported in Ankerberg, Op. cit., p. 340.

problem here is that the signals of the optic nerve only go to the brain. There is no signal traveling from the brain back up the optic nerve to the eye. In spite of the lack of scientific proof for a basis by which it can work, or of true accuracy in its use, iridology is still very popular.

> Iridology can be traced to ancient Chinese astrological practices, however according to Dr. Carter; the first precursor published on iridology was Phillippus Meyen's *Chiromatica Medica. (*Germany, 1670).[324]

Iridology was introduced to America in 1904. The most recent leader of iridology in America was the late naturopath, Bernard Jensen (1908-2001).

> ....Jensen is not a scientist but is a New Age Healer, a fact revealed in his various works, such as *Iridology; Science and Practice in the Healing Arts*. In this text, he discusses his belief in reincarnation, astral travel, psychic development and other occultic practices and philosophies.[325]

He claims that:

> Iridology can be used in conjunction with any other form of analysis and diagnosis.[326]

The iridologist believes he can:

> ...determine the inherent structure and the working capacity of an organ, can detect environmental strain, and can tell whether a person is anemic and in what stage the anemia exists...He can determine the constructive ability of the blood... He can determine the nerve force, the responsive healing power of tissue, and the inherent ability to circulate the blood.[327]

The same belief says that the iris of the eye can show acute, subacute, chronic, and destructive stages in the body.

> Many other factors are also revealed such as organic and functional changes...It foretells the development of many conditions long before they have manifested into disease symptoms.[328]

---

324 Ankerberg, John, Weldon, John, *Can You Trust Your Doctor?*, Wolgemuth and Hyatt, Brentwood, TN, (1991), p. 341.
325 *Ibid.*, pp. 343–344.
326 *Ibid.*
327 *Ibid*
328 *Ibid.*

We are told that:

> No other science tells so accurately the progress from acute to chronic states. Only iridology is capable of directing attention to impending conditions; only iridology reveals and evaluates inherent weaknesses.[329]

> In using iridology you need ask no questions yet you can tell where pain is, what stage it is in, how it got there, and when it is gone.[330]

There is no truth to these claims, as emphasized by the following test of iridology. In 1979, Bernard Jensen and two other practitioners of iridology were given 143 photographs of irises of patient's eyes to view and determine which individuals had kidney impairment. (48 had a diagnosis of kidney disease as revealed by standard blood tests; the rest had no kidney disorder.) These iridologists were not able to separate the diseased from the normal. One iridologist had picked out 88 % of normal patients as having kidney disease; another examiner found that 74% percent of those patients that had severe kidney disease were identified as normal. This test was reported in the *Journal of American Medical Association*, 242, 1385-1387, 1979.

The *British Medical Journal* 297:1578-1581, 1988, carried an article of a test given to five leading Dutch iridologists. They received a stereo color slide of the right iris of 78 people, half of whom had a diagnosis of gallbladder disease, and the other half were free of any disorder. The five practitioners were not able to differentiate the diseased from the normal, and were not able to agree among themselves as to who were diseased or not. This typifies the results of many tests given to iridologists.

Another problem that exists in iridology is that there are no standards in the charts used to represent the eye, from which the diagnosis of the health condition of the person being examined is made. The following quote presents this problem.

> For example, there are some twenty *different* iridology charts that a practitioner may choose from in his practice.[331]

Does iridology have an astrological basis for existence? Does it have its base in the "universal energy" concept? Like much of New Age medicine, iridology makes use of the concept of mystical energy. In fact, the pupil of the

329   *Ibid.*
330   *Ibid.*
331   Ankerberg, op. cit., pp. 346–7.

eye is held to be a repository of sorts for the body's *energy*, according to many iridologists.

> Most iridologists agree that the integrity of the body's energy is reflected by the quality of energy in this (pupil) hub, or core.[332]

As to astrology, iridologist Brint sums it up this way.

> From an Eastern point of view, the eye may be viewed as a *Mandala*... The Mandala links the microcosm and the macrocosm... Through the Mandala man may be projected into the universe and the universe into man... In iridology, the macrocosm and the microcosm are linked in our eyes... Iridology may be summed up as the observation of the change that arises from the interplay of various levels of consciousness and results in one's unique evolution into greater (occult) truth and light.[333]

---

332 Berkeley Holistic Health Center, *The Holistic Health Hand Book,* Berkley, California Press; Berkley, CA, (1978), p. 159.

333 *Ibid.,* pp. 155, 162.

CHAPTER 12
REIKI—CRANIOSACRAL THERAPIES

Reiki is a popular "body-mind-spirit" therapy performed by the application of hands. The palms of the hands will gently touch the body, or might not touch, in various anatomical areas for three to five minutes and in a set of up to 20 locations for a full treatment. There is no massage; the treatment will last from 60-90 minutes. Treatment schedule may be weekly with 2-4 visits. With use of Reiki, no diagnosis is needed or made. Any type of physical or mental disorder is considered as a disturbance of a *universal energy,* believed by Eastern neo-pagans and Western occultists to permeate and flow through our bodies. (Note: It has been reported that there are one and one half million American Reiki therapists in USA.)

The name "Reike" is defined by the following synonyms: "spiritual power," "mysterious atmosphere," "intelligence," "divine," "miraculous force," etc. Rei refers to ghost, spirit, soul, supernatural, miraculous, divine, etc.; while ki refers to spiritual energy, vital energy, life force, etc. It is the same meaning as qi, chi, prana, mana, vitalism and the other hundred names used to refer to this imagined force. Reiki has been defined further as a non-physical healing energy made up of *Life force energy* that is guided by a Higher Intelligence, or is spiritually guided life force energy. This is not referring to Jesus Christ, the Divine Son of God that the Christian follows.

The Oxford English Dictionary adds to our understanding of the alternative healing method of Reiki:

> Hence: therapy, apparently based on an ancient Tibetan Buddhist technique, developed in Japan in the late 19th or early 20th cent. By Dr. Mikao Usui (1865–1926), in which the therapist channels this energy from him or herself into the patient by the gently laying on of hands, to activate the natural healing processes of the patient's body and restore physical and emotional well-being.[334]

Mikao Usui is credited with re-discovering this healing method in 1922. It was believed to have existed in Tibet in the 1800's. Usui made it popular in Japan beginning in 1924 and continued teaching this method to others until his death in 1926. From then on one of his students, Chujiro Hayashi, carried on

---

334 Simpson, J., Weiner, M., Proffitt, et al., Oxford English Dictionary, (1989), 2nd ed.

the training of practitioners. Hawayo Takata, trained by Hayashi, came to the United States and has been the prime mover of the therapy in this country. She died in 1980. Reiki branched into several divisions in Japan as well as here in the U.S.A.

The difference between Reiki and many other New Age healing techniques is that treatment is not supposed to unclog, or balance universal energy. Reiki simply facilitates moving the energy from the cosmos through the therapist, and on into the client where it is then said to heal physically, mentally, emotionally, and spiritually. The teaching is that the energy has intelligence which can seek out and heal anywhere there is disorder making diagnosis unnecessary.[335]

It is reported that the recipient often feels warmth or tingling in the area being treated, even when a non-touching approach is being used. A state of deep relaxation, combined with a general feeling of well-being, is usually the most noticeable immediate effect of the treatment, although emotional releases can also occur.

> What sets Reiki apart from other hands-on healing modalities is that to become a channel to receive the energy you must be attuned by a Reiki master. The Attunement (**initiation into the occult**) opens you to receive and channel Reiki energy to others.[336]

Training to be a practitioner is divided into three levels.

First Degree level: This involves four "attunements," by a Reiki Master, in four sessions activating the "chakras," creating an open channel for the energy. The attunement methods are not made known and it is a secret to be held by those receiving the attunement. At the end of the four attunements the new therapist is ready to apply treatment. It is reported to be a very pleasant experience to receive Reiki, as a feeling of warmth and security pervades. It is said that once you become a Reiki therapist you never lose the ability.

Joyce Morris, in *The Reiki Touch* carried in *The Movement Newspaper*, October 1985, tells of a woman who received Reiki therapy. After the first session she remarked:

> I don't know what this is you've got but I just have to have it.

Another business lady remarked the following:

> Reiki should be available through every medical, chiropractic and mental health facility in this country. Your fees are a small price to pay for such impressive

---

335   Roberts, Llyn and Levy, Robert, *Shamanic Reiki*, O Books, (2008), pp. 2-5.
336   *Ibid.*, p. 2.

results. I don't know how Reiki works, but it works; that's all that counts in my book.[337]

The Reiki Magic Guide to Self-Attunement text by Brett Bevell speaks to the first attunement:

> I have sent a Reiki attunement across all time and space to all individuals who say the Reiki First degree Attunement Chant revealed later in this chapter....If you say this chant with the intent of being attuned to the First degree of Reiki, you will be attuned in the act of saying the phrase. This works because the attunement has been sent out across time and space to intersect with anyone who says the Reiki First Degree Attunement Chant while intending to be attuned.[338]

Second Degree Level: This level of training intensifies the Reiki energy, allowing the practitioner to channel energy at a distance and to effect deeper healing. It also introduces three symbols used to increase the power of the practitioner's healing ability. When completing this level of training the practitioner can heal over long distances.

Third Degree Level: (Reiki Masters) In Third Degree Reiki, you are attuned and trained with the capacity to attune others to Reiki. Another symbol is learned which is said to add power to the person having attained to this level.[339]

Why so many words and space discussing Reiki? It is a power that can be used to transform another person into New Age consciousness (thinking). It accomplishes what the meditative path does for others; it changes the way people think and what they believe is reality. They may embark thereafter upon learning yoga, meditation, and other spiritual transformation practices. Old values change, and truth is no longer truth.

In many physical therapy clinics different New Age practices are common, especially with massage therapy. The therapist may be combining Reiki and other energy balancing methods without the patient even being aware. Reiki seems to be the most exciting therapy practiced and appears to be spreading the fastest. A leading Reiki master made the following comment:

> When I looked psychically at the energy, I could often see it as thousands of small particles of light, like "corpuscles' filled with radiant Reiki energy

---

337 Barbara Ray, Ph.D., *The Reiki Factor, Smithtown,* NY: Exposition Press, (1983), p.63.
338 Bevell, Brett, *The Reiki Magic Guide to Self-Attunement,* Crossing Press, Berkeley, CA, (2007), p. 9.
339 *Ibid.,* p. 76.

flowing through me and out of my hands. It was as though these Reiki 'corpuscles' of light had a purpose and intelligence.[340]

A Reiki master explains *attunement*:

> Reiki attunement is an initiation into a sacred metaphysical order that has been present on earth for thousands of years ...By becoming part of this group; you will also be receiving help from the Reiki guides and other spiritual beings who are also working toward these goals.[341]

Again a Reiki master shares her experience in practicing this modality:

> For me, the Reiki guides make themselves the most felt while attunements are being passed. They stand behind me and direct the whole process, and I assume they also do this for every Reiki Master. When I pass attunements, I feel their presence strongly and constantly. Sometimes I can see them.[342]

Is Reiki compatible with Christianity? Isn't it natural healing? Check out this quote:

> During the Reiki attunement process, the avenue that is opened within the body to allow Reiki to flow through also opens up the psychic communication centers. This is why many Reiki practitioners report having verbalized channeled communication with the spirit world.[343]

The foundation of spiritualism (contact with the dead) is to believe the lie told in the Garden of Eden, you will not die, your eyes will be open, and you will be wise like God knowing good and evil. (Genesis 3:4, 5) Reiki is a fast track to make that connection with the spirit world. Ponder this next quote from another Reiki Master:

> Nurses and massage therapists who have been attuned to Reiki may never disclose when Reiki starts flowing from their palms as they handle their patients.

---

340 Rand, William Lee, The Nature of Reiki Energy, The Reiki News, Autumn, (2000), p. 5.
341 Rand, William Lee, Reiki: *The Healing Touch,* SouthÞeld, MI: Vision Publishing, (1991) p. 48. Reported in Youngen, Ray,A Time of Departing, Lighthouse Trails Publishing, (2006) p. 95.
342 Stein, Diane, Essential Reiki, (Berkley, CA: Crossing Press, 1995), p. 107 Reported in Youngen, Ray, *A Time of Departing,* Lighthouse Trails Publishing, (2006), p. 95.
343 Desy, Phylameana lila, *The Everything Reiki Book,* Avon, MA: Adams Media, (2004), p. 144. Reported in Youngen, Ray, *A Time of Departing,* Lighthouse Trails Pub., (2006), p. 97.

Reiki will naturally "kick in" when it is needed and will continue to flow for as long as the recipient is subconsciously open to receiving it.[344]

Reiki has become popular in several Catholic convents and some have conducted training in attunements. It has spread throughout protestant circles as well.

A systematic review of randomized clinical trials in 2008 assessed the evidence for effectiveness of Reiki. The conclusion: efficacy had not been demonstrated for any condition.[345]

In March 25, 2009 the Committee on Doctrine of the United States Conference of Catholic Bishops issued (Guidelines for Evaluating Reiki as an Alternative Therapy) halting the practice of Reiki by Catholics including Reiki therapies used in some Catholic retreat centers and hospitals. The bishops concluded (rightly) that the procedure was not compatible with either Christian teaching or scientific evidence, it would be inappropriate for Catholic institutions, such as Catholic health care facilities and retreat centers, or persons representing the church, such as Catholic chaplains, to promote or to provide support for Reiki therapy.[346]

CRANIOSACRAL THERAPY

Craniosacral therapy is another body—mind—spirit therapy quite like Reiki in its application, using a very soft touch to the head and neck area. Reiki is said to initiate a flow of cosmic energy through the therapist to the patient; however, therapists of *craniosacral therapy* tell us that they are correcting the clogged, sluggish, unbalanced flow of cerebrospinal fluid about the brain and spinal nerves. The disturbance of cerebrospinal fluid flow is proclaimed by those practicing craniosacral therapy to be the source of most disease and disorders of the human body. Such a concept is not recognized by medical science; indeed there is no evidence to support such a hypothesis.

At the time of the origin of this craniosacral hypothesis and resulting therapy, phrenology was popular. Phrenology was established upon the hypothesis that pressure to areas of the skull would alter the function of the brain and personality. Diagnosis was done by feeling the skull's shape and in turn therapy for the mind, personality, and character was performed by

---

344   *Ibid.*, p. 270.
345   Lee, MS, Pittler, MH, Ernst, E., Effects of Reiki in clinical practice: a systematic review of randomized clinical trials, *International Journal of Clinical Practice* 62 (6): 947. doi:10.1111/j.1742-1241.2008.01729.x. PMID 18410352. (2008) Retrieved 2008-05-02.
346   Committee on Doctrine of the United States Conference of Catholic Bishops, *Guidelines for Evaluating Reike as an Alternative Therapy*, March 25, (2009).

applying pressure to specific areas of the skull. Large hoods were used to cover the head and contained adjustable protrusions (which could be screwed in or out to different lengths) and when worn, applied pressure to selected points on the head for "mind-cure" treatment.

Craniosacral therapy had its origin in the United States through William Sutherland (1873-1954), an osteopathic physician. Sutherland would have been well acquainted with phrenology which may explain what motivated him to do some strange testing. Around 1901, he experimented on himself by placing belts around his head and then tightening those belts in certain positions about the head. He experienced headaches, disorientation and gastro intestinal distress from these tests. At times when he tightened belts in other positions on the head, he might feel relief and wellbeing. From this experimentation Sutherland developed the hypothesis that the cranial bones have motion one upon another and by pressure they can be moved, this, in turn, alters the flow of cerebrospinal fluid flow surrounding the brain, spinal cord, and spinal nerves, thus restoring health. He did not limit his description of disorders caused by improperly flowing cerebrospinal fluid to physical, but also included mental and emotional health.[347]

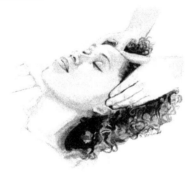

Figure 35. Cranio-sacral therapy

Dr. Sutherland eventually sensed a *power,* which he called *The Breath of Life* that arose from within the patient *without* his touch as the therapist. He believed that this Breath of Life carried a basic Intelligence (he capitalized the word "Intelligence") which the therapist could employ for delivering health. Sutherland and his associates considered the Breath of Life to carry a subtle yet powerful "potency" or force, which produces subtle rhythms which are transmitted around the body. He believed that this power—Breath of Life—came from the body's inherent life-force itself (chi, prana, universal energy). He theorized that the cerebrospinal fluid distributed the Breath of

---

347 http://www.craniocean.com/what_is_cranial.html://www.craniosacral- therapy.org/ History_02.htm

Life throughout the body. Dr. Sutherland took his hypothesis to osteopathic schools in the 1940's. This new teaching was labeled "Osteopathy in the Cranial Field."[348] The concept of cerebrospinal fluid flow being related to all diseases has never been verified by science, nor has a soft touch to the head been shown to alter the flow of spinal fluid. It is one man's hypothesis which a few others accepted without verification. This treatment modality does not fit the scientific explanation of the physiology of the nervous system, so how does it fit into spiritualism? How do we explain "The Breath of Life" that has Intelligence and arises from within the patient? Let us explore further.

In the mid 1970's another osteopathic physician, John Upledger, who had accepted Dr. Sutherland's hypothesis, began to teach the technique to non-osteopaths. Upledger is actually the one who coined the term "craniosacral therapy," as he was not allowed to use the term "cranial osteopath" for those who were not osteopaths. Dr. Upledger became the mover behind craniosacral therapy as we know it today.

Dr. Upledger added some techniques to Dr. Sutherland's original method. One contribution is referred to as *Therapeutic Imagery and Dialogue*. By use of this contribution Dr. Upledger may see a response he calls *Somato Emotional Release*, whereby the patient and therapist can engage together directly with the patients "*inner wisdom*" (Breath of Life) to receive knowledge about the patient that is unknown to either patient or therapist.[349]

Part of the hypothesis of craniosacral therapy is that the body develops what Upledger calls "*energy cysts*," which are said to be located at various locations of the body, especially in the connective tissue, such as ligaments, joints, and muscle. These so-called energy cysts are said to be the result of some unresolved physical or psychological trauma of the past, which then allow a variety of clinical symptoms to form. By use of therapeutic imagery and dialogue these cysts can be resolved, along with whatever clinical symptoms are present. Present day science has not found any of the above hypotheses to be true.[350]

Stan Gerome, an instructor at the Upledger Institute wrote an article entitled; *Dialogue, Imagery, CranioSacral therapy, and Synchonicity,* explaining imagery and dialogue. Gerome gives an illustration and the following is similar: A patient, John, being attended by a craniosacral therapist complains of pain at a point in his back which has limited his activity for several weeks. The therapist will ask if an image wants to come from that spot. John replies:

---

348   http://goldbamboo.com/topic-t6725-al-6CranioSacral_Therapy.html
349   http://www.larsonwellbeing.com/craniosacral-therapy/
350   http://www.massagetherapy.com/glossary/index.php

"Yes, I see a stone." The therapist continues: what color is the stone? Answer, "It is brown." What is its size? "It is the size of a marble." What is its name? Answer, "Anger." Now the therapist asks John permission to speak directly to the stone. The question is, how long have you been there, who put you there, and does this person know you are there? Answer: "I have been here for years, Ben put me here, and he does not know I am here." Therapist: John now knows you are there, and tell us why you are there. Answer from Anger "I am here so I could protect him from events in life he did not want to admit to." Anger, do you want to be free? "Yes." What will free you, Anger? "For John to see me as his anger."

When John accepts this dialogue as truth the energy cyst is said to relax and dissolve and John's problem of back pain heals. This is spoken of as *synchronistic,* where both the cyst and the physical problem resolve. What is the origin of such philosophy? Gerome credits Carl Jung (a famous spiritualistic psychiatrist) with the concept of synchronicity. Jung founded analytic psychology, and while working with people's conscious mind, proceeded to develop the unconscious concepts of psychology. A report of a belief of Jung's is of interest:

> It appears that many of Jung's beliefs were derived from *The Tibetan Book of the Dead.* It had been his constant companion ever since its first publication in England in 1927, and Jung considered its content the quintessence of Buddhist psychological criticism, an initiation process the purpose of which was to restore to the soul the divinity lost at birth....This is a very strong confession of faith in a book, the *Bardo Thodol*, that gives instructions to the dead and the dying and serves as a guide to the dead during the heavenly and hellish journey of forty-nine days between death and rebirth.[351]

Stan Gerome, a promoter of craniosacral therapy, in his article *CranioSacral Therapy* stated that he believes Jung's concept of sychronicity is at work in craniosacral therapy.[352] Synchronicity is a word Jung formed to explain connections between events or happenings that seem related. For instance if a person uses telepathy to communicate a message to someone else in a far distant location and the message somehow gets through, etc., this is synchronicity by Jung's definition. Similarly, the illustration continues. If a disturbance of flow of universal energy through the body at some location caused a psychological disturbance in the personality, correcting the flow by

---

351   Fodor, Nandor, *Freud, Jung, and Occultism,* University Books, Inc., New Hyde Park, New York, (1971), p. 157.

352   http://www.iahe.com/images/pdf/stan.pdf http://www.terrarosa.com.au/cst

whatever method would clear the personality defect. That connection between energy flow and a personality flaw is Jung's *synchronicity*.

Synchronicity is best explained by understanding there are agents of Satan, fallen angels, that can influence, carry messages, and be the power in Jung's sychronicity. Jung was a known spiritualist and also a theosophist. E.G. White warned us to have no connection to theosophy (a blend of oriental religions and mysticism), as it was, in essence spiritualism.[353]

In 1999, the British Columbia (Canadian) Office of Health Technology Assessment (BCOHTA) published an article entitled, *A Systematic Review and Appraisal of the Scientific Evidence on Craniosacral Therapy.* Their conclusion was that the theory is invalid and that practitioners cannot reliably measure what they claim to be modifying.

A physicist, Eugenie V. Mielczarek, Emeritus Professor of Physics at George Mason University in Fairfax, Virginia presented a paper, with the help of Derek C. Araujo, Adam Magazine, and Lori Sommerfelt representing the Center of for Inquiry, concerning the physics proclaimed by distant healers to be involved in Reiki, Craniosacral Therapy, Therapeutic Touch, Qi Gong, or any so-called distant healing. The summary of her paper follows:

Summary: Alleged distance healers justify their claimed abilities in terms of an unsubstantiated bio-magnetic field of about two milligaus emanating from the hands of certified distance healers. However, a two milligauss field strength is 18 orders of magnitude below the energy needed to affect any biochemistry. The postulate of an unknown energy field width eludes all science-based investigations and measurement, but nevertheless causes a transmission of energies large enough to affect the chemistry of cell cultures flies in the face of all micro and cellular biology experimentation and well tested theories of physics. This postulate of a medically healing energy field, which can only be generated by certain individuals, fails all test of medical science.[354] ...

We can count our blessings in the wisdom God has shared with us through the author E.G. White.

Satan a student of the Mind. ---For thousands of years Satan has been experimenting upon the properties of the human mind, and he has learned to know it well. By his subtle workings in these last days he is lining the human mind with his own, imbuing it with his thoughts; and he is doing this work in so deceptive a manner that those who accept his guidance know not that they are being led by him at his will. The great deceiver hopes so

353   White, E.G., 13 *Manuscripts Release* 1.3.
354   Mielczarek, Eugenie V., *A Fracture in our Health Care: Paying for Non-Evidenced Based Medicine,* Center for Inquiry, Office of Public Policy Washington D.C., June (2010).

to confuse the minds of men and women that none but his voice will be heard.[355]

Misuse of Sciences Pertaining to the Mind.—in these days when skepticism and infidelity so often appear in a scientific garb, we need to be guarded on every hand. Through this means our great adversary is deceiving thousands and leading them captive according to his will. The advantage he takes of the sciences, sciences which pertain to the human mind, is tremendous. Here serpent like, he imperceptibly creeps in to corrupt the work of God.

This entering in of Satan through the sciences is well devised. Through the channel of phrenology, psychology, and mesmerism he comes more directly to the people of this generation and works with that power which is to characterize his effort near the close of probation. The minds of thousands have thus been poisoned and led into infidelity.[356]

---

355 White, E.G., 1. *Mind, Character, Personality*, Southern Publishing Assoc., Nashville, Tenn., (1977) p. 18.1.
356 *Ibid.*, p. 19.

CHAPTER 13

"MYSTICAL HERBOLOGY"

Ever since man was restricted from partaking of the *Tree of Life* in the Garden of Eden, he has been searching for that magic sustainer of life. The plant kingdom has been the main source of his investigation for this *Elixir of Life*, with some additional interest in minerals. In the search for health, the field of *herbs* has had a long history. Winston J. Craig, Ph.D. , gives a cursory review of ancient civilizations involvement with herbs and minerals in his text *The Use and Safety of Common Herbs and Herbal Teas*. An herb is a plant that is valued for its flavor, scent, medicinal properties and often for its perceived *spiritual* values.

Records found from ancient civilizations such as from Mesopotamia, Egypt, India, China, have revealed the use of various herbs as medicinals. The oldest records date to near 3000 B.C. These oldest records show a rational approach to treatment of disease, but by 1500 B.C. almost all civilizations had reverted to an irrational and mystical approach. The emphasis for herb use became primarily spiritual and/or mystical combined with *astrology* in application as therapy for disease, without understanding of biochemical action. The same combination of spiritual, magical, and astrological relationships is a common belief in herb use today. The belief in a combination of properties of plants has led to a concept that plants have a *personality, a spirit*, a *consciousness,* which is on a very high plane—electrical magnetic frequency, and in turn, has a pronounced effect upon the human mind and emotions.[357]

The use of herbs has been a fundamental practice in all ancient health and healing systems. Herbs are considered helpful in *bridging* the cosmic energies which are said to be internal and external to the body. In Ayurvedic practice, herbs are always to be used in conjunction with meditation, diet, and other Ayurvedic approaches to health. Benefit from herbal therapy in Ayurveda from herbal therapy in Ayurveda medicine will depend upon its being added to other therapies. Little to no benefit is to be expected when it is used alone.

The herbal remedies of the past were not chosen for medicinal use because of their biochemical properties, but for their supposed properties to bring about positive or negative effects on universal energy, or due to their

---

357 Tisserand, Robert B., *The Art of Aromatherapy*, Healing Arts Press, Rochester, VT, (1977) pp. 45-49.

relationship to the zodiac, so as to bring balance to an unbalanced individual. Out of this use, however, it was recognized that certain plants had a variety of effects upon people, and over time, many plants began to be used as a result of their biochemical effects. Many present-day medicines are derived from herbs. More will be found by ongoing research. The use of some herbs in small amounts (such as tumeric) is of value as they contain many powerful chemicals that are healthful.

Ayurveda also used minerals in its treatment methods for thousands of years. Substances such as arsenic, antimony, and mercury were in common use until this past century. Mercury was the most popular mineral used and was given almost as a universal antidote for illness. Mercury, in the Hindu's understanding, is "semen from Shiva" one of their prominent gods.

The ancient apothecary, or pharmacy, had minerals and a variety of plant substances. Some of these pharmacies grew their own plants and prepared minerals for administration. Of particular note in alchemy is the mineral *mercury*, a silver white element derived from the red cinnabar ore, and is a deadly poison. The use of mercury continued down through the centuries, and in the early 1800's mercury, in the form of *mercurous chloride* (calomel), was given for almost all ailments. When I began the study of medicine in 1955, there were several forms of mercury still being used in medical care. It was quite effective as an ointment to treat fungus infections of the skin. Injections of *mercuhydrin* were used as a diuretic. Gradually, physicians began to understand its long-term toxicity and its use faded.

Plant lore and much of herbal use is based on the doctrine of pantheism, "one is all, all is one"; "as above, so below." The pagan's story of creation is that a blending of a two part (yin and yang) universal (life force) energy to a point of perfect balance created all material things. It also supposedly gave to living plants a high level frequency of cosmic energy, *a soul*. It is *this teaching* that is believed in the neo-pagan culture to give plants and herbs ability to have an influence upon the mind of man. For millennia herbologists have believed that there is a spiritual power connected with herbs. In more recent years this spiritual power has been expressed as electric-magnetic energy with a high wave *frequency*. There is always this attempt to explain *mystical power*, *life force energy*, in the terms and concepts of modern physics, making it more acceptable to the nonbeliever of mysticism. Such teaching is also more deceptive to the unwary.

In chapter 5 of this book, Universal Energy, explanation is given to the teaching promoted in New Age/Neo-Pagan belief systems concerning seven levels of perceived vibrational—frequencies of universal energy. Energy traveling at the speed of light is said to become material substance forming the cosmos, earth, and all that is on it. The higher (hypothesized) frequencies (subtle energies) are said to promote higher levels of consciousness. Herbs are believed to possess high frequency energy; therefore herbal treatment is believed to be most effective on the mind of man and is useful for therapy on emotions and mental conditions.[358]

The field of herbalism has much that is good but also opens a *chasm* that many fall into, thinking they are following a "natural" method. User beware, one can easily be led into a spiritual trap, accepting a false science, that of Satan's counterfeit system of healing and so giving him homage. The emphasis in this book's section on herbal use will be to expose this counterfeit of God's healing methods. Some of these false aspects are very difficult to ferret out, as the explanation of the application and use of certain methods sounds so beneficial and can blend so closely with the true. This is especially so in aromatherapy.

Most people will make their judgment as to whether a method is proper to use or not by whether they receive apparent benefit. This is never a test to be used to determine if a therapy is free of being Satan's counterfeit. Satan is not going to waste his efforts on a therapy that does not bring changes or *apparent* improvement. The Bible tells us he has power to do miracles, not just fake miracles; is given power to bring about real miracles. Author, E.G. White, makes an interesting observation of Satan's ability to perform miracles.

> No mere impostures are here foretold. Men are deceived by the miracles which Satan's agents have power to do, not which they pretend to do.[359]

The greatest use of herbs in the past was guided mainly by a *world view* that saw their influence upon humans not by biochemical action, but as substances containing *life-forces* by which man supposedly increased his own life-force. The New Age Movement of today looks to herbs both as a spiritual power—energy and as active biochemical agents. This will be better demonstrated in the following comments on flower and aromatherapy therapy.

"INTRODUCTION TO A PAGAN PHILOSOPHY OF HERBS"

> Herbs are 'Magick.' They have been the primary source of medicines for people of every culture and were considered 'magickal' or spiritual by many of them. An ancient *earth based* spiritual belief system concerning herbs appears in many ancient cultures and civilizations such as Celtic, Chinese, Indian, and

358 *Ibid.*, pp. 10-12, 92-103.
359 White, E.G., *The Great Controversy,* Pacific Press Publishing Association, Mountain View, California, (Now Nampa, Idaho) (1888, 1939, 1950), p. 553.

Native American philosophies just to name a few. Their religious beliefs shaped their view and relationship with the 'Great Spirit,' and the relationships between their citizens. This was a belief system which also demonstrated a wholistic view of illness, and utilized herbs according to religious belief.

You could say that an earth centered-nature religion still permeates herbalism today. We believe that herbalism is part of the **RELIGION of NATURE**, representing a balance of mind, body, and spirit and relies on intuition as well as science. (Emphasis added)

Pagans work with Nature, respecting and worshipping the spiritual forces they observe. Nature is perceived as the domain of the gods and of spirits. Nature religions teach a philosophy of *divine linking* between all of the earth's inhabitants.[360]

Exploring what Pagans believe about relationships said to exist between plants and man gives us more understanding as to why they have interest in the use of herbs, plant essences, essential oils, and aromatherapy for healing. This relationship is said to be that all plants have *souls* and *spirits* that guard and protect the species. Many plants are said to have also *animal spirits* attached.

Cachora (Indian Shaman) is quite plain about the underlying principle of healing herbs. He says that healing takes place when a person connects into the plant spirit, becoming the plant and understanding its personality. Using spirit as the method of transference, the plant's energy or healing properties are transmitted to the person....healing can take place by calling on the spirit and taking into one's mind the spiritual essence of the plant.[361]

In following paragraphs we will explore more concerning the belief in and use of plants, their essences, essential oils, and aromas as used by many today for health and healing.

Herbs have a proper use for their taste and biochemical properties. I recommend the book *Nutrition and Wellness, A Vegetarian Way to Better Health,* written by Winston J. Craig, Ph.D., R.D. , Professor of Nutrition at Andrews University, which covers much of the presently known benefits and information on the biochemical properties of herbs.[362] A second book I recommend is *Drugs, Herbs, & Natural Remedies,* by Mervyn Hardinge M.D.

360 http://www.purifymind.com/PhilosophyHerb.htm
361 Worwood, Valerie Ann, *Aromatherapy for the Soul,* New World Library, Navato, California, (1999), p. 9.
362 Craig, Winston J., Ph.D., R.D. , *The Use and Safety of Common Herbs and Herbal Teas, Second Edition,* Golden Harvest Books, 4610 Lisa Lane, 'Berrien Springs, MI, (1996).

, Dr. P.H., Ph.D., long-time instructor in pharmacology at Loma Linda School of Medicine, and also founder of the School of Public Health at Loma Linda.[363]

FLOWER THERAPY Flower therapy is a component of herbalism.

> Various flower remedies are also typically involved in the world of the occult, such as the *Vita Florum* and *Bach Flower Remedies* which claim to operate on the basis of cosmic forces and permit psychic diagnosis, prognosis, and other forms of guidance....[364]

The occultist Douglas Baker discusses the underlying theory in the use of flower remedies in his book, *Esoteric Healing*. He states that:

> Dr. Bach had discovered that dew which accumulated on the petals of wild flowers before sunrise, was changed dramatically by the presence of sunlight so that it now had an energy potential within it...each plant's dew had a quality of its own, a type of energy absorbed into the dew that could be used as a specific remedy. We should not be surprised, after our careful examination of the occult forces, a plan...that these could be applied to correct imbalances in the astral and mental auras of Man.[365]

Flower essences are prepared by placing the petals in water and in the sunlight. The water is then said to contain the flower's essence. The water is administered by placing drops of it on the tongue at various times each day over an extended period of time. It may be that the person prescribing the flower essence will make the diagnosis and then choose the proper flower for treatment by use of a pendulum.[366] Applied kinesiology is another method of choosing the proper flower essence to prescribe. This is done by having the person being tested hold a flower essence vial in one hand and with the other arm outstretched, downward pressure is made on the arm. The arm will increase in strength when the **best** essence is held. It is a popular form of divination.

Dr. Bach, an English homeopathic physician, a psychic, a believer in subtle energies, started the use of flower remedies. He developed thirty-eight

363 Hardinge, Mervyn G. , *A Physician Explains Ellen White's Counsel on Drugs, Herbs, & Natural Remedies,* Review and Herald Publishing Association, Hagerstown, MD (2001).
364 Ankerberg, John, Weldon, John, *Can You Trust Your Doctor?* Wolgemuth & Hyatt, Publishers, Inc. Brentwood, Tennessee, (1991), p. 260.
365 Baker, Douglas; Esoteric Healing Vol. 3, part 2, of *"The Seven Pillars of Ancient Wisdom: The Syntheses of Yoga, Esoteric Science and Psychology,* Herts, England, (1976). Reported in Ankerberg, *Can You Trust Your Doctor?* Wolgemth & Hyatt, Publishers, Inc., Brentwood, Tennessee,(1991), p. 260.
366 Pfeifer, Samuel M.D., *Healing at Any Price,* Word (UK) Ltd. Milton Keynes, England , (1980), p. 124-125. Reported in Ankerberg, op. cit., p. 259.

different flower essences which are still available after more than eighty years. Since the death of Dr. Bach in 1936, many other flower essences have been added to the treatment protocol. At least five hundred different essences are available for treatment of a variety of maladies.

How are these flower essences discovered for use in a specific ailment? Richard Gerber in his book *Vibrational Medicine,* page 512 explains:

> ...The information guiding their usage, like the information on previous Pegasus Products, comes from *channeled* sources.[367]...

Flower essences are directed mainly at treatment of emotional imbalances and personality dysfunctions.

> ...Unlike conventional drug therapies which impact solely at the level of physical cellular pathology, the energetic patterns contained within the flower essence work at the level of the emotional, mental, and spiritual vehicles.[368]...

Bach believed that the illness-personality link was an out-growth of dysfunctional energetic patterns within the subtle bodies. He felt that illness was a reflection of disharmony between the physical personality and the Higher Self or soul....Bach links this relationship of the physical personality to the Higher Self (Godhood of man) via a re-incarnational philosophy.[369]

ESSENTIAL OILS & AROMATHERAPY

Another part of herbology that has grown very popular is that of *Aromatherapy*. It, too, has its ancient origin in Ayurveda medicine. Its use is an attempt to heal through use of fragrances of botanical origin. The fragrances are extracted from plants by removing oils, called *essential oils.* Oils are obtained from plants by *compression* or by various *distillation* methods. *Life force*, *universal energy,* is believed to be contained within the oils and fragrance. By the application of the fragrance internally or externally this life force is believed to be transferred to an individual.

The scientifically non demonstrable concept of electrical magnetic *frequency* or *vibration* of a plant is proclaimed to be within the fragrance and is said to be of a frequency faster than light, affecting the *higher consciousness* of an individual so as to be useful for healing emotional and mental faculties.

---

367 Gerber, Richard, M.D., *Vibrational Medicine, the # 1 Handbook of Subtle-Energy Therapies,* Bear and company, One Park Street, Rochester, VT, (2001), p. 512.
368 *Ibid.,* p. 247.
369 *Ibid.,* p. 244.

The fragrance is considered to be the *personality* or *spirit* of the plant. It is believed to balance *subtle energy* flow (universal energy of high frequency).

Aromas are used in Ayurveda to calm aggravated doshas (vata, pitta, kapha), three forces, taught in Ayurveda, that govern biological processes. Topical application with oil or creams containing the fragrance is said to affect the organ or organs in close proximity to where the application was made, imparting increased flow of energy. The fragrances are also used in baths and by inhalation.[370]

The chemistry of the fragrances is complex, consisting of alcohols, esters, ketones, aldehydes, and terpenes. They do not dissolve in water, only in oil, ether or alcohol. Aromatic oils are used in three classes of consumer goods: food, toiletries, and medicines. *Foods*: as natural flavorings, such as oil of lemon, lime, and orange; *Cosmetics*: perfumes, tooth paste, etc.; *Medicine*: for flavoring of medicinals, as therapeutics of their own right, such as oil of wintergreen, clove oil, peppermint oil and eucalyptus oil used in steam inhalations and ointments for topical applications.[371]

I can hear your thoughts!

> First, you tell me in the first paragraph above that use of essential oils and the fragrances they contain is spiritistic, and then you list many common scents and fragrances used in foods, cosmetics and medicinals. Are you trying to tell me that their use is spiritistic also? You just lost me! Bye.

No! No! No! There is a difference, a distinct difference. Yet, this is a very difficult subject to make clear and of which to have a correct understanding. I am not sure I can give an answer applicable in all situations discerning which use is proper and which is not. I will try to give principles, and each person will have to use caution, wisdom and prayer to make that choice.

Let us look first at the principles of use for these scents, flavorings and therapeutic substances that are not considered a part of *aromatherapy*. The reason for their use is to utilize their *biochemical properties*. The chemicals in an aroma such as eucalyptus oil are soothing to an irritated throat and bronchus and are used for respiratory infections. We are not using it because of some vibration of high frequency or due to its spirit connection. Oil of peppermint is useful for simple gastrointestinal distresses, due to its biochemical properties.

Most anesthetics are gasses used for their effect on the central nervous system to allow painful procedures to be done without experiencing pain. Using these substances would not come under the definition of aromatherapy as the term is understood by holistic medicine practitioners. The above-mentioned

---

370   Tisserand, op. cit., p. 8.
371   *Ibid.*, p. 13.

examples and many other substances have been safely used for ages totally apart from any religious spiritistic connotation.

Let us go back and look again at principles proclaimed in the use of aromatherapy by holistic healers. The following quotation is taken from the text *The Art of Aroma Therapy* by Robert Tisserand , a frequently quoted author on the subject of aromatherapy:

> Aromatherapy belongs to the realm of natural therapeutics. As such it is based on certain principles which are shared by acupuncture, herbal medicine, homeopathy, etc. These principles are complementary, and are based on man's interpretation of nature from his understanding of life. Surely the universe was created and is sustained on one set of principles, so there can only be one truth. .The main principles of our therapy are: *Life Force, Yin—yang, Organic foods*[372]

Life Force: synonyms are chi, prana, mana, logos, orenda, the innate, animal magnetism, XE "animal magnetism" odic force, bio plasma, monism, self, higher self, divine self, purer consciousness, XE "purer consciousness" creative principle, essence, supreme ultimate, etc., etc. I refer the reader back to chapter 5 on Universal Energy.

Tisserand continues elaborating on life force by telling us it is the same all-pervading force that is continually bringing about a state of health and harmony in the body. He tells us that it is the only power which can produce health for us. What the author does here is to describe the sustaining power of the Creator God, but separates God from His power and makes the power *god itself*. It is part of the pagan's counterfeit story of creation in contrast to the true creation by the Son of God, Jesus Christ, in harmony with the Holy Spirit and God the Father.

Yin—yang: Yin and yang are words taken from the Chinese and used since there are no English words for direct translation. They are intrinsic to the Chinese story of creation, a story that removes a personal Being as the Creator and applies credit to a *force,* or as now referred to as an *energy.* This is seen in the following quote.

> The physical universe was created when Oneness became duality, and we can see this duality, this yin and yang, everywhere in the universe, in every atom, every action, and in every function of the human body. Yin and yang are manifest everywhere, except at the very centre of being, the perfect point of balance, at that infinite moment when the future becomes the past." "Every single function of a living organism manifests these two forces"

372 *Ibid.*, p. 45.

...."To know which oil is predominantly yin or yang gives a basic guide to their application in sickness.[373]

Organic foods: When we think of people choosing to purchase and/ or eat only "organic" food, our understanding is that this involves a desire to avoid as much as possible contaminants in food such as the chemicals used in insect control, etc. It is also a thought that organic foods will have a better balance of the constituents of which they are made when not pushed in growth by various added minerals. The reason for choosing organic by many is all of the above, but also for some people there is a pagan religious belief involved. They believe that any interference with the growth of the plant will alter its *Life Force*. The fragrances—essences of a plant are considered organic and work in harmony, to organize the body and its chemistry. They recognize the *Life Force* as the only power which can produce health. Aromas are a constituent of plants and are considered to be a concentration of *Life Force*

I wish to share with the reader a few more comments made from a text on aroma therapy:

> Essential oils contain this mystery of life; they have powerful inexplicable energies too....Plants are the interface between cosmic energies and the earth, upon which we depend.[374]

> From a brain biochemistry point of view, the pursuit of spirituality through aroma makes a great deal of sense, as the mechanics of smell are but one short biological step away from consciousness, including higher consciousness (godhood). Thinking of it in terms of light, essential oils are captured light, passed from the heavens, by plants, to us. From a vibrational, electromagnetic, and energetic point of view essential oils are in harmony with life.[375]

I wish to share one more comment from this text of *Aroma Therapy for the Soul*:

> Twenty years ago in aromatherapy, there was an unwritten rule that we would not be open about the spiritual side of the essential oils we worked with. We talked about their anti-infectious qualities and their beautifying effects on the skin or about any number of benefits to body and mind. The positive spiritual changes were recognized, but silently. It seemed far too bold to suggest light and wisdom of the universe flowed through them, their

---

373   *Ibid.*, p. 49.
374   Worwood, op. cit., p. xviii.
375   *Ibid.*, p. xix.

fragrance like messengers from heaven, aromatic angels that come and touch us with the positivity and love of the deity....

With an etheric quality, essential oils activate the receptors of love, compassion, and empathy. They are an informational network, carrying messages and crossing boundaries, operating on many different levels. Through them, we can contact the wisdom of nature, the power of light, the energy of the universe and the love in our hearts.[376]

This comment opens to us the deceptiveness of the holistic movement. These healers capture the minds of people by the teachings that holistic healing therapies are actually effective on the biochemistry and physiological functioning of our bodies, that their actions can be explained by the sciences of physics and chemistry. This is a charade. That which gives power to these holistic methods, is the act of giving our *will* (power of choice) to that power. The physical methods of therapy are meaningless; it is the acceptance of the method and its perceived power which then allows Satan to exercise his control over us.

Ayurvedic medicine and the Hindu religion of which Ayurveda is a component were established more than 3500 years in the past. Aromatherapy is an integral part of Ayurveda and Hinduism. The aromas are used to pacify aggravated doshas. Doshas (rajas—tamas), the dualism of prana is the equivalent words in Sanskrit language to yin—yang in Chinese. Aroma therapy is used to balance doshas.[377]

A question arises, how and by what means are these different aromas selected for use in treatment of various disorders? An answer comes from the book *Vibrational Medicine, The Handbook of Subtle-Energy Therapies.* Here in Dr. Gerber, the author is speaking of flower essences, but his words apply to aromas as well. Note the following quote:

A number of flower-essence practitioners are learning to combine the knowledge and techniques of acupuncture, herbal medicine, and homeopathy with their use of flower essences, some practitioners use flower essences potentized as high homeopathic dilutions in order to release a higher energy and stronger life-force pattern to the patient."...He is now producing a new class of vibrational tinctures that are made from the captured light of stars and planets. Most flower essences and gem elixirs are produced utilizing the light of our local star, the sun, to imprint the various life-energy patterns into the storage medium of water (and alcohol). However, unlike conventional

376   *Ibid.*, p. xix.
377   Gerson, Scott M.D., *Ayurveda, The Ancient Indian healing Art,* Element Books Limited (1997), p. 104.

vibrational essences, these *intuitively* created star elixirs carry the energy and informational patterns of various stars and planets that can be ingested for particular vibrational and healing benefits. The information guiding their usage, like the information on previous Pegasus Products, comes from *channeled sources* (by spirits through mediums).[378] (Emphasis added)

Clearly, there are two purposes in use of aromas that come to us in oils or a tincture. One uses them to utilize their *biochemical properties* in foods, cosmetics, and medicinals; the other use seeks to use them so as to *partake of their spiritual power*. I think that after considering all of the information presented in this chapter, few Christians are going to choose to use aromas in order to gain a higher spiritual experience. We would not desire to have contact with spirits in our quest to secure healing. However, it is not uncommon for sincere devout Christians to seek out flower essences, essential oils, and aromas to find healing for some discomfort and or ailment. Often the purchase of these substances is done from a shop carrying all sorts of New Age merchandise. By entering into aromatherapy do I place myself in a position to be deceived even if I am aware of Satan's counterfeit and my desire is to only use the biochemical properties of the essential oil or aroma? Important question!

How can I know that I am not choosing the power of spirits when I partake of aromatherapy? If I am a person who seeks to be a consultant or therapist in *natural healing* and wants to be sure of avoiding entanglement in a method that is a counterfeit and is one of Satan's deceptions, how can I recognize and avoid such? People tell me that when they purchase the essential oil containing a certain aroma, that they in no way believe in, or accept the spiritistic background associated with aromatherapy. They just want to get the *good* out of it and do not accept it as being spirit-discovered and/or empowered for its effectiveness. They use it because *it works* and they want no part in the rest of its trappings. They say they are strictly partaking of its biochemical properties to treat their malady.

How do we know if an essence, essential oil, or its aroma really is able to do what we take it for? Has it been tested on thousands of people for those same symptoms, tested against a placebo? Has the aroma been tested by being exposed to the patient without his or her awareness and it gave the same relief even when one was not aware of receiving it? Does it do the same for most everyone with the same symptoms? Does it create the same response in animals when it is feasible to so test? Does it give immediate results when we are exposed to it or does it take time and repeated application for it to begin to give relief? These are a few of the questions we need to ask when considering

---

378 Gerber, op. cit., pp. 511,512

as to whether the relief we receive from its use is really physiologic or an influence from a spirit.

Am I spiritually safe to go to the New Age store to buy, to try out the different essences, from the many varieties of aromas to find the one that heals me? Has someone chosen the aroma for my therapy by use of the pendulum, the sway test, or muscle testing? I believe that there are spirits and that they have power but I am not going to have anything to do with them, I just want to get the substance that is helpful for me and I reject any spirit connection. That should prevent any spirit influence over me

I ask: is that possible? Let us consider the first great deception in the Garden. Adam and Eve were told to avoid going near the Tree of Knowledge of Good and Evil, as that was the only place Satan could tempt them; which was *his ground*. If they stayed away from there, Satan would have no influence on them. When Eve found herself near the tree she reasoned that she was capable of recognizing and resisting this fallen angel. She had no concept that the voice speaking to her was from Satan, the foe of God. Her protection vanished as she began to parley with the serpent. We, too, have been warned to stay off Satan's ground, as our protection will be diminished.

> Satan, the fallen prince, was jealous of God. He determined through subtlety, cunning, and deceit to defeat God's purpose. He approached Eve, not in the form of an angel, but as a serpent, subtle, cunning, and deceitful. With a voice that appeared to proceed from the serpent, he spoke to her. . . . As Eve listened, *the warnings God had given faded from her mind.* She yielded to the temptation, and as she tempted Adam, *he also forgot God's warnings.* He believed the words of the enemy of God[379]. . .

> The lie that Satan told Eve, "Ye shall not surely die," has been sounding through the centuries from generation to generation. Thus Satan tempted our first parents, and thus he tempts us today[380]. . . .

Where and what is Satan's ground? It was my understanding that he is able to roam the whole earth. Yes, that is true, but there are places we may visit or frequent, attitudes we harbor, mistrust of God's leading, looking outside of His plan for aid, etc., that causes our guardian angel to separate from us. At that point, the warnings for our protection that God has given may well fade from our memories, leaving us on our own to face the tempter. And we are no match, no match at all. In Appendix H are listed many situations and

---

379 White, E.G., Truth Triumphant, Page 26.2 (E.G. White Writings DVD 2007 Edition)
380 *Ibid.*, p. 26.4.

conditions, but by no means all, that are said to be Satan's ground. It would be well to review them.

As we near the close of this chapter I wish to quote a paragraph from a book that contains an excellent review of the source and power behind aromatherapy:

> But in almost all these systems which claim to utilize herbs, plants, and their etheric energies for diagnosis, healing, psychic development, altered states of consciousness, etc., the herbs and plants themselves possess no mystical power. As in crystal healing and similar methods, they are merely implements behind which spirit powers can work. They are no different than dowsing rods, crystals, radionic devices, Tarot cards, I Ching sticks, rune dice, or the Ouija board. No power resides in any of these implements themselves; they merely become a focal point behind which the spirits secure their goals.[381]

Can Christians, safely, partake of a healing method that Satan invented for his use, and for 3500 years has been an integral part of pagan religions as a component of his counterfeit healing system, then give it a new face of proclaimed scientific properties, and incorporate it into our healing system, by saying "I do not take of the belief system, I just take the good from it?"

The answer for me is *No*! The reader will make his or her own decision.

Postscript:

The writing of this chapter had been concluded and I was planning to send it to the editor for a professional touchup. I received email correspondence from an individual unknown to me, asking me to defend my position of naming the alternative therapeutic discipline of *essential oils—aromatherapy* as being spiritistically deceptive. This individual was a spokes-person for a large company which grew various herbs and plants from which they extracted *essential oils* and in turn marketed them. She had displeasure with me because my book *Spiritualistic Deceptions in Health and Healing* had a few paragraphs that referred to essential oils and aromatherapy. She felt that my stand on this subject was detrimental to their company's "*mission*" of teaching people of the benefits of essential oils as medicinals for health.

I will share with you some of our correspondence as it did bring up a few issues I had not included in this chapter. I believe it to be important to write a brief of our interchange of correspondence. Points she used to justify use of essential oils—aromatherapy were presented to me in a way that I had not previously heard from individuals attempting to justify their use of

---

381   Ankerberg, op. cit., p. 261.

aromatherapy. Covering some of these teachings and beliefs may be of value to others.

It is not unusual for proponents of and especially marketers of various holistic therapeutic disciplines and/or products to attempt to tie in their use as being *Biblical.* So did my correspondent, I was informed that the Bible referred to essential oils 188 times. Frankincense and myrrh were aromatic oils and were given as gifts to the infant Jesus. (Actually they are resins not oils.)

Twelve different aromatic oils are mentioned in the scriptures, with references to different uses for oils, cooking oils, oil for lamps, anointing, incense, etc. I checked all those verses. Out of 188 references to oil there was one mention of being used as a medicinal and that was the parable of the man who was beaten and robbed on his way to Jericho. The scriptures tell us that the Good Samaritan who took care of him placed oil on his wounds. It did not state which type of oil. Many medical therapeutic practices have been standard over time, yet that does not establish that they were effective.

I searched the writings of E.G. White for comments about the *Twelve Oils of Ancient Scripture* listed in the web site of this company that the young lady represented. These oils are aloes/sandalwood, cassia, cedar, cypress, frankincense, galbanum, hyssop, myrrh, myrtle, onycha, rose of Sharon/cistus, and spikenard. When God directed the style of treatment to be used in Western Health Reform Institute in 1865 there was no mention of essential oils— aromatherapy. Yet aromatherapy had been used in Ayurveda for 3500 years prior.

In the website given to me to check out, I found a very interesting article on essential oils entitled *Twelve Oils of Ancient Scripture.* The author Judy DeRuvo elaborated on each of the twelve. Listed in the next paragraph is a brief of the proclaimed uses and effects of using these aromatic oils. It is interesting that in the first sentence on the first oil, *aloe/sandalwood,* she refers to India, and thereafter the explanations are tied into Ayurveda (Hindu) vocabulary and principles. I will list some of her *quips* below, referring to the actions of these twelve oils she listed as being mentioned in Biblical scripture.

Enhancement to meditation; allows mind to move into the deepest states of meditation; connects with the great cosmic prayer; affects chakra energy; links the kundalini energy at the base chakra with the crown chakra; aligns all the chakras and subtle bodies; keeps you grounded, close to your divine essence; empowers the will; supports the sacral chakra; helps release emotional toxins lodged in the subtle bodies; aligns the heart chakra of the mental body to the physical; cypress has frequencies that are in transition between the physical and spiritual (etheric) plane; clears blockage in energy flow; cypress oil disconnects spleen energy attachments.; spiritual and karmic implications; operates beyond the auric field; frankincense helps each of us to connect to that part of us which is eternal and divine; promoting clairvoyance; it opens the 3ʳᵈ eye for connection; sheds light on life's purpose and on the inner self; it clears the aura and energy fields; it transmutes dense thought forms.[382]

The many paragraphs that contain these remarks also contain Bible verses attempting to blend them with the above Hindu terms and concepts.

My first response to give answer to the question as to how I could include essential oils in my book on exposing spiritualistic deceptive practices in the medical field was to send this book's chapter on *Mystical Herbology* to the individual contesting my writing. The response back was that my chapter is only "RHETORIC writing." "It did not line up with scripture."

Another teaching that seems common in *aromatherapy lore* is that at the time of the great Black Plagues in the fourteenth century, physicians put certain essential oils in a face mask in such a way that air breathed through a cloth soaked in essential oils which would protect from the infectious plague. This practice did occur but it was to offset the stench of death. Medical history books records this practice. There are no comments in the history books that it was protective from infection by destroying bacteria. The cause of the plague was then totally unknown. Bacteria were not discovered until the nineteenth century, 500 years after the plagues. I have a copy of an ancient drawing of this practice of a physician using a nose piece soaked in perfume.

In the above dialogue two books were recommended in support of essential oils and aromatherapy being based in Judeo Christian scripture. *The Chemistry of Essential Oils Made Simple: God's Love Manifest in Molecules*, and *Healing Oils of the Bible* by David Stewart, Ph.D. Recently I received an e-mail request to give my opinion on these two books by an individual who has dabbled in essential oils and has a serious question, as to where is the border between the mystical aspect of use of essential oils and aromatherapy and a non-mystical use. This question is not new and has been difficult to answer.

I have just finished reviewing the book on chemistry of essential oils. The author David Stewart has had significant education in physics and chemistry and lays out the chemical structures of many aromatic molecules and gives a synopsis of organic chemistry in an attempt to make clear to students of essential oils their molecular structure. He shares that he also is a Methodists minister. Stewart expresses his belief in a Creator God, One that made man in the image of God. I did not find a sentence establishing for certain his belief in a six day creation yet I gathered that such is his belief. There are direct comments made, however, that reveal a belief akin to pantheism (*panentheism*) concept of God's

---

382 http://www.siohealthynaturally.com/YoungLiving/120OilsOfAncientScripture.html web site altered since correspondence) (https://www.youngliving.org/oils4wellness) present web site

creation—*i.e., a spark of divinity in man and all creation.* His discourse on the action of essential oils influence on the chemistry and physiology of man definitely include the concept of plants and their oils containing a *divine* attribute.

> When molecules of essential oils are inhaled, swallowed, applied to the skin, or internalized into your body in any way, they resonate with your bodily tissues at the frequencies intrinsic to their molecular spectrum as well as their resultant harmonic and beat frequencies. This will increase your own natural electromagnetic vibrations and restores coherence to your electric fields to produce healing and maintain wellness....[383]

Science does not recognize such harmonic and beat frequencies. Such expressions are found only in the writing of New Age—Neopagan literature. Essential oils also are said to respond to prayer/words and negative—positive thoughts, demonstrated by their changing frequencies. Even the *intent* of the therapists or patient will guide the molecules of essential oils to the location in the body where they are to restore health.[384] Molecules of essential oils are purported to contain *subtle electromagnetic properties* which allows them to communicate directly with *cellular intelligence*, similar to homeopathy remedies.[385] Stewart presents support for these concepts by referring to the book *Vibrational Medicine* by Richard Gerber M.D.

If you read "Appendix C" in this book, which is a critique on the book, *Vibrational Medicine,* mentioned above, you will read a comment made by its author Dr. Gerber, wherein he states that much of the information in that book came from *channeling of spirits.* Some other books that David Stewart recommends are from authors with similar beliefs. As I read further in Dr. Stewart's writings it seemed to me he has attempted to blend pantheistic concepts with Christianity and applied it to the scientific world. There is nowhere in the book any reference to scientific studies that substantiate his concepts.

Healing Oils of the Bible another book by David Stewart follows a similar pattern of thought as the first book. I share with you my analysis of that text. In response to requests for me to write an appraisal of the book, *Healing Oils of the Bible* by *D*avid Stewart Ph.D. , it is necessary to again understand the author's *world view* as expressed throughout the text of his book. Vocabulary used by authors of different world views may be similar but with significantly different meanings. This is especially true of religious terms.

---

383   Stewart, David, Ph.D., *The Chemistry of Essential Oils: God's Love Manifest in Molecules,* Care Publication, Marble Hill, MO, (2005), p. 181.
384   *Ibid.,* p. 183.
385   *Ibid.,* p. 229.

David Stewart, says he is a Methodist minister who has had advanced education in biology, chemistry and physics. He freely expresses belief in creation by a God of the universe, *by the breath of His mouth* as recorded in the Bible. However he blends the Biblical account with the *panentheistic* concept—*God in everything*—divinity in all; that even plants have *divinity within* of which they can impart. He attempts to blend Eastern view of *Reality* with Biblical world view and they do not mix.

In the Introduction of the book, a statement is made that plants and their essential oils contain an *essence*, have *Life force, divine intelligence,* and *vibrational energy*. Words that at first view might not be recognized for what the author is saying. The correct understanding of his use of these terms is ascertained more clearly as one reads through the book. They have definitely been used in the setting of a *pantheistic* world view.

Stewart's intrigue continues as he explains that plants were brought into existence by the Thought and Word of God. No argument, however, he then tells us that the plants are also *responsive* to our thoughts and will respond accordingly.[386] Essential oils are said to have:

Theological applications:
1. purification from sin[387]
2. spiritual up lifting[388]
3. possess divine intelligence[389]
4. Impossible for God to lie therefore essential oils are truth[390]
5. demons are repulsed by essential oils' molecular high vibrational energies[391]

Psychological responses:
1. enhance spiritual state in worship[392]
2. bring emotional releases[393]
3. essential oils can release, unblock emotional congestion stored in various tissues other than brain[394]
4. open up subconscious mind to release deep seated emotional trauma[395]

---

386 *Ibid.,* p. xxi.
387 *Ibid.,* p. 19.
388 *Ibid.,* p. 34.
389 *Ibid.,* p. 92.
390 34 *Ibid.,* p. xvi.
391 *Ibid.,* p. xxi.
392 *Ibid.,* p. 26.
393 *Ibid.,* p. 79.
394 *Ibid.,* p. 79
395 *Ibid.,*

5. elevate spiritual consciousness[396]
6. balance electrical energies within the body giving courage, confidence, and self-esteem[397]

Paranormal influence:
1. cause growth up to one inch in height of person[398]
2. rapid correction of scoliosis and or kyphosis[399]
3. able to repulse demons[400]
4. able to be directed by thought or word to the part of body desired[401]
5. possess divine intelligence[402]
6. use of oil by priests in ceremonial cleansing of a leper purported to be reflexology practice in Bible days[403]
7. able to determine disease causing bacteria, virus, or parasite, from non-disease causing and eradicate the pathogenic (disease causing) ones[404]

Dr. Stewart blends science with Eastern religious concepts to the degree it is hard to know which he is relating to. He gives zero references to back up any conclusions he makes. Never did I find any reference to scientific studies to support his hypothesis and conclusions. He did mention that science at times has to use supposition and that he is free to do the same. The difference here is science gathers all the evidence that it is able to secure which came about by rigorous testing and evaluation and then makes a judgment call, willing to change with new evidence. I do not find such trend in his text.

Is use of essential oils medically dangerous? Not likely. However, there needs to be an accurate diagnosis made before treatment with any method. To not treat a serious illness with a known beneficial treatment method presents a danger, especially when we seek out medically untrained to give us care. The most danger of all, however, is the participation in a proclaimed healing technique that has its roots in the Eastern dogma of reality. This association over time blurs our concept of origins and the mind more easily accepts the explanations given for healing by Eastern thought. We get caught in the web of false theory and give Satan homage and think we are honoring the Creator God. I believe it leads us into Satan's trap.

---

396 *Ibid.*, p. 80.
397 *Ibid.*
398 *Ibid.*, p. 90.
399 *Ibid.*, p. 80.
400 *Ibid.*, p. 19.
401 *Ibid.*, p. 51.
402 *Ibid.*, p. 19.
403 *Ibid.*, p. 51.
404 *Ibid.*, p. 77.

Also the chemicals shown to have biological beneficial effects in animal and man as outlined in the book can be found in a variety of foods. It is not necessary to extract them by distillation to have access to such; they are referred to as *phytochemicals*. I close this chapter with a short quote from David Stewart and then you decide if use of essential oils is Biblical.

> Oil molecules are both receivers and transmitters of thought. They can receive and respond to our thoughts and, in turn, broadcast messages back to us and to our bodies. In fact, the best way to learn about essential oils is to talk to them and let them teach you as you use them. Sleep with them and pray with them and they will reveal their secrets to you…"[405]

---

405   Stewart, op. cit., *Chemistry of Essential Oils,* p. 733.

CHAPTER 14
CRYSTAL HEALING, TALISMANS, AMULETS

God added luster to His creation when he made thousands of different types of precious stones and gems. Even before the creation of this world the Bible tells of God's creation of decorative stone:

> ...every precious stone was thy covering, the sardius, topaz, and the diamond, the beryl, the onyx, and jasper, the sapphire, the emerald, and the carbuncle, and gold: the workmanship of thy tabrets and of thy pipes was prepared in thee in the day that thou wast created. (Ezekiel 28: 13, 14)

At the time of Exodus from Egypt and building the sanctuary in the wilderness, explicit instructions were given by God concerning the garments of the high priest Aaron and his breast plate. First, two onyx stones were to have engraved on each the names of six tribes of Israel, then set in ornaments of gold, placed on an ephod worn on the shoulders. A breast plate was crafted with twelve gemstones, four rows of three stones: Row 1. sardis, topaz, carbuncle; Row 2. emerald, sapphire, diamond; Row 3. ligure, agate, amethyst; Row 4. beryl, onyx, jasper. On each stone was engraved the name of a tribe.

The names of gemstones were often used to emphasize a description of some scene or event. Job spoke of precious stones to make scripture the emphasis between material and spiritual riches.

> It cannot be valued with the gold of Ophir, with the precious onyx, or the sapphire. The gold and the crystal cannot equal it: and the exchange of it shall not be for jewels of fine gold. No mention shall be made for coral, or of pearls: for the price of wisdom is above rubies. The topaz of Ethiopia shall not equal it; neither shall it be valued with pure gold. (Job 28: 16-19)

The prophets Ezekiel and John were both shown scenes in heaven and the throne of God, with the names of precious stones used in their descriptions of it.

> And I looked and, behold, a whirlwind came out of the north... and a fire enfolding itself...as of the color of amber...The Appearance of the wheels and their work was like unto the color of a beryl...and the likeness of the firmament

upon the heads of the living creature was ...the color of the terrible crystal, stretched forth over their heads above...And above the firmament that was over their heads was the likeness of a throne, as the appearance of a sapphire stone... (Ez. 1)

John's vision of the New Jerusalem coming down from heaven to earth also described a variety of gemstones:

Having the glory of God: and her light was like unto a stone most precious, even like a jasper stone, clear as crystal;...And the building of the wall of it was of jasper: and the city was pure gold, like unto clear glass. And the foundations of the wall of the city were garnished with all manner of precious stones. The first foundation was jasper; the second, sapphire; the third, a chalcedony; the fourth an emerald; The fifth, sardonyx; the sixth sardis; the seventh, chrysolyte; the eighth, beryl; the ninth, topaz; the tenth a chrysoprasus; the eleventh, a jacinth; the twelfth an amethyst. And the twelve gates were twelve pearls: every several gate was of one pearl: and the street of the city was pure gold, as it were transparent glass. (Rev. 21)

God truly loves beauty in all His creation. His adversary, the devil, takes God's creative beauty of gemstones and applies it to his use in deceiving mankind. Let us now turn our attention to a masterful deception in health and healing by Satan, in crystals and gemstones.

Simon Lilly, in *The Complete Illustrated Guide to Crystal Healing* p. 190, states that the oldest written recordings of the use of precious stones for healing comes from a variety of writings recorded in India. Their use was closely associated with beliefs and practices of astrology. Gemstones were believed to absorb and transmit energy radiating from the planets and to facilitate balancing of negative and positive energy in man. If the position of the planets were not satisfactory according to a person's birth chart, then crystals and gems were supposed to be able to improve the relationship of energies coming from the planets to man. The teachings from India spread across the world and left its influence in most civilizations.

Even civilizations that had little contact with, or influence from India or other advanced civilizations, developed some type of use of precious stones in the practice of health and healing. This concept is clear when one reads the history of shamans, medicine men of the Americas, witch doctors of Africa, native healers of Australia, and elsewhere. Michael Harner, present day shaman and instructor of shamans, shares with us some of the history of shaman use of crystals and gemstones. In his book, *The Way of the Shaman*, he quotes Jerome Myer Levi:

The wide spread employment of quartz crystals in shamanism spans thousands of years. In California, for example, quartz crystals have been found in archaeological sites and prehistoric burials dating as far back as 8000 years[406]

Harner summarizes this history of the shaman's use and belief in crystals with the following statement.

> ...Western science has obviously advanced to the point that it recognizes the quartz crystal as a power object, something the shamans have known for thousands of years.[407]

Stone has been an integral part of man's history—in building structures, as tools, in ornamentation, and in healing through shaman (witch doctors). Quartz crystal is the favored stone for healing by a shaman. The shaman is closely connected to the spirit world and its gods. In Australia and Southeast Asia, the supreme god is *Baiame*, the power believed to be behind healers and magicians who use quartz crystals. The indigenous people of Australia associate quartz crystals with the Rainbow Serpent, a fertility god.

> ...Here are the associations with rainbows, water, rain, clouds, and heaven that link to quartz as belonging to the upper world of the *spirits* and ancestors.[408]

The quartz crystal is considered by the shaman as solidified light. To be initiated into the shaman's domain it is necessary to be filled with solidified light of quartz. The apprentices will have quartz crystals put into their bodies by rubbing ground quartz into their skin and will drink water in which crystals have been placed, ostensibly enabling them to see *spirits*. The initiate is taken to a grave where the dead come and give him magical stones. Afterward, a snake appears as an ally and ushers him deep into the earth where he meets more snakes. From there he goes to the Supreme Being (Baiame) and receives crystals for his own healing.

In Malaysia shamans believe that spirits in the air cut quartz crystals out of the sky in order to use them in healing. Similar stories of crystals and spirits are common with the ancient healing practices. North American natives were

---

406   Levi, Jerome Meyer, "Wii'ipay: The Living Rocks—Ethnographic Notes on Crystal Magic Among some California Yumans." *Journal of California Anthropology* 5 (1): (1978), p. 42. Reported in Harner, Michael, The Way of the Shaman, Harper Collins Publishers, New York, NY, (1990), p. 109.

407   Harner, Michael, *The Way of the Shaman,* HarperCollins Publishers, New York, NY, (1990), p. 112.

408   Lilly, Simon, *The Complete Illustrated Guide to Crystal Healing,* Element Books Inc., Boston, MA, (2000), p. 184.

closely allied with quartz crystals for healing and higher spiritual power. The crystals are kept in leather pouches and consulted frequently by the shaman in order to better understand and work with the world of spirits. Rattles used in dance and healing ceremonies to summon helpful spirits are often filled with pieces of quartz.

In the Southwestern United States, Indian tribes valued turquoise as a stone possessing power. In Central America as well, the turquoise stones were thought to connect heaven and earth, to give protection and strength via the *spirit* world. The various natives of the world all had their witch doctors; "shaman" is a name coming from the witch doctors of Siberia.

Crystal and gemstone healing has the longest history in the Ayurvedic system of healing. The explanation for their power and healing is tied in with astrology, as is all of Ayurveda. Health is maintained as the body remains in balance with its energies' three divisions or doshas: pitta, vata, and kapha (similar to yin and yang). Imbalance equals illness, and powdered gemstones given in water mixed with honey or cream are prescribed to balance doshas.[409]

The shaman of all cultures treated their crystal with special reverence by keeping it in a special container separate from the other objects in his medicine bag. He avoided talking about it lest it lose power. The crystal was viewed as a *spirit helper* and a special partnership might be entered between the shaman and his crystal; it was considered as *living*, or a *live stone*.

The Yuman tribe shamans of California felt they must feed their crystals, hence placement in tobacco water.[410]

In the last 35 years we have seen a public explosion of practices and beliefs that were for centuries kept in the quiet. Neopaganism/ Western occultism has ushered into our midst the nature worship of ancient paganism from the pagan societies of the East, African animism, and American Native practices under the title of *holistic medicine*. Harner expresses it this way:

> The burgeoning field of holistic medicine shows a tremendous amount of experimentation involving the reinvention of many techniques long practiced in shamanism, such as visualization, altered state of consciousness, aspects of psychoanalysis, hypnotherapy, meditation, positive attitude, stress-reduction, and mental and emotional expression of personal will for health and healing. In a sense, shamanism is being reinvented in the West precisely because it is needed.[411]

---

409   *Ibid.*, pp. 184-191.
410   Harner, op. cit. p. 109.
411   *Ibid.*, p. 136.

Crystal work is a component of both ancient and modern shamanism. In Native American healing, the shaman will utilize the crystal as a method for both diagnosis and treatment; the crystal is believed to be a vehicle through which the healing spirits work.[412]

What is so special about crystal that has brought it so much attention? First let us look at its chemical and physical properties. Nearly all of the rocks on the crust of the earth are crystalline with most being formed of oxygen and silicon. Aluminum, iron, calcium, sodium, potassium, and magnesium combined with oxygen comprise the rest. Every crystal consists of a single chemical molecular compound; one molecule is repeated throughout, forming a geometric internal structure. A crystal is defined by its internal structure. It is made up of atoms that have bonded together creating molecules forming regular repeating patterns. These patterns, arranged in precise geometry, create a crystal's solid form with flat faces. The internal repeating molecule forms a crystal lattice. A lattice would be similar to stacking boxes of the same size and shape in the exact same position in relationship to all other boxes, and so filling a room or warehouse.

When electricity is delivered to a crystal it expands in regular pulses. A quartz crystal when compressed will emit a measureable voltage, called the *piezoelectric effect*. Crystals are used in most electric instruments, for example watches are dependent on crystals for their accurate timing. A crystal's internal geometric form determines its physical properties and its *healing*.

Seven geometric forms of lattices are found among crystal formations: cubic, tetragonal, hexagonal, trigonal, orthorhombic, monoclinic, and triclinic. This would be analogous to having seven shapes of boxes, with each group of shaped boxes filling a separate room and stacked in a repetitive manner leaving no free space. It is this internal *lattice* formation that determines the type of crystal and its physical properties.

When a quartz crystal lattice is distorted by heat, pressure, light, or friction, electrons flow creating electricity. Electricity delivered to a quartz crystal creates expansion of the crystal in regular pulses. This physical property makes it possible with a perfect crystal to create time pieces that are exactly accurate. Thus, most watches today have a quartz crystal with a battery connected to it causing impulses in absolute regularity, enabling the watch to show time.

Crystals have many properties. One is the ability to transform and transmit light. Glass fiber optics (crystals) transmits communication by light. Small quartz crystals have the ability to possess vast amounts of memory. The first laser was formed by using a ruby gemstone. Light usually diffuse in nature, was

---

412   *Ibid.*, pp. 108-112.

concentrated on the ruby which then emitted a single beam of light carrying intense energy. Most electrical kitchen appliances will have a crystal involved in their functions. Solar cells are dependent upon crystals. The electronic industry also is dependent upon crystals for the function of computers and similar instruments. The understanding and ability to manufacture perfect crystal has revolutionized our electronics world.

I have mentioned only a little of the understanding of crystal formation and the physics involved; we now turn to the subject of the use of gems and crystals for healing. Shaman and similar healers did not have the knowledge of a crystal's physical properties as we have now; however, they did believe that precious stones had the ability to transmit, transform, and amplify energy. They believed that a *universal energy/life force,* underlying the powers of the universe, was transmitted by the planets to earth. This life force power was accepted as that which replenished, transformed, and renewed all things in the universe. The so-called *universal* energy is described as being composed of a light layer, and a dense layer. The dense layer transformed itself into material substance encompassing all material things of the universe, including earth and all life on earth. The lighter forms of the *universal life force* formed the elements of the spirit world.[413] Author Henry Mason explains further:

> "So, the universe is energy. That energy is the universe, and the source of everything manifested in our universe: the stars, our sun in particular, our planet, our lives, and our selves. We are part and parcel of the universe. We are dense, self-aware energy beings. We are part of the Universal Life Force, and we live on a planet that is a part of the Universal Life Force. We came from the same place. We are made of the same elements, coalesced from the same energy."[414]

You may have noticed that no mention of a Creator God is made in this description of the universe. Satan's counterfeit story of creation is what is depicted above. God's power of creation and of sustaining creation is *hijacked* and the personality of the Creator is taken out. The power is divided into spiritual and material, and again divided into positive and negative energy. As explained in a previous chapter, it is also divided into seven different electromagnetic frequencies. The first level, the slowest frequency, is said to be the material physical substance of the universe—planets, earth, man. The remaining six increasing levels of energy frequency comprise the spiritual division of the so-called universal energy. Richard Gerber M.D. , in his book

413	*Ibid.,* pp. 108-112.
414	Mason, Henry M. , *The Seven Secrets of Crystal Talismans,* Llewellyn Worldwide, St. Paul, MN, (2008), p. 11.

Vibrational Medicine, makes the following comment about the proclaimed higher levels of energy:

> To most individuals, the higher dimensional energies are in the realm of invisibility. To a fortunate few with *clairvoyant* perception, the beauty of these invisible realms can be perceived with great ease. The only thing that seems to limit human potential is its definition of itself. As technology makes visible what was previously seen only by clairvoyants, the invisible becomes visible.[415]

The false creation story continues: life force energy comes to earth from three sources, namely the sun, the moon from its reflection of the sun, and the perceived molten mass from the center of the earth. The claim is made that this is pure science and not religion. I disagree; it is religion from ancient Babylon. Author Henry Mason continues:

> In a like manner, the sun projects tremendous spiritual energy to the earth. Virtually all cultures with recorded history have a sun god or goddess or the equivalent that embodied their understanding of that *spiritual strength and power*. He is Tonatiuh to the Aztecs, Horus to the ancient Egyptians, Apollo the Romans, Tsohanoai to the Navaho, and Freyr to some Norse. She is Sol in Norse mythology, and Sunna to the Germans. But whatever the name and whatever the culture, we instinctively understand the sun as the source of *spiritual* strength....

> Like the sun, the moon is also a source of spiritual strength to Earth. The moon has been worshiped, like the sun, since recorded time. While in some cultures the moon was a god, in many it takes the feminine form. For example, to the Chinese she is Shin Moo, to the Celts she is Morgana. Again, different names in different cultures, but a universal recognition that the moon is a power in the affairs of men and women, and one that should be respected and honored.[416]

> The earth also absorbs the Universal Life Force from the sun and moon, uses it, and transmits it to the wind, the waves, and the life-giving atmosphere we need. In a like manner, it absorbs the spiritual energy of the Universal Life Force from the sun and moon, uses it to nourish itself, and transmits that *spiritual* energy through its elements and compounds into the plants and animals that absorb it to sustain life....[417]

---

415   Gerber, Richard, *Vibrational Medicine the Number One Hand Book Subtle Energy Therapies,* Bear and Company, One Park Street, Rochester, Vermont, (2001), p. 325.

416   Mason, op. cit., pp. 12, 13.

417   *Ibid.,* p. 13.

The apostle Paul discusses this subject of worshiping the created instead of the Creator:

> The wrath of God is being revealed from heaven against all the godlessness and wickedness of men who suppress the truth by their wickedness, since what may be known about God is plain to them, because God has made it plain to them. For since the creation of the world God's invisible qualities—his eternal power and divine nature—have been clearly seen, being understood from what has been made, so that men are without excuse. For although they claimed to be wise, they became fools and exchanged the glory of the immortal God for images made to look like mortal man and birds and animals and reptiles." (Romans 1:18-23)

A *Talisman* is a *gemstone*, a *crystal* worn about the body in the belief that this object can aid us in our life; it is considered to act as a charm. This *aid* comes from the stone, supposedly, by amplifying our own powers, by focusing our feelings, thoughts, actions, and habits, thus benefitting us in reaching our goals. Secondly, it is taught that a talisman is a source of energy and power in and of itself due to its mineral nature, and its ability to amplify our own power by channeling in more universal life force from the sun, moon, and *earth*. The mineral crystals have seven fundamental structural arrangements in their molecular lattice and each type will have a specific type of influence on a person. Example: a triclinic crystal system produces a talisman that is believed to have *barrier* properties. A barrier talisman supposedly is protective against illness and injury. The monoclinic crystal system is considered to produce a talisman that is *protective* physically and spiritually. It then is called an *amulet*.

Not only the molecular structure and lattice type, but the color, and even the shape of the gem is considered to influence its effect. Talismans and amulets are used to maintain the optimum function of the physical and spiritual attributes of man.

We now turn to the use of crystals in illness and disease. The discipline of crystal healing is totally dependent upon the hypothesis of *universal energy* and it's believed negative and positive characteristics. This teaching is out of *astrology*. Subtle energy system concepts, such as electrical polarity, meridians, pressure points, chakras, aura, and subtle bodies, are used to assess and correct what are perceived as energy imbalances.

Crystal healers view the human body in totally different ways than orthodox scientists and doctors. Completely different languages and terms are used respectively in each system.[418]

---

418   Lilly, op. cit., p. 34

A most important aspect of crystal healing is for the healer to be *grounded* and *centered* prior a healing session.

Grounding means total focus. All energy believed to be passing through the body will remain in balance, but if any excess energy flows it will *go into the earth* where it is safely dissipated. Grounding is accomplished by the use of gems, usually dark colored; the best place to set them is near the throat and coccyx. Grounding can be done by Hindu-type meditation, guided imagery, and visualization (using the imagination to create a view of the change desired), by tree meditation (visualizing a tree and its roots with the tree representing the healer and the roots the *ground* connection with mother earth).

Centering happens when all physical, mental, and emotional energies are integrated and balanced. Centering can be done by imagery and visualization such as drawing the *earth energy* up through your body by deep breathing focus, sight focus, or voice focus, or by sounding *Om* or *Aum*," or by *tapping in*. Tapping in is done by tapping lightly with the finger tips on the chest below the clavicle on either side. It is said to bring into balance all of the *meridians* of the body (meridians are energy flow channels of Chinese Traditional Medicine and not recognized to exist by science).[419]

When *grounded* and *centered* the healer will then proceed to the therapeutic act of using the crystals and gemstones. The following are examples of ways that the healing sessions are to be conducted. By these descriptions we recognize the absurdity of crystal therapy, and spiritually dangerous to partake of the practices.

1. Place stones in positions upon or about the body, where disease or distress is felt to present, in arrangement, so as to depict the Seal of Solomon or Star of David, thus symbolizing a connection between heaven and earth.

2. To recharge your body and spirit do the following: place a crystal over a pulse point such as the wrist; when done in the sunlight it will supposedly increase the therapeutic benefit.

3. Healing by use of crystals and breathing techniques could be as follows: Inhale to bring energy into your aura; hold your breath several seconds as you focus your thoughts on the crystal held in your hand. With a forceful effort expel your breath out thus causing the energy within the crystal to be expelled through the top of the crystal as it is pointed toward the area of the body in need of healing. This effort must be repeated several times to be effective.

4. One technique for self-healing is as follows: place a crystal over a *chakra* area of the body. While inhaling, place both hands on top of the stone being used and draw energy through it into the chakra. Hold the breath for

---

419   *Ibid.*, pp 45-47.

5-6 seconds concentrating energy in that location, then exhale forcefully while throwing your hands out to each side of your body, thus dispersing negative energy. As you inhale bring the hands back to the same location on the body, then repeat.[420]

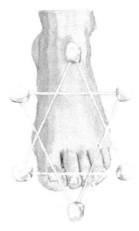

Figure 36. crystals in form of Solomon's seal

Water is believed by crystal healers to be able to hold a memory of an energy pattern of some object placed within it. The following practices are based upon this concept. Take a crystal and grind it into a very fine powder, place in a bowl of spring water for several hours, transfer the water into a dark glass jar and refrigerate. Or, one may place the ground stone in a bowl of tap water and expose it to sunlight for several hours; this creates an *essence* of sun energy/universal energy. Next withdraw the water from the bowl and place it into a jar with 50% brandy; this becomes a *mother tincture*. In turn place a few drops of the mother tincture into another small bottle of 50% brandy. It is then ready to be consumed by drops as a medicinal, or placed in bath water, in steam inhalation, etc. Both solutions of regular spring water or the essence water can be used similarly.

The particular crystal that is selected for therapy may be chosen due not only to its lattice structure, but also due to color. The color of the gem is contingent upon the crystal formation and its atomic structure which in turn, bends the rays of sunlight. Some colors depend upon the basic mineral while others are colored by impurities. When all colors are absorbed in the stone it is then black; when all light is reflected, the stone white.

Different colors are believed, by crystal healers, to affect different aspects of health. Each color represents a specific wavelength of light and may be

420   *Ibid.*, pp. 52, 53.

referred to as "vibration" of energy, of creativity, of balance, etc. Different colors are said to affect the body in different ways. Examples: orange is supposed to influence physical rigidity, restricted feelings, digestive disorders, lack of focus, lack of vitality, unable to let go of past memories, etc.; green is equated with abnormal growths, sense of claustrophobia, being trapped, unfulfilled, restricted, dominated, a need to be in control or to be controlled, invasive illness, etc.

Problems occurred in the past due to use of ground gems, as not all gems are safe. Minerals have been used since ancient times as source of colored pigments. Their colors do not fade due to sunlight but may change with extensive time due to oxidation. Some of these colored pigments are toxic and are no longer used. Red was from mercuric oxide and arsenic oxide— toxic. Orange is also from toxic minerals, yellow from arsenic and sulfur, etc. Another practice in crystal healing involves *chakra balancing*. The Indian Ayurveda system of healing believes that there is a network of subtle energy channels that run through the body. This network said to be composed of a central channel along the spine and which is made up of seven centers of energy called chakras.

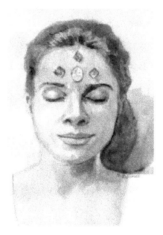

Figure 37. Crystals over forehead chakra)

The seven chakras are proclaimed to be linked to the seven colors of the rainbow, with each chakra being of one of the seven colors. The chakra system is also believed to be influenced by a set of associated symbols, use of sound, color, shape, animal and god forms, as well as the senses.

The goal of chakra crystal balancing and healing is to empower each chakra to its optimal function as well as to the system as a whole. *The most fundamental chakra balancing act is Hindu-type mediation*, but the crystal healer supplements that act with use of his crystals. Choice of crystals for healing is determined by the problems the individual may have, or it may be just to maintain health. Once the chakra felt to be most associated with a health situation is determined, then it is necessary to select more specifically the optimum crystal needed to place over the chakra as therapy. Selection of a color, and mineral type of stone to match the chakra, is done by visualization, intuition (divine inspiration), applied kinesiology (divination by muscle testing), color meditation by visualization, or by dowsing with a pendulum.

WAND

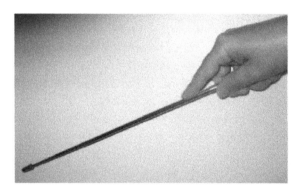

Figure 38.

"Wand" is a word that we do not often hear in the health and healing arena, yet it is still being used and promoted as if it was of great value. At a large religious assembly in June 2010, I was sitting at a table signing copies of the book *Spiritualistic Deceptions of Health and Healing.* The book exposes spiritualism in certain health and healing methods. I was approached by an individual who with enthusiasm presented to me his healing *wand* as an instrument that would remove pain by use of *life force energy.* A wand is an object, usually a thin rod or stick ranging from a few inches in length to several feet long. A dictionary definition explains it as a "staff of a diviner, a fairy, or a magician."

This wand I was shown was the size of a ball point pen, platinum in color, and was said to be filled with crystals. Its magic was promoted as a *reliever of pain.* Point it at pain anywhere on the body and the pain was said to vanish. I asked if it worked on chronic low back pain; the answer was slow in coming but the advocate of the wand had to admit defeat for this malady, yet was claiming great success for headaches, small joint pains, soreness and minor discomforts. This person was truly sincere in his belief of the wand; in fact, he was a distributer of such. He shared with me that some members of his church were concerned about his use of this healing wand therapy and had even suggested to him that he might be partaking of occultic power. He told me this in a manner and tone that led me to believe that he felt those who had warned him about the wand really did not understand the value and true scientific power he felt was truly within his wand.

A dictionary definition explains a wand as a "staff of a diviner, a fairy, or a magician." It has been a tool of the magician for thousands of years, its use is often found in stories of magic and fantasy. Great power is often attributed to the wand in these stories.

In the popular *Harry Potter novel* extensive references are found pertaining to the use of the wand. Through it a wizard might affect great power for good or for evil. Harry Potter was born into a family of wizards; his father and mother were such. In this fantasy novel his parents were obliterated by the power from a wizard, Lord Voldemort, the most powerful of all wizards. Harry eventually attends a school for wizards and witches where he receives a wand. He observes his headmaster using his wand to blast through a door and knocks another powerful wizard flat.

In the most recent popular fantasy story of Harry Potter, he, as a student wizard, goes to a store that sells wands. After inspecting many different ones for size and feel, he chooses the one best for him. As he raises this wand in the air and quickly presses the tip toward the floor, sparks and light flash from the distal end of the wand and Harry receives a feeling of exhilaration.

There is a claim made by some that the use of the wand is Biblical! How can anyone make that claim? There is the story of Moses and Aaron using their shepherd staffs as a magic wand and with great power. The story starts in the fourth chapter of Exodus as Moses was talking to God at the burning bush. God told him He would give to Moses a sign he could use to impress Pharaoh that he, Moses, was sent to Pharaoh by the God of the Hebrews. At the bush encounter in the desert by Mt. Horeb God told Moses to cast his staff to the ground; it became a moving snake and Moses ran from it. He was told by God to pick it up by the tail and it became a staff again.

The story continues as Aaron cast down his staff at the feet of Pharaoh, and it became a snake. Pharaoh's magicians were able to do the same, but Aaron's rod—snake, swallowed up the magicians' snakes.

The staff of Aaron was used to bring on several of the ten plagues that God placed upon the Egyptians so they would understand that the God of the Hebrews was the God of the universe. Aaron's staff was used to strike the Nile river to turn it to blood, stretched over the river to cause it to bring forth frogs, and struck on the ground and covered the nation with gnats. Moses stretched out his rod to bring on the plague of locusts, pointed it skyward causing a great hail storm, and used it to bring darkness over the land. When Moses came to the Red sea and Pharaoh was behind them with his army, Moses stretched his staff over the sea and it parted (Ex. 14:16). After crossing to the other side,

Moses held up his staff and pointed toward the passageway between the walls of water and God allowed the water to come together, covering the Egyptians. As they journeyed in the dry desert and water had vanished, God directed Moses to strike a rock with his staff. The rock split open and water gushed out. (Ex. 17:6)

At a later time when Israel was traveling in the desert and water was not obtainable God asked Moses to speak to a rock to cause it to give forth water (Numbers 20:10-12). But Moses in his anger with the people for their complaining said "Hear now ye rebels; must *we* fetch you water out of this rock?" Moses struck the rock two times with his rod: and the rock gave forth water in abundance.

> The Lord spake unto Moses and Aaron, Because ye believed me not, to sanctify me in the eyes of the children of Israel, therefore ye shall not bring this congregation into the land which I have given them. (vs. 12)

The rock from which water flowed at Mt. Horeb, and the water which flowed from the rock as they journeyed represented the living water of grace which flows from Christ, the Son of God. When Moses was told to speak to the rock, it represented our privilege to ask of God for the water of life, to be given in abundance. Moses assumed that *he and Aaron* had the power to bring forth the water with his staff. For this error he and Aaron were not permitted to enter Canaan. It was God directing Moses and through the use of his staff that God's power was made manifest; there was no innate power from Moses or the staff.

When a person takes up the *magic wand* he is assuming he has power within himself to project power through the rod to accomplish some feat. There may well be some response but it is not power of one's own self; it is the power of Satan working through the person and the wand.

Divination is a common component of crystal work and healing practices. It is often done by the use of a crystal pendulum, or may be done by muscle testing called *applied kinesiology*. Healing may be performed using a pendulum made of crystal.

Geomancy, an ancient practice of *casting stones*, then reading the resulting patterns as the stones came to rest, was practiced in many civilizations on many continents. The stone may be cast on a cloth with areas of the cloth demarcated to mean certain things and the stones also pre-chosen to represent various meanings. As the stones come to rest, the diviner will interpret the fall of the stones.[16]

Scrying is crystal ball gazing. It is a way to access the unconscious, or subconscious, mind.

A crystal, or some other polished surface, is used to amplify or act as a screen for knowledge held in symbolic form within the mind." "The mind dives down into itself, leaving the familiar clear coordinates of time and space experienced as an individual wave, and centers the deep ocean of consciousness where collective and universal currents are to be found. [421]

The warning God gave the nation of Israel just before they were to enter the Promised Land, as recorded in Deuteronomy 18: 9-12, should be a warning to us as well and help us choose to have nothing to do with crystal healing or any aspect of the crystal, gemstone, and precious stone false premise.

When thou art come into the land which the Lord thy God giveth thee, thou shalt not learn to do after the abomination of those nations. There shall not be found among you any one that maketh his son or his daughter to pass through the fire, or that useth divination, or an observer of times, or an enchanter, or a witch, or a charmer, or a consulter with familiar spirits, or a wizard, or a necromancer. For all that do these things are an abomination unto the Lord: and because of these abominations the Lord thy God doth drive them out from before thee. (Deut. 18: 9-12)

Absent healing with crystals is done, with permission, for those who may be long distances from the healer. This permission can be obtained by dowsing, intuition, or meditation if the individual has not previously given permission. A *witness* will be used, that is a picture or lock of hair, a signature, drop of blood, or something the person has handled. The witness is said to carry the energy pattern of the individual desiring healing.

The Complete Illustrated Guide to Crystal Healing tells us no one understands how long-distance healing works, but that it works. As with all crystal healing acts, it is important to have been grounded and centered (in a meditative state) before attempting the art of distant healing using a pendulum over the witness. Also, simply placing chosen gems on a mirror that lies next to a witness may work.

Belief in *astrology* and its signs and symbols is very popular. Ancient Indian healing tradition, Ayurveda, developed a complex system of the relationship of the planets to stones and their use in health and healing. Today Eastern and Western theories of astrological crystal relationships have merged, so that there are stones for each month, each planet, and each zodiac sign. Wearing of copper is believed to reduce the effects of planetary forces on health. Dowsing for a stone to use in dealing with astrological influences is also a common practice.

---

421   *Ibid.*, p. 176.

The quartz crystal has entered the mind—control field of therapy as well. Marcel Vogel, senior scientist with IBM for 27 years, concludes that the natural energies of a healer can be amplified and directed to heal another's mind problems. His quote is below:

> The crystal is a neutral object whose inner structure exhibits a state of perfection and balance. When it's cut to the proper form and perfection, the crystal emits a vibration which extends and amplifies the powers of the user's mind. Like a laser, it radiates energy in a coherent, highly concentrated form, and this energy may be transmitted into objects or people at will.

> Although the crystal may be used for *mind to mind* communication, its higher purpose...is in the service of humanity for the removal of pain and suffering. With proper training, a healer can release negative thought forms which have taken shape as disease patterns in a patient's physical body.

> As psychics have often pointed out, when a person becomes emotionally distressed, a weakness forms in his subtle energy body and disease may soon follow. With a properly cut crystal, however, a healer can, like a surgeon cutting away a tumor, release negative patterns in the energy body, allowing the physical body to return to a state of wholeness.[422]

John Ankeberg and John Weldon present an in-depth discussion of the use of crystals in their book *Can You Trust Your Doctor?* Therein, we learn that the real power from crystals is derived from the spirit world and many who become involved in crystals for health move on to channeling with spirit guides. Crystal healers claim that the crystals are mere devices for attracting the spirits, who then supply the real power. Even when the crystals are not used, the occult power remains.[423]

> According to the nature of the illness, the crystal will become hot or cold as it is passed over the person's aura. The crystal is absorbing the bad energy out of the body, according to these teachings. It is important to remember that "the crystals are your teachers. Hold one in your hand. Be open to its power. It will teach you.[424]

422   Miller, R., *The Science of the Mind,* The Healing Magic of Crystals: an Interview with Marcel Vogel, August (1984): Reported in Gerber, op. cit., pp. 338, 9.

423   Ankeberg, John, Weldon, John, *Can You Trust Your Doctor?,* Wolgemuth and Hyatt, Brentwood, TN, (1991), p. 243, 249.

424   Newhouse, Sandy, Amoeda, John, *Native American Healing,* [Holistic Health Handbook, "A Tool for Attaining Wholeness of Body, Mind and Spirit" Berkeley California Press, Berkeley, CA, (1978), p. 67. Reported in Gerber, op. cit., p. 243.

There is danger in consulting cultist physicians:

> ...Angels of God will preserve His people while they walk in the path of duty; but there is no assurance of such protection for those who deliberately venture upon Satan's ground. An agent of the great deceiver will say and do anything to gain his object. It matters little whether he calls himself a 'spiritualist', an 'electric physician,' or a 'magnetic healer.'...[425]

Isaiah 8:19, 20 make it very plain:

> And when they shall say unto you, Seek unto them that have familiar spirits, and unto wizards (diviners) that peep and that mutter: should not a people seek unto their God? For the living to the dead? To the law and to the testimony: if they speak not according to this word, it is because there is not light in them.

This system of deception that Satan has devised starts very innocently. When our interest is developed, we are led on to more involved practices. This in turn, can lead to developing psychic powers and communicating with spirit entities, animal entities, etc. This *channeling* allows for demonic possession of our minds and souls. The end result is loss of eternal life.

Clearly the whole practice of crystal healing and crystal divination is *spiritualism*. What is spiritualism? It consists of the doctrine of the immortality of the soul. It is also the belief that the dead can communicate with the living. A spiritualist is one who holds such belief and may practice it as a medium.[426]

> Satanic agents claim to cure disease. They attribute their power to electricity, magnetism, or the so-called sympathetic remedies, while in truth they are but channels for Satan's electric currents. By this means he casts his spell over the bodies and souls of men.[427]

> ...Through satanic delusions, wonderful miracles of human agents will be urged. Beware of all this Christ has given warning so that none need accept falsehood for truth. The only channel through which the Holy Spirit operates is that of truth.[428]

---

425   White, E.G., *Evangelism*, Pacific Press Publishing Association, Nampa, ID, (1887), p. 607.

426   Shorter, Gen and Rick, *Jewelry, Ornaments, Personal Decoration and More...The Spiritualism Connection,* Homeward Publishing, Yorba Linda, CA, (2008), p. 61.

427   White, op. cit., p. 609.

428   White, E.G., *Selected Messages,* Book 2, Review and Herald Publishing Association, Washington D.C., (1958), p. 49.

CHAPTER 15

HOMEOPATHY

SAMUEL HAHNEMANN M.D.

Samuel Hahnemann MD (1755–1843) was a German physician who was appalled at the results of conventional medical care and refused to prescribe the drugs and bleeding treatments used by physicians of his day.

> Hahnemann attacked the extreme medical practices of the day, advocating instead, good public hygiene, improved housing conditions, better nutrition, fresh air, and exercise.[429]

He believed that if a healthy person was given enough of a substance to produce symptoms similar to the symptoms of a particular illness, then by diluting that substance to minute doses and ingesting, the body would be stimulated to heal itself of the illness. This *presumed* phenomenon he called *homeopathy*.

Homeopathy is a discipline of therapy for illness that Hahnemann initiated and which subsequently became popular in his day. The use of this therapy has continued ever since. It is a method of treatment utilizing an extremely diluted preparation of a "mother tincture" of a plant, mineral or animal substance. It began in Germany and spread throughout Europe, being brought to the US in the early 1800's. It became very popular and was commonly practiced until the ascendancy of scientific medicine. After the turn of the century and in the early part of the 20th century, there were 22 medical schools following this type of discipline in the US. There were more than 100 hospitals, and over 1000 pharmacies devoted to homeopathic medicine.[430] It was commonly practiced in the United States since people were able to purchase a home kit of homeopathy remedies and treat themselves. I have in my library a home medical text dated 1918, which has instructions and guidelines for homeopathy treatments for home use. However, by the mid 1900's, the use of homeopathy had almost

429 Lockie, Andrew, MB, ChB, MRCGP, MF Hom. Dip obst RCOG, *Natural Health Encyclopedia of Homeopathy,* Dorling Kindersley, London, New York,) 2000), p. 14.
430 Ankerberg, H. John,Weldon ,John, *Can You Trust Your Doctor?* Wolgemuth & Hyatt, Brentwood TN., (1991), p. 264.

died out in the US. Yet, in the last 40 years there has been a rapid resurgence of the practice among various practitioners.

Hahnemann once took a large dose of Peruvian bark (quinine) while he was healthy and said that he developed symptoms similar to malaria. He thereafter initiated a theory that if very small doses of quinine were administered, standard doses would not be necessary for treatment of malaria. To understand how Hahnemann arrived at this conclusion we need to understand his concept of disease.

In his text, *Organon,* paragraph 11. he defines the bodily condition we call *disease*. First, he states that all disease manifests *subjective* and *objective* symptoms. This situation, in turn, is caused by *vital energy* being in an "*untuned spirit-like dynamis*"—unbalanced universal energy status. He reasoned that if disease was a result of spirit-like energy being "*out of tune*," then it could only be corrected by "*retuning*" through the action of another spirit. He further reasoned that if the "*spirit*" of animal, plant, or mineral when given in large doses would create similar symptoms as the disease under consideration then this same spirit taken in a very minute quantity would correct the unturned—unbalanced spirit causing the disease, thereby, effecting a cure.

Symptoms, is the key to understanding his reasoning. When disease was present, symptoms were present. To eliminate the symptoms would, he believed, cure the malady. These correcting spirits were found by trial and error. A mineral or plant substance would be taken by a healthy individual in sufficient quantity—dose to bring on symptoms. If those symptoms were similar to symptoms peculiar to a disease then this substance under test would be considered the *remedy* for that particular disease. This whole concept was built upon belief in the *spirit dynamis* of vital energy—life force. Every plant, mineral, or animal was considered to have its specific spirit dynamis.

The cause of, and correction of disease, was considered to be by action of *spirit*. Biochemical, infectious agents, lack of or insufficient nutrients, toxic substance ingested causing biochemical interaction, etc., were not understood and had no part in the thinking of Hahnemann. Today, individuals accepting homeopathic therapy as being legitimate therapy are thinking in the terms of correcting a disorder by a biochemical adjustment or interaction; however, there is no scientific evidence to substantiate the remedying claims of homeopathic substances.

It is very important to understand Hahnemann's *world view* in order to comprehend the rationale of his conclusions regarding disease, its cause, and treatment. Understanding his belief in man's origin will help to clarify why he formed certain conclusions.

First Hahnemann was a follower of the powerful spiritist and medium Emanuel Swedenborg. Those familiar with the occultic philosophy and theology of Swedenborg, such as his blending of the world of nature and the occult, can recognize the parallels in Hahnemann's thinking. Andrew Weil received his M.D. from Harvard Medical School, is a research associate in Ethnopharmacology at Harvard, and is somewhat sympathetic with aspects of new age medicine. He observes that Hahnemann was 'steeped in the mysticism of Emanuel Swedenborg.'[431]

Hahnemann was also a Freemason, and as the authors have demonstrated elsewhere, the study of Freemasonry presents an excellent opportunity for delving into mysticism and the occult.[432]

Hahnemann was also an admirer of the occultists Paracelsus and Mesmer.[433]

He was a believer in the concept of animal magnetism, which is the same power behind psychic healing. In his *Organon* (text book on homeopathy) Hahnemann confessed similarities between the practice of homeopathy and mesmerism. He wrote:

I find it yet necessary to allude here to animal magnetism, as it is termed, or rather Mesmerism... It is a marvelous, priceless gift of God...by means of which the strong will of a well-intentioned person upon a sick one by contact and even without this and even at some distance, can bring the vital energy of the healthy mesmerizer endowed with this power into another person dynamically...The above mentioned methods of practicing Mesmerism depend upon an influx of more or less vital force into the patient...[434]

Hahnemann was also influenced by animism and Eastern religion. In discussing Hahnemann's writings and that of other leading homeopaths, Dr. H. J. Bopp, in his book, *Homeopathy*, comments:

As a matter of fact the vocabulary is esoteric and the ideas are impregnated with oriental philosophies like Hinduism. The predominant strain of pantheism

431 Weil, Andrew, *Health and Healing: Understanding Conventional and Alternative Medicine,* Houghton Mifß in, Boston, MA, (1983), p.14. Reported in Ankerberg, John, Weldon, John, *Can You Trust Your Doctor?* p. 315.

432 Ankerberg, John, Weldon, John, *Can you Trust Your Doctor?,* Wolgemuth & Hyatt, Brentwood TN., (1991), [sold to Word] p. 316.

433 Gumpert, Martin, *Hahnemann: The Adventurous Career of a Medical Rebel,* L.B. Fisher, (1945), NewYork, NY, p. 25. Reported in Ankerberg, John, Weldon, John; *Can You Trust Your Doctor?* P. 316.

434 Hahnemann, Samuel, *Organon of Medicine,* 6th edition, reprint, B Jain Publishing, New Delhi, India, (1978), pp. 309, 311.

would place God everywhere, in each man, each animal, plant, flower, cell, even in homeopathic medicine.[435]

Dr. Samuel D. Pfeifer, in his book *Healing at Any Price,* mentions the influence of Eastern thinking upon Hahnemann by quoting a biographer who reveals that

> ...he is strongly attracted to the East. Confucius is his ideal.[436] Dr. Pfeifer continues:

On Confucius, Hahnemann himself writes in a letter:

> This is where you can read divine wisdom, without (*e.g.,* Christian) miracle–myths and superstition. I regard it as an important sign of our times that Confucius is now available for us to read. Soon I will embrace him in the kingdom of blissful spirits, the benefactor of humanity, who has shown us the straight path to wisdom and to God, already six hundred sixty years before [650 B.C.] the arch enthusiast.[437] (*Jesus Christ, Divine Son of God).*

His reverence for Eastern thought was the fundamental philosophy behind the preparation of homeopathic remedies. Hahnemann claimed inspiration, as seen in a letter he wrote to the town clerk of Kothen in 1828. He said:

> he had been guided by the invisible powers of the Almighty, listening, observing, tuning in to His instruction, paying most earnest heed and religious attention to this inspiration. [438]

Hahnemann believed in universal energy or *vital force* as some called it. He believed that the power, or effects, of his minutely diluted remedies resulted from the working of vital force. Hahnemann's vital force, which is believed to *rule* the physical body, is similar to the soul, or the *etheric* and *astral bodies* of many occult disciplines. [439], [440]

---

435 Bopp, H.J. , *Homeopathy,* Down, North Ireland, Word of Life Publishing, (1984), p. 9. Reported in Ankerberg, John, Weldon, John; *Can you Trust Your Doctor?* p. 317.

436 Fritsche, A., *Hahnemann – Die Idee der Homoeopathie,* Berlin, (1944), pp. 235-37. Reported in Pfeifer, Samuel M.D., *Healing at any Price, The Hidden Dangers of Alternative Medicine,* Word Limited, Milton Keynes, England, (1988), p. 68.

437 Pfeifer, Samuel M.D., *Healing at Any Price,* Word Limited, Milton Keynes, England, (1988), p. 68.

438 Bopp, op. cit., p. 3; Ankerberg, op. cit., p. 318.

439 Pfeifer, op. Cit., pp. 68–69

440 *Ibid.*

What does this mean? In chapter 5 we learned about vital force and the division of universal energy into seven frequencies or levels. Level one is said to be our material world and our physical bodies. The belief is that the level of energy above the first is in a plane with frequencies faster than light, and, that the *etheric body* is an electromagnetic template of our physical body. The *astral body* is said to be an even higher level of frequency from which we can have *out of body* experiences and astral travel.

From the above paragraph we understand the belief that the vital force in the remedies of homeopathy is purported to be actually influencing and treating the higher levels or bodies of energy rather than just the physical body. This is truly *mysticism*.

Because homeopathists operate in the realm of the invisible and not in that of the visible and material, many of them admit to the belief that homeopathic medicines really work upon the etheric or astral bodies.

> This is where disease begins and spreads outward into the physical body presenting as *symptoms.*[441]

> This is why a number of occultic religions such as Hinduism and anthroposophy employ homeopathy. Its philosophy fits well with their occultic views of man and health.[442]

The power that is transmitted directly in psychic healing through the laying on of the healer's hand, or from a distance, is no different than the power to heal that occurs in the homeopathic remedy. Homeopathic practitioners claim that a cosmic *vital force* is transferred from the homeopathic *medicine* into the patient. But the same effect is supposedly accomplished by radionic devices (see section "Radionics" in chapter 16) which employ spiritistic power.[443] Using these devices, it is said, makes the use of homeopathic remedies unnecessary.

LAWS OF HOMEOPATHY This system is built on the theory that:
1. Most diseases are caused by an infectious disorder called the *psora,* (itch); (see glossary)
2. Life is a spiritual force (vitalism) which directs the body's healing;
3. Remedies can be discerned by noting the symptoms that substances produce in overdose (proving), and applying them to conditions with

---

441 Kent, James Tyler, *Lectures on Homeopathic Philosophy,* (1999),; Reported in Ankerberg, op. cit., p. 326.
442 Ankerberg, op. cit., p. 326.
443 Weldon, John, Levitt, Zola, *Psychic Healing An Exposé of an Occult Phenomenon,* Moody Press,)1982), pp. 53–65.

similar symptoms in highly diluted doses (laws of similia);
4. Remedies become more effective with greater dilution (law of infinitesimals), and become more potent when containers are tapped on the heel of the hand or a leather pad (potentizing). [444], [445]

Proving is a term used to describe the process used by homeopathic practitioners to select new substances for inclusion in the list of therapeutic remedies. A substance will be tested by taking it in high doses, then recording the symptoms it creates. It may be taken daily in high doses for as long as a month, and any type of sensation or supposed change is recorded during this time.

> Consider the alleged 'symptoms' of chamomilla as given by Hahnemann in his *Materia Medica Pura* [1846, Vol. 2, pp. 7—20]: "Vertigo... Dull...aching pain in the head...Violent desire for coffee...Grumbling and creeping in the upper teeth....Great aversion to the wind...Burning pain in the hand....Quarrelsome, vexatious dreams... heat and redness of the right cheek."[446]

One author, writing about Hahnemann, said he (Hahnemann) documented thirteen pages of symptoms from taking chamomile. If such is the case when healthy people take this substance, how can we expect it to cure sick people?[447]

A very interesting comment about proving of the remedies, is made by Ankerberg in *Can You Trust Your Doctor?* (p. 273). We are told that the remedies that are listed in the homeopathic *Materia Medicas,* when tested or proved over the past 150 years by non-homeopaths, have never given the responses found by homeopaths.

CHOOSING THE PROPER REMEDY

In a pharmacy with inventory of more than 2000 homeopathic remedies, how do I select the proper substance that is closest to my symptoms? This is the decision the homeopathic doctor has to make when prescribing for a patient. Homeopathy teaches that it is important to get the exact medicinal for

---

444 *Position Paper of National Council Against Health Fraud,* Feb 1994; p. 5. http://www.ncahf.org/pp/homeop.html
445 *Ibid.,* pp. 3–4.
446 Stalker, Douglas, Glymour, eds.; *Examining Holistic Medicine,* Buffalo, NY, Prometheus books, (1985), p. 32, Sobel, David S., ed.; *Ways of Health: Wholistic Approaches to Ancient and Contemporary Medicine,* Harcourt Brace Jovanich, New York, NY, (1979), pp. 295–297 Reported in Ankerberg, op. cit., p.. 274.
447 Ankeberg, *Can you Trust Your Doctor?,* op. cit., pp. 275–276.

the specific illness and the patient's constitution. The following procedures may be used to choose a specific substance for therapy.

1. Astrological signs or other modes of astrology may be used to determine the proper diagnosis and therapy.[448]

2. Dr. Bopp writes about the use of the pendulum in choosing the proper remedy for homeopathic treatment. Dr. A. Voegeli, a famous homeopathic doctor, has confirmed that a very high percentage of homeopaths work with the pendulum.[21] Dr. Pfeifer also notes the use of pendulums by homeopaths because "it is easier to take a short cut with the radionic pendulum."[449]

3. John Weldon, author of *PSYCHIC HEALING An Exposé of an Occult Phenomenon,* reports that many homeopaths today have spirit guides with research on homeopathy being done in séances. There are groups whose (homeopathic) research is carried out during séances, through mediums who seek information from spirits.[450]

Dr. Bopp tells in his book, *Homeopathy,* about a woman who worked in a homeopathic laboratory in France. She personally related the story of an interview she had on applying for a job in a specific homeopath laboratory. She was asked about which astrological sign she was born under, and whether or not she was a medium. She told the sign and answered "yes" to the question about being a medium. She was then informed that new treatments to be produced by the laboratory were researched in séances.[451]

As *conventional* doctors of the past used large doses of toxic drugs, *eclectic* physicians discontinued the use of mercury and the heavy toxic substances and tended to be better at diagnosing, but, prescribed small doses for every symptom. The *homeopathic* physician, though ridiculing conventional doctors, continued to use toxic drugs in his treatments. He simply used extremely weak dilutions. The following are examples of drugs used in homeopathy: "Nux vomica (strychnine), sulphur, lobelia (nicotine), phosphorus, ipecac, hydrochloric acid, alcohol, lead, arsenic, colchicine, jalap, senna, mercury, aconite, belladonna (atropine), podophyllum, camphor, veratrum, staphysagria, opium, quinine, cantharides, croton oil, phosphoric acid, tartar emetic, iodine, and numerous other agents."[452] The solution made by repeated dilution often surpasses the point of having any molecules of the original substance left, yet

448 Bopp, op. cit., p. 5.
449 Pfeifer, op. cit., pp. 79–80.
450 Ankerberg, John; Weldon, John; op. cit., pp. 328–329.
451 Bopp, op. cit., p. 8.
452 Marcy, E.E. and Hunt, F.W.; *The Homeopathic Theory and Practice of Medicine,* (1877), Vol. I, pp. vii–xxxii; Reported in Hardinge op. cit., p. 82.

the homeopathic doctor claims these extreme dilutions are the most potent of the preparations. How can this be? Let us consider the process of dilution.

When each dilution takes place, the solution is shaken vigorously by hitting the hand that holds the dilution on a hard surface, so as to *thump* the solution. This is called *succession.* It is claimed that this process causes the remedy to be more *potent*. This is believed to be the critical part in preparation of the remedies. Notice the following comments by leading homeopaths Dana Ullman and Stephen Cunnings:

> Homeopaths have found that the medicines do not work if they are simply diluted repeatedly without vigorous shaking or if they are just diluted in vast amounts of liquid. Nor do the medicines work if they are only vigorously shaken. It is the *combined* process of dilution and vigorous shaking that makes the medicine effective...[453]

How can the medicine get stronger and stronger with increasing dilution? The homeopathic practitioner says that the solution (water) receives an *imprint* or *signature* from the original substance (mother tincture) and this is passed along, thereby increasing the potency. Chemists and physicists find no scientific evidence to support this theory.[454]

There have been homeopaths who claimed that homeopathic remedies act similar to vaccinations, a theory that was quickly and unwisely accepted by some adherents of homeopathy. When a vaccination is administered, the immune system manufactures protective proteins, and stimulates specific white blood cells to respond to the organism or allergen contained in the vaccination. A memory is created within the immune system which allows it to respond powerfully to this specific organism or allergen should it be encountered at another time.

The proponents of homeopathy claim that the small homeopathic dose will trigger an immune response. This is not true. The quantity of active ingredients in the homeopathic remedy usually is too small to trigger an immune response. A vaccination will have far greater concentration of an organism or allergen. The response of the body from an immunization can be measured chemically. The high-dilution homeopathic remedies do not produce measurable responses. Vaccines are used as prevention, not as a cure. Homeopathic remedies have no relationship to immunization science.

---

453 Ullman, Dana; Cummings, Stephen; *The Science of Homeopathy,* New Realities, [journal] Summer of (1985) p. 20. Reported in Ankeberg, op. cit., p. 330.
454 *NCAHF Position Paper on Homeopathy, pp. 3,4 (1994),* http://www.ncahf.org/

PREPARATION OF HOMEOPATHIC REMEDIES

Materials for use in remedies are finely ground or dissolved in water. They are then mixed with a solvent, and the mixture is allowed to soak. The fluid containing the original substance is then filtered or strained. The filtered solution–the *mother tincture*–is placed in a dark jar for keeping.

One drop of the mother tincture can be diluted one of two ways; using either a nine part solvent or a ninety-nine parts solvent, and then shaken vigorously and the solution banged down firmly on a hard surface after each dilution, a process devised by Hahnemann. The *thumping* after the dilution is believed to transfer the spirit from the remedy substance into the solvent. Homeopathy teaches that the *essence* (spirit—remedy) can be carried by water even after all molecules of the original substance are diluted out of the solution. Once the mixture has reached the required strength and potency, a few drops of it are added to lactose tablets, pills, granules, or to a powder so as to impregnate the carrier with the remedy. It is then stored in dark glass bottles.

Dilutions are most often made by using one part of the mother tincture and nine parts solvent, (1–X). With each additional dilution the labeling would be 2–X, 3–X, etc. When dilutions go beyond 24–X there may not be one molecule left of the original remedy substance in the solution. Homeopaths do not depend on molecules of the original substance to effect healing. They are looking to the *signature/energy— imprint/spirit* of the original substance to be passed on and magnified by dilution. This signature or imprint said to be in the solution has not been scientifically demonstrated.

Given below are examples of common remedies as listed in *Natural Health, Encyclopedia of Homeopathy*, by Dr. Andrew Lockie, (2000):

Mercury: found in cinnabar ore from Spain, Italy, US, Peru,China
Rx for symptoms of:
 a. Foul smelling discharge
 b. Reserved, suspicious state of mind
 c. Insecurity
 d. Copious perspiration that does not relieve condition
 e. Person feels worse at night

Hellborus: Southern Europe–extremely poisonous
Rx for symptoms of:
 a. Mental dullness
 b. Chilliness
 c. Tendency to drop things

    d.   Person feels worse between 4 pm and 8 pm

Aconite: Europe, Central Asia–deadly poisonous, handling root can cause poisoning
Rx for symptoms of:
    a.   Symptoms triggered by shock or cold wind
    b.   Panic attack and fear of death
    c.   Acute infection with sudden onset

Nux Vomica: (strychnine) (poison nut tree) India, Burma, Thailand, China, Australia
Rx for symptoms of:
    a.   Irritability
    b.   Over-critical nature
    c.   Tendency to be highly driven and ambitious
    d.   Chilliness
    e.   Desire for rich foods

Carcinosin: Cancer cells usually from breast
Rx for symptoms of:
    a.   Workaholic, of passionate nature
    b.   Conditions that are affected by being at the beach
    c.   Desire for travel
    d.   Desire for butter or chocolate
    e.   Sleeping difficulty

    Remember, there are more than 2000 remedies in the homeopathy pharmacy! In review, homeopathy came from the concept of one man's beliefs which were not scientifically verified. However, it had a great advantage over the common medical care of his day. He did not advocate the use of harmful drugs in large doses. He promoted not only good personal hygiene, but also good hygienic conditions for the home and its surroundings. Diet, fresh air and exercise were also part of his regimen. The remedies (substances given in minute doses) were given credit for the improvements in health, without any scientific evidence to verify that they had anything to do with improvement.

HAS HOMEOPATHY BEEN VERIFIED?
    Studies have been done to test the value of these remedies but there is no clear proof that they have any effect on the body in minute doses. Larger (more concentrated) doses have shown some effect on the system. This effect may

not always be good. Some remedies available may contain regular modern drugs added to them so they will have an effect on human physiology.

There has been a strong effort on the part of believers in alternative therapeutic modalities to scientifically explain the perceived effects of such methods as acupuncture, homeopathic, therapeutic touch, Rolfing, osteopathic, chiropractic, hypnosis, and many other therapy techniques. James Oschman, in his book, *Energy Medicine The Scientific Basis*, makes a strong argument for the scientific explanation. He presents the recent advances in the understanding of electromagnetic physiology in biology. Some researchers, who are adherents of the concept of *vitalism,* have reported advances in laboratory research of electromagnetic discharges of body, organs, cells and molecules. Other researchers are unable to reproduce these same laboratory results. The gap is still wide between hypothesis and true scientific proof of cause and effect. Many believers in alternative medicine, or energy medicine, tend to proclaim that energy medicine is now proven to be scientific. They have ignored this gap of proof in a presumptuous manner.

Controlled studies of homeopathic remedies, when done by the homeopaths, tend to show positive results. However, most other stud- ies do not support these positive results. Studies should be repeated by objective investigators, with independent analyses of the homeopathic formulations employed, to ensure that they have not been adulterated with active medications.

A recent meta-analysis of 107 controlled homeopath trials appearing in 96 published reports also found "the evidence of clinical trials is positive but not sufficient to draw definitive conclusions because most trials are of low methodological quality and because of the unknown role of publication bias." The reports also concluded that there is a legitimate case for further evaluation of homeopathy, "but only by means of well performed trials." (Kleijnen, 1991) [455]

In the British medical journal *Lancet* August 27, 2005, a large study made by the University of Berne in Switzerland reported the results of a meta-analysis of 110 trials, each of homeopathy and conventional medicine. No convincing evidence was found that the homeopathic approach to illness was any different from using a placebo. Conventional medicine did significantly better.

April 19, 2010 Med J Aust. 192(8):458-60 carried an article *Homeopathy: what does the "best" evidence tell us?* The author Edzard Ernst of Peninsula Medical School, University of Exeter, Exeter, United Kingdom summarized his study of homeopathy as follows:

---

[455] *Ibid.*

The Cochrane Database of Systematic Reviews (generally considered to be the most reliable source of evidence) was searched in January 2010....DATA EXTRACTION: Each of the six reviews was examined for specific subject matter; number of clinical trials reviewed; total number of patients involved; and author's conclusions. The reviews covered the following conditions: cancer, attention-deficit defect, hyperactivity disorder, asthma, dementia, influenza and induction of labour. DATA SYNTHESIS: The findings of the reviews were discussed narratively (the reviews; clinical and statistical heterogeneity precluded meta-analysis). **CONCLUSIONS**: The finding of currently available Cochrane reviews of studies of homeopathy do not show that homeopathic medicines have effects beyond placebo. http://www.cochrane. org/evidence

WORLD HEALTH CONDEMS HOMEOPATHIC Rx

Homeopathy not a cure, says WHO. Homeopathic remedies often contain few or no active ingredients. People with conditions such as HIV, TB and malaria should not rely on homeopathic treatments, the World Health Organization has warned. It was responding to calls from young researchers who fear the promotion of homeopathy in the developing world could put people's lives at risk.[456]

The group, Voice of Young Science Network, has written to health ministers to set out the WHO view. Objective evidence that homeopathy is effective on these infections does not exist says Dr. Nick Beeching, Royal Liverpool University Hospital by letter June 2010, to WHO. The doctors from the UK and Africa said:

We are calling on the WHO to condemn the promotion of homeopathy for treating TB, infant diarrhea, influenza, malaria and HIV. Homeopathy does not protect people from, or treat, these diseases. Those of us working with the most rural and impoverished people of the world already struggle to deliver the medical help that is needed. When homeopathy stands in place of effective treatment, lives are lost.[457]

A researcher in bimolecular science at the University of St Andrews, Dr. Robert Hagan, and a member of Voice of Young Science Network, part of *Sense About Science* promoting "evidence-based" care said:

---

456 http://news.bbc.co.uk/2/hi/8211925.stm
457 *Ibid.*

We need governments around the world to recognize the dangers of promoting homeopathy for life-threatening illnesses. We hope that by raising awareness of the WHO's position on homeopathy we will be supporting those people who are taking a stand against these potentially disastrous practices.[458]

Dr. Mario Raviglione, director of the Stop TB department at the WHO, said:

Our evidence-based WHO TB treatment/management guidelines, as well as the International Standards of Tuberculosis Care do not recommend use of homeopathy.[459]

Physicians also complained that homeopathy was being promoted as a treatment of children with diarrhea. A representative of the WHO department of child and adolescent health and development said:

We have found no evidence to date that homeopathy would bring any benefit. Homeopathy does not focus on the treatment and prevention of dehydration - in total contradiction with the scientific basis and our recommendations for the management of diarrhea.[460]

Dr. Nick Beeching, a specialist in infectious diseases at the Royal Liverpool University Hospital, said:

Infections such as malaria, HIV and tuberculosis all have a high mortality rate but can usually be controlled or cured by a variety of proven treatments, for which there is ample experience and scientific trial data. "There is no objective evidence that homeopathy has any effect on these infections, and I think it is irresponsible for a healthcare worker to promote the use of homeopathy in place of proven treatment for any life-threatening illness."[461]

In June 2010 Delegates to the British Medical Association's conference were expected to support seven motions opposing the use of public money to pay for remedies which they claimed have no place in modern medicine and health care. Hundreds of delegates called for a ban on funding homeopathic remedies by the National Health Service. The British Medical Society's position comes as a result of an absence of evidence that use of homeopathic remedies are more effective than placebo.

---

458   *Ibid.*
459   *Ibid.*
460   *Ibid.*
461   *Ibid*

In the first half of the 20th century, the 22 homeopathy medical schools in the United States closed or converted to regular medical schools. With the advance of scientific evaluation in medical care, the old harmful way of using dangerous drugs slowly changed. The homeopathic doctor was no longer having better results than the M.D. The public turned to *science-driven* medicine. There is now a resurgence of homeopathy among New Age adherents and some others that consider it to be more *natural.* Its return in America is not based on science, but is the end result of the belief in *Vitalism.* A man's belief in his origin has great influence in his choice of healing methods.

I refer again to James L. Oschman, a biology scientist, who, in his book *Energy Medicine, The Scientific Basis,* speaks of his belief in alternative medicine therapies and of having felt the electrical charges enter his body as applied by *energy therapists.* He expresses his belief that these electrical charges are explained by electromagnetism. He writes that the electromagnetism of one person can restore balance to the electromagnetism of another. He tells of laboratory testing of healers using therapeutic touch and other methods with tools for measuring electromagnetic charges. He admits to the problem of the reproducibility of these experiments by other investigators.

We have received wise counsel regarding the type of medical care we choose, following God's *"will"* versus gain and life itself:

> ...Those who give themselves up to the sorcery of Satan may boast of great benefit received thereby, but does this prove their course to be wise or safe? What if life should be prolonged? What if temporal gain should be secured? Will it pay in the end to disregard the will of God? All such apparent gain will prove at last an irrecoverable loss. We cannot with impunity break down a single barrier which God has erected to guard His people from Satan's power.[462]

I wish to share with you the words of a Christian physician who has written on this subject.

There are to be sure some honorable and conscientious ones seeking to utilize homeopathy detached from its obscure practices. Yet, the occult influence, by nature hidden, disguised, often dissimulated behind para-scientific theory, does not disappear and does not happen to be rendered harmless by the mere fact of a superficial approach contenting itself simply with denying its existence. *Homeopathy is dangerous.* It is quite contrary to the teaching of the word of God. It willingly favors healing through substances made dynamic, that is to say, *charged with occult forces.* Homeopathic treatment is the fruit of a philosophy and religion that are at the same time Hinduistic, pantheistic

462   White, E.G., *Testimonies for the Church* Vol. 5, Pacific Press Pub. Assn., Mountain View, CA, (1882), p. 199.

and esoteric.[463]

When God led Israel from Egypt to Canaan He gave them health laws and statutes. Israel was the only nation in the history of the world that had a medical and health system that was based on prevention. The Mosaic health code is medically and scientifically reliable, based on sound physiology and proven principles of hygiene.[464]

When God led Seventh-day Adventists in health reform starting in 1848, He gave directions and guidance that are based on the physical laws of the universe. These directions are in harmony with today's understanding of physiology and hygiene. They are built on the principle that we were created and placed under the laws of the physical universe, and that our bodies operate according to those laws. It is not from an imbalance of spirit energy, I repeat:

> Disease is the effort of nature to free the system from conditions that result from a violation of the laws of health.[465]

God gave specific directions for developing a healing center so that His methods could be practiced. In 1866, such a center was started and in the space of 40 years, was one of the greatest health centers of its type in the world. It prospered so long as it followed the directions God gave. At that time, homeopathy was in its zenith in the United States, but God did not direct His people to use homeopathy in the health institutions. I conclude this chapter with the following comment made by Ellen White with regard to the practice of regular medicine and homeopathic medicine:

> When the great question of health reform was opened before me, the methods of treating the sick were plainly revealed to me. The old-school cruel practice (use of mercury, antimony, arsenic, strychnine, bleeding, cathartics, etc., these were called drugs in that day) and the sure results, where one claimed to be benefited, thousands were made lifelong invalids who, had they never seen a physician, would have recovered of themselves without implanting in their system diseases of a most distressing character.

> Eclectic (medical doctors using same drugs but very small doses) was less dangerous. The *homeopathy*, which creates so deadly opposition from the regular practice, was attended with far less evil consequences than the old-school practice, but *did much harm* because it could be resorted to so easily

---

463 Bopp, op. cit., p. 9. Reported in Ankeberg, *Can you Trust Your Doctor?*, p. 336.
464 Hubbard, Reuben A., *Historical Perspectives of Health,* Printed by the Department of Health Education School of Health Loma Linda University, Loma Linda, CA, (1975), pp. 23-38.
465 White, E.G., *Temperance*, Pacific Press Pub. Assn., Mountain View, CA (1877), p. 85.

and used so readily with so little expense. Many practice upon themselves and fall back upon this without real knowledge of their ailments, and do great harm to themselves. Proper regulation of their diet, abstinence from tea, coffee, and all spices and flesh meats, gaining an intelligent knowledge of temperance, would be medicine above all drugs. (Emphasis added)

But Dr. Maxson... I told him (that) after the whole system of drug medication had been laid open before me, I was shown of God that we should have an institution, conducted on hygienic principles, and in that institution lectures should be given not on how to use drugs, not to lead minds and educate them in the methods of drug using, but to teach people the better way—to live healthfully and do without drugs. The words were repeated, Educate! Educate! Educate!

I then saw that an intelligent knowledge of pure air, and use of it wisely and abundantly, and simple healthful food taken into the stomach temperately, eating and drinking to the glory of God, and ten thousand would be well who are now sick. Then I was taken from room to room and shown disease and its causes, and the result of drug medication. I was then shown through rooms of a hygienic institution that was conducted on hygienic principles and these simple means–sunlight, pure air, healthful habits. Constant instruction needs to be given, line upon line, precept upon precept, in regard to the necessity of clean bodies, clean houses and clean premises. Breathing clean air would preserve health without the use of drugs.[466]

---

466 White, E.G., *Manuscript Releases/20MR* No. 1497; Ellen G. White Estate Inc. Washington DC, pp. 373–374.

CHAPTER 16

DIVINATION AS A DIAGNOSTIC TOOL

A young American woman had been living in a Southeast Asian country. She developed an earache and sought medical care at a modern hospital in an Asian city. One complaint led to another and an abdominal ultrasound (exam of the abdomen by use of sound waves) was ordered, then an abdominal CT scan (machine that makes computer generated pictures of the insides of the abdomen). A diagnosis was made of a cancerous fatty tumor surrounding the right kidney that had spread to other areas of the abdomen. The woman was devastated with this diagnosis. The attending physicians desired to proceed with surgery, but she elected to return to America.

Her American doctor ordered a PET–CT scan (a $5000+ test which is better able than the CT scan to determine if cancer is present). The test indicated active tissue in the abdomen that could be cancer. A laparoscopic surgical procedure (looking in the abdomen by optics) was scheduled to be done. A blood test prior to this procedure revealed severe anemia (low number of red blood cells) which made it unsafe to proceed with surgery. Additional blood studies and another ultrasound were ordered in a further attempt to define the disorder. A repeat ultrasound exam of the abdomen did not add any new information. At this point the expenses had reached nearly $10,000. and the doctors were still not able to determine the exact diagnosis.

Study results to this time could not differentiate between a malignancy and endometriosis, a non-malignant disorder. A laparoscopic procedure was done, which revealed tumors spread in various areas inside the abdomen. Biopsy of the tumors revealed cancer. Extensive surgery to remove as much cancer as possible was performed. Following surgery, treatment would be needed for many months in an attempt to control the disease.

So goes the story for many people seeking definite answers to medical problems in an age of very sophisticated diagnostic equipment and highly-trained physicians. Thousands of dollars can be spent, yet the question still remains as to the exact diagnosis which is so important in order that the proper treatment can be given, in the best sequence, to receive the best results.

Why not seek out some *alternative* style practitioner with a *Homo Vibra Ray,* or the Mora machine, or the Rife machine, or some similar type instrument to make the diagnosis and treat at the same time with little expense? These machines are said to be able to read energy wave frequencies or vibrational energy of the cells of the body. (*Such energy frequencies and/or vibrations from cells cannot be demonstrated by physical science.*) However, this is a belief of some alternative medicine practitioners. By tuning in to those frequencies, the machine is said to compare them to the assumed normal frequency. Then, by the operator spinning a few dials, frequencies are said to be sent back into the body to correct the body's cell frequencies, thereby correcting disease and restoring health.

Another choice is to find a holistic medical doctor who can pass his hands over the abdomen, or hold a pendulum above the abdomen in order to localize tumors. Questions can be asked of the pendulum, as it is held above the spot where it has located a tumor, as to whether or not the tumor is a cancer. The pendulum can spin clockwise if a positive answer is given, or counter-clockwise if it is negative. Any question under the sun can be asked and a *yes* or *no* answer can be obtained. The pendulum can be asked what type of therapy would be best. Should the answer be homeopathy, the pendulum can pick out the proper remedy.

This alternative method is quick, non-invasive, and inexpensive compared to the above-described conventional medical tests and treatment. Is the machine or the hands-on technique accurate? Can they be trusted? Why are scientifically trained physicians not using these techniques? Is it because more money can be made doing many tests? Let us proceed in a search for answers to these questions.

Let me give a definition at this point for the word *alternative therapy*: therapy that is not shown to be evidence-based by quality scientific testing. When an *alternative* method of treatment is shown to be evidence-based it then becomes scientific medicine.

The General Conference Manual for Seventh-day Adventist institutions updated in 2009 contains the following comment: GC Health Institutions Working Policy-2009, FH 20 Statement of Operating Principles for Health Care Institutions:

> Adventist health care and ministries are to promote only those practices based upon the Bible or the Spirit of Prophecy, or evidence based methods of disease prevention, treatment, and health maintenance. "Evidence-based" means there is an accepted body of peer reviewed, statistically significant evidence that raises probability of effectiveness to a scientifically convincing level.

The following paragraph tells of incidences involving Christian church members and church institutional workers, as was related in a special report, *New Age Movement and Seventh-day Adventists,* written by the Biblical

Research Institute, General Conference of Seventh-day Adventists, July 1987, for general reading by Seventh-day Adventist members (see APPENDIX E).

- A nurse corrected chronic constipation by repeated application of her hands to her abdomen during the day, to correct *electrical currents*.
- A mother swings a pendulum over her son afflicted with cancer to determine the herbs he needs for healing.
- A young person was tied to a tree so his back was against "its window" to effect healing; the window had been located on the tree by use of the pendulum.
- Women shopping for groceries use a pendulum to select the best products.
- Books on iridology, a method for diagnosing disease through the iris of the eye, were on sale in a college-operated supermarket. Another popular volume on the same shelf was *Magnetic Therapy: Healing in Your Own Hands*, by Abbot George Burke. The author refers with approval to the studies of Dr. Franz Mesmer (from whom the term "mesmerism" derives) and traces his research through pagan thought to Isis, a famous goddess of ancient Egypt.[467]

The nation of Israel was admonished by God just as they were about to enter the Promised Land:

> When thou art come into the land which the Lord thy God giveth thee, thou shalt not learn to do after the abominations of those nations. There shall not be found among you any one that maketh his son or his daughter to pass through the fire, or that useth *divination*, or an observer of times, or an enchanter or a witch, or a charmer, or a consulter with familiar spirits, or a wizard, or a necromancer–for these nations, which thou shalt possess, hearkened unto observers of times, and unto *diviners*: but as for thee, the Lord thy God hath not suffered thee so to do.[468]

Caution was also given in regard to false prophets and their proclamations:

> They have seen vanity and lying *divination*, saying, The Lord saith: and the Lord hath not sent them:" "And mine hand shall be upon the prophets that see vanity, and that divine lies: they shall not be in the assembly of my people....[469]

In studying the history of divination it soon becomes obvious that every civilization used various forms of divination in an attempt to obtain knowledge

467   *The New Age Movement and Seventh-day Adventists,* Biblical Research Institute, General Conference of Seventh–day Adventists, Hagerstown, MD, (1987), p. 3.
468   Deuteronomy 18:9–14.
469   Ezekiel 13:6–10.

not obtainable by the usual means. It is of ancient origin. Reading of omens is recognized as a very early divining practice. A child born with an abnormality might well be looked upon as revealing something of the future. Reading the stars and using the zodiac were common. Tarot cards, palm reading, crystal balls, and séances all contributed to the use of divination in daily life.

Dictionary definitions of divination are:

> The act or practice of trying to foretell the future or explore the unknown by occult means.[470]

> A general term for various false systems for seeking supernatural aid, either for information regarding the future or for guidance in present affairs...[471]

And from the Catholic Encyclopedia.

> Divination is a form of occultism wherein the person uses objects such as tea leaves, a crystal ball, tarot cards, Ouija board, or any superstitiously interpreted object as the means of attempting to gain or elicit knowledge or information that is beyond ordinary human intelligence. The attempts to contact the dead through a séance, for example, are spiritistic divinations that have been contested by parapsychological testing and proved false. Likewise astrology, witchcraft, zodiac readings or horoscopes are forms of divination. Although it is natural for human beings to attempt to 'lift the curtain' and see beyond the present, the tendency should be controlled lest it distract from the unfolded and true vision of God contained in His revelation to mankind.[472]

> But Laban said to him, 'If I have found favor in your eyes, please stay. I have learned by *divination* (some versions use the word experience) that the Lord has blessed me because of you.' (Genesis 30:27).

The Bible records the use of divination, but it does not always say what method was used. Does the Bible promote the use of divination by these stories?

Joseph had his cup placed in the sack of grain belonging to his brother Benjamin. He called it his *divining cup*. Joseph's servant said to the brothers:

---

470 *Webster's New World Dictionary, 3rd College Edition,* Published by Webster's New World dictionaries A Division of Simon & Shuster, Inc., (1988).
471 *Seventh-day Adventist Bible Dictionary, Review and Herald Publishing Association, Washington D.C.,*(1979).
472 *The Catholic Encyclopedia,* Thomas Nelson Inc. Publication, Nashville, TN, (1976), p. 168.

> Isn't this the cup my master drinks from and also uses for divination? This is a wicked thing you have done. (Genesis. 44:5).

When his brothers were brought to Joseph, he said to them:

> What is this you have done? Don't you know that a man like me can find things out by divination? (Genesis. 44:15).

E.G. White, in *Patriarchs and Prophets*, page 229, states that Joseph never claimed the power of divination, but he was willing to have them believe that he could read the secrets of their lives.

Over 400 years later, God told the descendants of Joseph and his brothers that He was going to give them a land that others possessed because those people were practicing divination along with other acts of which God did not approve. Their degree of iniquity had come to its full. But Israel did not heed God's command to abstain from divination for we read that the divining rod was in use in Hosea's day.

> My people ask counsel at their stocks, and their staff declareth unto them: for the spirit of whoredoms hath caused them to err, and they have gone a whoring from under their God. (Hosea 4:12).

King Ahaziah of Israel sent messengers to Ekron, a city of the Philistines, to inquire of Baalzebub, the god of Ekron, as to whether or not the king of Israel, Ahaziah, would recover from his injuries of falling through the lattice. When Elijah was sent of God to intercept those servants of the King, he asked them this question:

> ...Is it because there is no God in Israel that you are going off to consult Baal-Zebub, the god of Ekron? (II Kings 1:3 NIV)

The servants returned to the King who then sent 50 soldiers to bring Elijah to him. When the soldiers came near Elijah God sent fire down from heaven and consumed the Captain and the 50 soldiers. The king sent another 50 and again fire consumed them. The Captain of the next 50 asked Elijah for mercy, where upon God told Elijah to go with him to the King with a message from God. Elijah told the King that he would not get up from his bed because he inquired of Baalzebub rather than inquiring of the God of Israel. (II Kings, chapter 1).

King Nebuchadnezzar, while traveling with his army came to a division in the road. He could proceed to Egypt, or he could travel toward Jerusalem.

He did not know which way to go first, so he had an animal killed and "read the liver" as a method of divination.

> For the King of Babylon stands at the parting of the road, at the fork of the two roads, to use divination: he shakes the arrows, he consults the images, he looks at the liver. (Ezekiel 21:21 NKJ).

The use of various methods of divining has been presented including the rod, cup, arrows, and liver. There are scores of other methods. Divination by astrology to establish medical diagnosis has also been a common practice.

Is divining used in medical practice today? In the scientific method of medical care divining is not used. It is used, however, by some of the alternative and holistic practitioners. This fact is to be found in the writings of those alternative disciplines.

Ankerberg and Weldon in their book, *Can You Trust Your Doctor?*, lists the names of several alternative healing disciplines that in their own literature state that some practitioners may use divination: these disciplines are psychic healing, reflexology, herbal medicine, naturopathy, dowsing, iridology, color therapy, chiropractic, homeopathy, astrologic medicine, and therapeutic touch. The pendulum is the most common method of divination.[473]

PENDULUMS

The practice of divining using a rod, wand, or pendulum is ancient. No exact history is available to pin-point the start, but some drawings found in China show evidence of this practice as far back as 1400 B.C. In the Bible (Deuteronomy 18:9–14) which is dated around 1450 B.C., strong words of warning were given to the people of Israel concerning divining as they were about to enter Canaan. Divination was recorded in the Bible as having been used 500 years prior to the writing of Deuteronomy 18. This passage does not state the method of divining that was practiced. In the Bible, it is recorded that *divining by a staff* was practiced in Israel around 750 B.C. (Hosea 4:12).

Divining with a rod can be considered the same act as using a pendulum. When was it first used in medical diagnosis? We do not know, but early in history the rod became connected with health and healing as evidenced by the following examples. Greek mythology shows ties to serpent power and the use of a *rod* when Apollo handed over to Hermes (Mercury) a magic wand. Homer, in his *Odyssey*, tells how this rod could send men's souls to Hades or return them; it had power to bring winds and storms. Another name for the rod

---

473   Ankerberg, John; Weldon, John; *Can You Trust Your Doctor?,* Wolgemuth and Hyatt, Brentwood, TN, (1991), pp. 100–101.

was *caduceus* and was depicted as entwined with snakes. The rod was passed on to Aesculapius, the Greek god of healing, and has since become the symbol of medicine.

The pendulum is one of the most frequently used methods of divination. It may be used in psychology to assess personality disorders, to make diagnosis in medical conditions, to choose treatments or medicinals, to find oil in the ground, to locate different metals in the earth, and most frequent of all, to find water underground.

Around 1900, a Catholic Priest, Alexis Mermet, who was a dowser for underground water and metals, concluded that dowsing should be amenable in medical diagnosis for humans and animals as well. He wrote the book, *How I Proceed in the Discovery of Near or Distant Water, Metals, Hidden Objects, and Illnesses.* He makes the following Statement:

I invented the method of pendular diagnosis.[474]

It is unlikely that Mermet was really the first to use the pendulum in medical diagnosis, but at least he thought so.

A question was asked, why does a pendulum appear to react to a metallic substance or an underground water vein as well as to a simple act of thought— an action of the mind? In 1806, a bright young German scientist, Johann Wilhelm Ritter, took up this question. While experimenting with a variety of pendulums on various metals, he noticed that the pendulum would swing in a specific pattern for each type of object over which it was suspended. He demonstrated that the swinging or rotating of the pendulum, when held at the top versus the bottom of an object, would give different directions of motion in the pendulum. He did this on the human body and mapped out different anatomical areas showing how the pendulum would spin in one direction, but at other places it would reverse its direction of spinning. Because this reaction reminded him of magnetic characteristics he called this *polarity*.

Today, there are healers who teach that illness is a result of an organ's or the body's polarity becoming disturbed and out of balance. They also teach that in order to bring healing, it is useful to apply magnets about the body. There are *magnetic healers* who apply magnets to the body to balance the polarity. Then there are other healers who do not consider polarity, but apply magnets in various places for almost any symptom common to man. They may not have a philosophy as to how it works, but they say it works and that is good enough for them. The philosopher, Frederick Wilhelm Joseph von Schelling, explained it as follows:

---

474   Bird, Christofer; *The Divining Hand;* New Age Press, Black Mountain, NC, (1979), p. 289.

There was a "force" in nature that could be revealed mechanically, chemically, electrically, magnetically, and also vitally. [475]

He concluded that when a pendulum is used by a "sensitive" operator it was possible to detect the force described. He believed there was a polarity throughout the universe which was the source of all substance. Ritter, a member of the Bavarian Academy of Sciences, in the early 1800's summarized it this way:

> What we have, then, are the celestial movements themselves here repeated in microcosm. Could it be that the whole organism of the universe is reflected in the human body?[476]

> The book continues: What Ritter had stumbled upon at the start of the nineteenth century was the fact that a pendulum or dowsing rod could be used to extract pure information from the universe about any subject no matter how abstract or nebulous.[477]

The dowsing instrument would respond to the questions or commands of the dowser as long as it could be answered by a *yes* or *no*.

Many people have had very little contact with dowsing, or pendulum exposure, and may only have heard of one or two styles. If their experience has been that they have witnessed or heard only of positive responses from this particular technique, they may be convinced that there is some physical explanation for its function. Knowledge of the various ways pendulums are used will undermine confidence in there being a true physical explanation for the information obtained by their use. In Appendix D, I have included material on water witching. If you read the information presented there you will better understand my above comment.

RADIONICS

Radionics, psychotronics, etc., involves the occult use of technology (various devices). It does not really deal in heretofore undiscovered areas of undetected energy, but rather is *dependent on the psychic ability of the operator, referred to as radiaesthesia.* For example, radionics is divination (not always recognized or admitted), and the same as using a rod or pendulum. Radionics is divination aided by a mechanical apparatus–Abrams box, black box, or any one of the numerous machines used for such work.

---

475   *Ibid.*, p. 126.
476   *Ibid.*, p. 128.
477   *Ibid.*, p. 129.

Some years ago I had a family come to my office in great distress. They had secured the services of a medical practitioner who had sent a saliva specimen of their little girl to a lab that used a radionic machine. The family was told that the machine made the diagnosis of acute leukemia. They were shaken and frightened. They asked for my help in determining if this was so. The child had no symptoms that would have caused a physician to suspect such an illness. A blood count was ordered and done at a hospital laboratory. It was normal with no hint of leukemia. Their medical practitioner had given them the diagnosis of leukemia, because the machine had diagnosed leukemia. The family did not understand what clinical and lab findings go with leukemia and my assurance that the child did not have the disease was not enough to relieve their fears. I sent them to a pediatrician who had advanced training in leukemia. He agreed with me, but their doubts lingered. It took many months of normal life before they were free of the fear caused by this wrong diagnosis.

What concept of science did this medical practitioner have that caused him to believe the diagnosis made by the machine? This introduces a belief that is common in the non-scientific world of health and healing, that of *vibrational medicine*. The radionic machine is said to be able to detect *vibrations* or *frequencies* from the saliva. If any disharmony is in the salivary vibrations, the machine can analyze in such a manner as to detect and diagnose the abnormality. Where does the idea originate that saliva has vibrations, or frequencies? How does vibration from saliva relate to an individual and make it possible for a machine to make a diagnosis of leukemia?

We have to return to the basic pagan belief that every existing thing has a common origin from a non-describable energy (*vitalism*) that is present throughout the universe. This energy is said to be manifest in every *living* substance (some authors, writing on this subject, include *inanimate* substances), and that there is an *aura* of radiating energy that emanates and surrounds those substances. This radiating energy is believed to have a specific vibrational or electromagnetic frequency. If the particular frequency is off normal, it indicates an imbalance of energy. Electronic machines have been made that are supposed to detect the vibrational imbalance, ascertain the reason for the imbalance, and make a diagnosis. It is simply another form of divination. It is not true science. *Vibrational Medicine* is simply a synonym for *Energy Medicine*.

A commonly used radionic machine is the EVA machine—Electro Acupuncture According to Voll (Reinhold Voll). Voll was a German physician engaged in acupuncture, starting in the 1950's. EVA technique is a form of radionics, with the concept of measuring by use of an electronic machine, hypothesized electric impulses from specific acupuncture points which, in turn, are said to have originated from an organ having *meridian connections* to that specific point. The machine is supposed to reveal low, normal, or high electronic vibrations from the organ. Low amplitude electronic vibration reveals a weak organ; a high signal reveals inflammation.

Then, if you find an organ that has a low energy, for example, you insert a medicine contained in a vial into that electrical circuit which also consists of the patient and the machine. If the medicine vibrates at the same frequency as the weak signal being tested, synchronizes, harmonizes, literally, electronically, with the low signal from the weak organ, the amplitude or strength of the signal will get higher as the two frequencies will superimpose and add together. Then you know that what is in the vial is the right medicine for that organ, for that patient. The person doing the testing must be *highly sensitive,* that is, have high occult powers.

The American Cancer Society, exposing non-scientific alternative medical treatments, lists the following synonyms regarding terms used by proponents of various alternative treatment methods: Electromagnetism, Bioelectricity, Magnetic Field Therapy, Bioelectromagnetics, Bioenergy Therapy, BioResonance Tumor Therapy, Energy Medicine, Black Boxes, Electronic Devices; Electrical Devices, Zapping Machine, Rife Machine, Cell com System.

These terms refer to names given by alternative healers to the energy they say comes from the body, which machines are said to be able to detect, diagnose, and use to treat for different medical disorders.

It is claimed by radionic practitioners that when electromagnetic frequencies, or energy fields, proclaimed to be within the body are unbalanced, disease and illness occur. The belief is that these imbalances disrupt the body's chemical makeup. By applying electromagnetic energy from outside the body, either by the hands of a *healer* or by electronic devices, practitioners claim they can correct the electrical imbalances in the body.

There are a variety of radionic machines for sale on the internet. You may find a practitioner that uses one but most physicians will not do so. What are these machines, how do they work? Why doesn't most medical doctor use them? Let me present my answer.

The machines are simply *galvanometers* that measure the electrical resistance of a person's skin. The machine will usually have two electrodes, one the patient will hold, or, someway be attached to the patient. The other electrode in the form of a pointed wand—probe, will be held by the operator of the machine and apply to *acupuncture points* on the body. The machine has a dial with a needle, or has a screen that shows some type of graph which will move in response to flow of electricity through the machine. The machine sends a current through an electrode held by the patient, the other electrode— probe, held on the skin by the operator, receives the electricity flowing through the body and carries it back into the machine which has a gauge. The needle on the gauge moves according to the strength of electrical flow which is determined by 1) amplitude of electricity generated by the machine, 2) the quality of contact on the skin of the two electrodes. If the probe is pushed hard making better skin contact the electrical flow increases, if a poor contact on the skin is made then less electrical flow. That's it! Nothing more!

A galvanometer is the same electrical tool as the "volt-meter" most men have in their tool boxes. I took my volt-meter, turned it on so it emitted a low amplitude electric current and then grasped an electrode in each hand. No swing of the needle. Then I moistened the fingers holding the electrodes and the needle moved, I squeezed harder and the needle moved further. I took one probe and touched a spot on my body and no motion of the needle, I moistened the skin and now the needle moved and the harder I pushed the probe the greater the swing of the needle in the dial.

An acupuncture point is considered by its proponents to connect to and reveal the status of energy balance of an organ, endocrine gland, immune system, or some other body response such as allergy etc. The results of the test really depend upon the operator, not some hypothetical energy balance. This type of testing is often promoted as being able to detect any and every type of disease, even before it manifests in the body. Machine testing is also proclaimed to be able to detect vitamin and mineral deficiencies or excesses, to check substances for allergic response, to select appropriate homeopathic medicinal remedies, and even to treat. Real science! NO! This is fraud or divination or both!

Let's look at some names applied to these radionic instruments: electroacupunctue according to Voll (EAV); electrodermal screening (EDS); bioelectric functions diagnosis (BFD); bioresonance therapy (BRT); bioenergy regulatory technique (BER); biocybernetic medicine (BM); computerized electrodermal screening (CEDS), electrodermal testing (EDT); limbic stress assessment (LSA); meridian energy analysis (MEA), or point testing. Additional names one may encounter are Dermatron, Vegatest, Accupath 1000, Asyra, Avatar, BICOM, BioTron, Biomeridian, Computron, Dermatron, DiagnoMetre, Eclosion, e-Lybra 8, ELAST, Interro, Interactive Query System (IQS0), I-Tronic, Kindling, LISTEN System, Mora, Matrix Physiques System, Meridian energy Analysis Device (MEAD), MSAS, Oberon, Omega, Acubase, Omega Vision, Orion System Phazx, Prognos, Prophyle, Punctos III, Syncrometer, Vantage, Victor-Vitalpunkt diagnose, Vitel 618 and ZYTO, Zapping Machine, Royal Rife Machine, Cell Com System.

What are the claims about the machines' capabilities? Let us look at an advertisement connected with the *Mora Machine*.

> The Mora technique can be likened to being a health detective. In the hands of the right practitioner it delivers a fascinating in-depth investigation of what

exactly is going on in your body on every level at that precise moment. It tests the body for imbalances as well as intolerances of foods and other allergens such as animal fur or dust, for example. It can be used to identify specific nutritional deficiencies and to find the correct homeopathic remedy.

The technique is, in fact, a form of painless electro-acupuncture; painless because there are no needles involved! Originally created for use by holistic skin therapists who continue to use it to treat disorders such as eczema, psoriasis and acne, it is now widely used to detect most disorders that manifest themselves physically, no matter what the cause.

The Mora machine itself picks up electromagnetic waves from the body and then manipulates those that have gone out of kilter by increasing or decreasing their amplitude before sending them back to the body to effect a cure. Where the detective work comes into force is in finding which nutritional or mineral deficiencies are responsible and which ones and what doses or cocktail mix of them will correct them....[478]

Bio-Resonance Frequency Therapy is vibrational technique of *recording a person's voice,* and submitting it to machine analysis. It is claimed to check for nutritional imbalances, stress, and illness. The acoustical vocal recording is claimed to provide information so that specific frequencies can be ascertained and returned, which are said to resonate and support the body. With this technique it is not necessary to make a diagnosis, as the frequencies imparted back to the body go to the core of the energy imbalance problem.

Practitioners claim that these above mentioned methods can treat ulcers, headaches, burns, chronic pain, nerve disorders, spinal cord injuries, diabetes, gum infections, asthma, bronchitis, arthritis, cerebral palsy, heart disease, and cancer. There is no scientific evidence to support any of the claims made for these devices.

VIBRATIONAL MEDICINE

I suggest that the reader do an Internet search for the term "vibrational medicine," and read some of the 900,000 web sites available under this heading. The heading on one entry I found is as follows: "*VIBRATIONAL MEDICINE, ENERGY MEDICINE, and VIBRATIONAL RESONANCE.*" As I looked through more than 300 web sites, I soon realized that the term, "vibrational medicine," is used in referring to any or all of the subjects I present in this book. The following definitions are from the Alternative Health Dictionary:

---

478   http://www.mora-akademie.org/mora-mglichkeiten.html?&L=1 (if site does not open try "mora machine")

Vibrational medicine (energetic medicine, energetics medicine, energy medicine, subtle-energy medicine, vibrational healing, vibrational therapies): "Healing philosophy" whose main "tenet" is that humans are "dynamic energy systems" ("body/mind/ spirit" complexes) and reflect "evolutionary patterns" of "soul growth." Its postulates include the following. (a) Health and illness originate in subtle energy systems; (b) These systems coordinate the "life-force" and the "physical body." (c) Emotions, spirituality, and nutritional and environmental factors affect the "subtle energy systems." Vibrational medicine embraces acupuncture, aromatherapy, Bach flower therapy, chakra rebalancing, channeling, color breathing, color therapy, crystal healing, absent healing, Electroacupuncture According to Voll (EAV), etheric touch, flower essence therapy, homeopathy, Kirlian photography, laserpuncture, the laying on of hands, meridian therapy, mesmerism, moxibustion, orthomolecular medicine, Past-life Regression, Polarity Therapy, psychic healing, psychic surgery, radionics, the Simonton method, sonopuncture, Toning, Transcendental Meditation, and Therapeutic Touch. The expressions "energy healing," "energy work," and "energetic healing work" appear synonymous with "vibrational medicine."[479]

These vibrations, frequencies, and auras that all objects are said to possess are not demonstrable by science despite the using of extremely sensitive instrumentation. This concept is found only in the writings of theosophy (pagan theology), occult writings, believers in *vitalism*, energy medicine, and New Age writings. True science is often quoted, with an attempt to blend it into the vital force concept so that it looks like true science, but the connection is just not there. Yes, sometimes the machine or pendulum makes a correct diagnosis, but mostly it is incorrect. If it is not true science, how can it be correct any time? How does divination give correct answers at any time or with any method? A power does direct divination—the power of demons or fallen angels. Because a machine gives a correct diagnosis at times does not prove it works by the laws of science. Because a method of treatment may seem to bring healing does not prove the method is following God's laws of physics.

It is worth noting the conclusions of the Theosophical Research Center in its publication, *The Mystery of Healing, page 63:*

It is now admitted by those who use the various types of diagnostic machines associated with radiesthesia that for successful work it is necessary to have present a human operator of a special type (*i.e.*, one with occult abilities). It is also well known that some operators are more proficient than others, while in the case of certain people, the machine will not work at all.[480]

---

479   http://www.experiencefestival.com/alternat health dictionary - v
(reference above is now off line).
480   Wilson, Weldon, *Occult Shock and Psychic Forces,* Master Books, San Diego, CA, (1980), p. 198.

In psychometry, an object that a person has handled such as a glass, book, or anything else, can be taken and *dowsed* (using pendulum or radionic machine) to answer questions or to determine the proclaimed energy imbalance in the person, thus giving answers as to how to treat for illness. A doll may be used to represent a person and the pendulum held over it to identify the location of illness.

OUIJA BOARD

The forms of divination used for medical reasons presented in the preceding pages are performed on, or for, someone. They are not designed to be used by one's self. The Ouija board allows a person to divine for himself. If there are questions concerning health relating to diagnosis or treatment, these questions can be asked so as to receive a yes or no answer. The Ouija board can spell out words and give numbers.

The Ouija board is flat with the words *yes* to one side (left or right) and *no* to the other. The letters of the alphabet are also on the face of the board, along with numbers zero through nine. There is a small heart-shaped board on which to place one's hands. When questions are asked of the Ouija board, the small heart-shaped board will slide on the surface of the Ouija board and point with its tip to *yes* or *no*, or to various letters and/or numbers so as to spell out words or numbers, thereby answering the question asked of the board.

The Ouija board is frequently used in parties or at other gatherings of people. This is a method of divination that began in Europe in the late 1700's or early 1800's. Baron von Reichenbach, a student of Mesmer, is credited by Garrison in *History of Medicine,* p. 369, with initiating it. However, almost all techniques have an ancient history of use.

This method of divination, like crystals, seems to be a fast-track for contact with the spirits. Where there has been use of the board, it is not unusual to hear of strange physical phenomena occurring in the home or location of use. This may manifest by objects moving around the house, doors opening and closing with no one present, and many other physical manifestations. A person repeatedly using the Ouija board is subject to demon possession.

The answers coming from divination are accurate and true many times, but at other times they lie. The devil uses these answers to his advantage; an accurate answer may be given in order to gain our interest and confidence. We can be sure that in the long run, his, Satan's, interest is in our destruction. The highest level and most deceptive divination is when man is led to believe he is communicating with the dead.

> For the living know that they shall die, but the dead know not anything....
> (Ecclesiastes 9:5).

There is danger in consulting cultist physicians. ...

> Angels of God will preserve His people while they walk in the path of duty, but there is no assurance of such protection for those who deliberately venture upon Satan's ground (see appendix H). An agent of the great deceiver will say and do anything to gain his object. It matters little whether he calls himself a 'spiritualist,' an 'electric physician,' or a 'magnetic healer.'[481]

Isaiah 8:19, 20 state it very plain:

> And when they shall say unto you, seek unto them that have familiar spirits, and unto wizards (diviners) that peep, and that mutter: should not a people seek unto their God? For the living to the dead? To the law and to the testimony: if they speak not according to this word, it is because there is no light in them.

Satan's systems of deception start very innocently, and then when our interest is developed we are led on to more involved practices. These in turn can lead to developing psychic powers and communication with spirit entities, animal entities, etc. Channeling allows for demonic possession of our minds and souls. The end result is loss of eternal life.

When so many different instruments and methods can be used to obtain answers to questions and to receive information that is requested, it becomes obvious that the instruments are only a ploy. The real reason is the connection between the mind of the one seeking information and the *intelligence* that gives the answers, namely Satan or his angels. This same situation is seen in the practice of the different martial arts derived from qi gong (manipulation of vital energy), or using a crystal to direct channeling of energy and spirits.

CONCLUSIONS ON DIVINATION

In the use of the pendulum, what can it do that scientific instruments cannot do? The pendulum can work from maps or dolls, and from long distances; it can find a vein of water or metal, making it possible to cover a considerable area in a rapid manner. It can diagnose and select the remedy. One can ask the pendulum questions and receive a *yes* or *no* answer. These are things scientific instrumentation cannot do.

---

481   White, E. G.; *Evangelism,* Pacific Press Pub. Assn., Mountain View, CA (1887), p. 607.

It is interesting to note that the dowser's ability may be blunted or turned off by his own doubts, or by the presence of someone who is a strong disbeliever.

> The rod must be held with indifference, for if the mind is occupied by doubts, reasoning, or other operation that engages the animal spirits, it will divert their powers from being exerted in this process, in which their instrumentality is absolutely necessary: from whence it is that the rod constantly answers in the hands of peasants, women and children, who hold it simply without puzzling their minds with doubts and reasoning. Whatever may be thought of this observation it is a very just one, and of great consequence in the practice of the rod.[482]

It is obvious that the power and intelligence involved is not operating under the rules of our physical laws which do not vary and do not depend upon a *sensitive* person to demonstrate or utilize them. Ben Hester, in his book, *Dowsing, an Exposé of Hidden Occult Forces,* shares with us his and his two friends' eight-year foray into searching for answers to the power behind these practices. He started as an avid believer that the power in dowsing could be explained and was seated in the science of physics that is yet unknown. His friends held the opposite opinion. They joined their talents, energy, and time to pursue an exhaustive study and examination of the subject.

They examined a large volume of the writing and history of dowsing. What stood out was that those writers believing in the subject of dowsing tended to exclude negative remarks and this same trait of presenting only biased views seemed to prevail in books against the practice. There is a 500 year history of writings in many languages telling of dowsing accomplishments, but also books showing the failures of the practice. Throughout this period, the explanation for the power that often did perform some outstanding feat of delivering knowledge could never be arrived at, or agreed upon, even by the dowsers themselves. Hester makes the following comment:

I had a nearly closed mind in favor of dowsing as a not-yet-understood physical phenomenon. The discovery of contradictions in the information from field interviews and written material on dowsing was the beginning. Once my eyes were opened to the fact of the truly supernatural aspect of dowsing and the fact that it had never been satisfactorily explained in the five hundred years of written material–even to the community of dowsers–my own questioning began.[483]

---

482 Hitching, Francis, *Earth Magic*, Morrow, NY, (1977), p. 196.
483 Hester, Ben, *Dowsing an Exposé of Hidden Occult Forces,* Leaves of Autumn Books, Payson, AZ, (1982), p. ix–x.

The answers found by Hester and his friends to the question of what power is involved in dowsing were "found to be shocking.[484]

> When all the theories were compared, all the opinions evaluated, and all the contradictions considered, the ancient biblical condemnation of *divination* began to make sense. In fact the biblical description of dowsing, the death penalty imposed for practicing it, and the exposing of its power source is the only reasonable consideration to be found. It is the only explanation avoided in all dowsing literature.[485]

The past 200 years have seen contention between dowsers and science. Those involved in divination want so much to be able to show that their work is scientific, yet the proof has been elusive. It is an accepted truth that dowsing organizations admit and write that they have no explanation for the feats that they perform. The dowser sees it as a power that has yet to be discovered but is in the physical world, or as some extra talent given to an individual as is music or other artistic ability.

The pagan and nature worshiper sees divination as an extension of his mind which has merely been expanded by a simple procedure. He believes that the intelligence of the universe rests within his mind and is only waiting to be released. The field of science that tests and observes for consistent results tends to see divination as trickery and chance, and to deny that a special power is involved.

There is a third explanation to be considered. As the Bible-believing Christian reads the Bible and he is told of the power of Satan and his angels. The Christian sees two conflicting powers, the devil and his angels, and Christ, the Divine Son of God, and His angels. The power of Satan does not always do evil; many times it will do good and marvelous acts to gain men's loyalty. Eventually, man will suffer the consequences for choosing to follow and utilize the directions and power of Satan, but it may not be until the judgment day. By accepting his power, we, in essence, choose him as our lord.

I believe the power and intelligence acting in divination to be of Satan. This power has intelligence to be able to answer "yes" or "no" to any question in the universe. It does not matter one twit as to the instrument used in the divination in obtaining the knowledge desired and sought. It has to do with giving the "will" of the diviner to this power. When the divining instrument "bobs," indicating one-foot distance in America, but a meter in Europe, and this measurement is actually set by the mind of the dowser, there can be no other answer. When dowsing can be done over an individual, or from a saliva

---

484 *Ibid.*, on back cover of book.
485 *Ibid.*

sample, a hair, or an object the individual has handled, from a thousand miles distant, there can be no other answer.

The Bible tells of the response of the Ephesians when they were converted and considered their interest in witchcraft prior to conversion. They made a bold move:

> ...Many of them also which used curious arts brought their books and burned them before all men: and they counted the price of them and found it fifty thousand pieces of silver.[486]

E.G. White shares the following comments on the acts of the Ephesians:

> When the Ephesians were converted, they changed their habits and practices. Under the conviction of the Spirit of God, they acted with promptness, and laid bare all the mysteries of their witchcraft. They came and confessed, and showed their deeds, and their souls were filled with holy indignation because they had given such devotion to magic, and had so highly prized the books in which the rules of Satan's devising had laid down the methods whereby they might practice witchcraft. They were determined to turn from the service of the evil one, and they brought their costly volumes and publicly burned them. Thus they made manifest their sincerity in turning to God....[487]

Further comments were made by the same author in her book *Messages to Young People*:

> Those on *divination* contained rules and forms of communication with evil spirits. They were the regulations of the worship of Satan, —*directions for soliciting his help and obtaining information from him.* By retaining these books, the disciples would have exposed themselves to temptation; by selling them they would have placed temptation in the way of others. They had renounced the kingdom of darkness, and they did not hesitate at any sacrifice to destroy its power. Thus the truth triumphed over men's prejudices, their favorite pursuits, and their love of money.[488]

---

486   *King James Bible,* Acts 19:19.
487   White, E.G., *Messages to Young People,* Southern Publishing Assn., Nashville, TN, (1930), p. 275.
488   White, E.G., *Life Sketches from the Life of Paul,* Review and Herald Publishing Association, Hagerstown, MD, (1974), p. 138.

CHAPTER 17

THOSE WHO PRACTICE MAGIC ARTS

In Greek Mythology, Odysseus learns that his men have just been turned into swine when given a *potion* by Circe. Hermes gives Odysseus a protective herb, and when Circe offers him the *potion* he drinks it without harm.

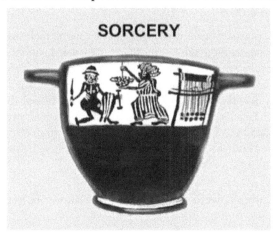

Figure 39. sorcery cup

In ancient times, the use of herbs, special concoctions for creating magic, and a variety of incantations were used to create mind-changing experiences. Plants with psychedelic properties are often used in Wicca (witchcraft), Satanism, occult magic, and shamanistic cultures to produce altered states of consciousness and to facilitate contact with the spirit world.[489] Today, many substances are commonly used to affect the mind; even though they are not taken for a psychic experience or to facilitate contact with the spirits, they actually do alter the mind to a varying extent. Mind-altering substances include tobacco, alcohol, marijuana, different narcotics, amphetamines (speed), cocaine, peyote, and other various plants such as certain mushrooms; even some prescription pharmaceuticals might be included in this list. Worldwide, there is "enchantment with the use of drugs." Should we also include caffeine?

---

489   Ankerberg, John; Weldon, John; *Can You Trust Your Doctor?*, Wolgemuth & Hyatt, Brentwood, TN, (1991), p. 257.

The *King James Bible* tells us what will be the end of those practicing *"sorcery."* The *New International* version of the Bible translates the same word from the original Greek, as *"those who practice magic arts."* They do not obtain eternal life and translation to heaven.

> Blessed are they that do His commandments, that they may have the right to the tree of life, and may enter in through the gates into the city. But outside are dogs, and *sorcerers (those who practice magic arts*, NIV) and whoremongers and murderers and idolaters and whosoever loveth and maketh a lie. (Revelation 22:14, 15).

What is their eventual end?

> ...sorcerers and idolaters and all liars, shall have their part in the lake which burneth with fire and brimstone, which is the second death. (Revelation 21:8).

Why does God destroy the sorcerers (those who practice magic arts)?

> ..for by their sorceries were all nations deceived. (Revelation 18:23-24).

> Neither repented they of their murders, nor of their sorceries, nor of their fornication, nor of their thefts. (Revelation 9:21).

What is *sorcery* and who is a *sorcerer*? In the book of Revelation in the King James version of the Bible, the word sorcerer has been translated from the Greek words "pharmakeia," "pharmakeus," and "pharmakos," all, according to *Young's Analytical Analysis*, have the meaning of "enchantment with drugs," "charm," and/or "remedy." *Webster's New World Dictionary Third Edition*, lists: "witchcraft," "magic," and enchantments," as synonyms for sorcery. It is defined as follows: "1) the supposed use of an evil supernatural power over people and their affairs: witchcraft, black magic." (Examples are: to cast a spell to cause harm to something or someone); 2) seemingly magical power, influence, or charm." This definition does not imply causing harm but influencing an event, situation, or person.

Young's Analytical Concordance of the Bible presents a broader definition of the word sorcery as it has been used in the King James Version. The Hebrew words *kashaph, kashap*, and *kashaphim*, meaning "wizard" or "witchcraft," are translated in the King James Bible as *"sorcerer,"* as is the Hebrew word *anan* which refers to *"observing the clouds,"* a form of divination. The Greek words *mageia* and *magos,* or "magic" in English, are likewise translated sorcerer. Witchcraft, one of the synonyms of sorcery, is given additional synonyms by the concordance: *divination, charm* and *remedy*.

Webster's New World Dictionary further expands the meaning of sorcerer by defining *magic* as use of charms, spells, rituals to control and/or cause events, or to govern forces–occultism, baffling effects and or illusions; truly, the practice of magic arts. In this chapter the word sorcery is used as defined by the synonyms and expanded definitions. I do not refer to black magic or to placing a curse on something or someone. The sorcerers will, in all probability, have as their goal to be helpful and to do well for others, yet the end result of following their advice or leading will be our loss.

A sorcerer could be one associated with alchemy, as the ancient alchemists concocted drugs and hallucinogens.[490] Manly Hall, in his book *The Secret Teachings of All Ages,* tells us that alchemy and astrology are the oldest sciences of the world. He tells us that mastery of these sciences would restore man from the curse of the forbidden fruit so that he could again enter the Garden of Eden.[491] Alchemy was considered a science of multiplication and a process of improving upon what already existed.

Not only was alchemy considered a science, it was a religion teaching that God is in everything, a Universal Intelligence, a Universal Spirit, found in all matter.[492] A common definition of an alchemist is one who tries to turn base metal into gold. Certainly that was one goal, but it also was a ploy to divert the attention from the true nature of the alchemist–that of bringing about a transmutation of material substance. This, in turn, would bring about a change of his spirit from being mortal to immortal.

During the middle ages, alchemy was forbidden by the universal church, and one practicing it could be sentenced to death. The common definition of an alchemist was a person who tried to turn base metal into gold; but many alchemists, in truth, practiced an occultist pagan religion. They were ridiculed because people really thought they believed that substances could be turned into gold, however, they were able to practice their occultic religion unrecognized. Alchemists were found all over the world working not only with metals, but experimenting with plants, and subsequently finding many drugs and psychedelic substances. Hallucinogens and mind-altering substances were used at times to facilitate contact with the spirit world. One author's definition of alchemy is:

> Our work ...is the conversion and change of one being into another being, one thing into another thing, weakness into strength, bodily into spiritual nature.[493]

490   Steed, Earnest; *Two Be One,* Logos International, Plainsfield, NJ, (1978), p. 95.
491   Hall, Manly P., *The Secret Teachings of All Ages,* Jeremy P. Tarcher/Penguin of Penguin Group Inc. New York, NY, (1928), p. 494.
492   *Ibid.,* p. 498.
493   Cirlot; *Dictionary of Symbols,* Philosophical Library, NY, (1962), p. 8 reported in Two Be One by Steed, p. 89.

The forerunner of a *chemist* was the alchemist. He not only looked for a way to transform one substance into another, he also was looking for some magical substance from mineral or herb that had the *secret of life, bringing immortality when consumed.*[494]

Earnest Steed, in his book *Two Be One*, makes the following statement.

> At the root of all alchemy was astrology with its macrocosm, microcosm, and transformation.[495]

Various secret societies, Cabalists, Masons, and Rosicrucians, adhered to the philosophy of alchemy down through the ages.[496] *Morals and Dogma of the Ancient Accepted Scottish Rite of Freemasonry* by Albert Pike, has twenty pages [772–792] on the philosophical doctrine of the alchemists.

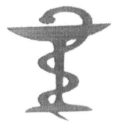

Figure 40. Thoth's sign

Manley Hall, a respected Masonic writer, tells us that alchemy was the secret art of the land of Khem (Ham), or Egypt.[497] Thoth (another name for Cush), was known as the moon god in Egypt. The same god, called Hermes in Greece, was also known as Mercury.[498] The Thoth sign is a flask with a snake coiled around it or a Y-shaped tree with the snake ascending it. This sign of a flask with the snake, can be seen on signs at pharmacies in many countries.

The symbol of snakes entwining a rod, staff, or tree (*caduceus*), is an ancient symbol associated with medicine and healing. Mesopotamians considered the intertwining of serpents as the god of healing. (A 4000-year-old beaker with a caduceus on its sides was found in Mesopotamia and is in the Louvre Museum in Paris. It is also shown in the book *Medicine: an Illustrated*

---

494   Steed, op. cit., p. 93.
495   *Ibid.*, p. 92.
496   Pike, Albert, *Morals and Dogma of the Ancient Accepted Scottish Rite of Freemasonry*, LL.H. Jenkins, Inc., Edition Book Manufacturers, Richmond, VA, (1871), pp. 772-792.
497   Hall, Manly P., *The Secret Teachings Of All Ages, Tarcher*/Penguin Books, 375 Hudson Street, New York, NY (1928), pp. 494–509.
498   *Ibid.*, p. 494; Hislop, Alexander, *The Two Babylons*, Loizeaux Brothers, Neptune New Jersey, (1858), p. 25 and footnote, p. 26.

History by Lyons and Petrucelli.) The Greek god of healing, Asclepios, had as its symbol *one* snake twined around a rod or staff (Thoth symbol).

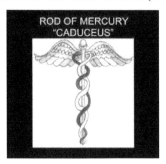

Figure 41 caduceus

I had the privilege of visiting the ruins of an ancient Asclepios temple of healing in Pergamum, Turkey. The temple still had in its ruins this symbol of a snake climbing a flask and entwining itself around the base. This temple was associated with an ancient medical school, at which the physician Galen was a professor. His concept of disease and healing dominated the *mind-set* of medical practice for more than 1500 years.

The alchemist, the pseudo-scientist in China, also searched for the elixir of eternal life, which he felt was needed in order to harness the energy that created all things, including life. The Taoist alchemist thought he could find a "potion" which contained the secret to life. Over thousands of years, as the alchemist looked for that secret to life, he tested a vast array of substances. He did not comprehend the biochemical aspects of the substance he tested, so the testing of the potions was not always free of danger. In the book, *Secrets of the Alchemist,* we are told of the ultimate goal of laboratory alchemy in China—to produce the elixir of immortality, and:

> According to Chinese records, a number of alchemists–and several emperors–succumbed to fatal doses of these mystical substances. Often the cause was mercury poisoning, since many alchemical recipes called for ingredients of pure mercury or mercuric compounds.[499]

Pharmaceutical science of today is the study of the biochemical properties of a substance and its interaction with the biochemistry of a living subject. The ancient alchemist had no comprehension of either the biochemistry of a plant, or understanding of living organisms. Since man sinned and was driven from the Garden of Eden and lost access to the tree of life, he has ever

---

499   Editors of Time-Life books, Secrets of the Alchemists, Time-Life Books, Alexandria, VA, (1990), p. 110.

been looking for the *secret of life*. He attempted to find it through alchemy by blending substances, transforming a substance, or creating a potion that would hopefully give eternal life. The ancient pagan pantheistic beliefs teach that there is constant transformation and change. The Pa Kua, (Chinese circle of harmony), is also a symbol of this concept.

The European alchemist sought to find and capture the *vital energy* that he thought gave life. It was very elusive. The Chinese alchemist looked for it in some herb or plant so as to make a potion that could then be administered. Perhaps this helps explain why the Chinese have so many herbs as medicinals– the constant quest to find one that would bestow eternal life.

Alcohol was called the *"water of life."* It was cold, but tasted hot; it was considered water and fire, elements that were regarded as creative.

> The words *whiskey* and *vodka* both mean, *water of life,* conveying the belief that opposites were blended to achieve life.[500]

Ancient medical treatment involved the use of a great many practices and substances in an attempt to relieve disease. It not only involved herbs and concoctions, but minerals, acts, dances, rituals of many types, and the many preparations the alchemists had made. *Hippocrates* (460-370 B.C., *and Greek medicine,* brought about a change to medical treatment and influenced the thinking of doctors for 400–500 years. He used very few of the usual treatment modalities and taught that disease was related to lifestyle. He believed in the cosmic forces, the four humors (fluids), and the dualism concept, yet he felt that *exercise* and *rest, nutrition* and *excretion*, were the great influences for health or for disease.[501]

After Hippocrates, the physician *Galen* (129-200 A.D.) changed the *mind-set* of medicine. Hippocrates' influence lasted 400 or more years, but Galen's influence lasted more than 1500 years. Galen was at the Asclepios healing center and medical school in Pergamos of Asia Minor (Turkey). Hippocrates had brought in a breath of fresh air to medicine and looked at lifestyle as the greatest influence on disease. He advocated living in such a way as to lessen illness. Galen turned the mind of physicians the other way. He advocated the use of many drugs. *Theriac* was a mixture of more than 70 minerals and substances (eventually over 200) that Galen advocated. These herbs and substances were blended together for use as a universal antidote for illness, snake bites, or any type of disorder.[502] Theriac as a universal treatment concoction was used until

---

500   Steed, op. cit. p. 93.
501   Lyons, Albert S. M.D., Petrucelli, H. M.D., *Medicine an Illustrated History,* Harry N. Abrams, Inc. Publishers, NY, (1978), p. 195.
502   *Ibid.,* p. 259.

the late 1800's in Europe. Today a similar popular medicinal is to be found in Russia. It is called *Mumio*, and contains approximately 50 different substances. Masonic writer Manley Palmer Hall, states the following:

> Upon the authority of Hippocrates, Galen, and Avicenna, medieval astrologers and physicians developed an elaborate system of correspondences between the planets and herbs, chemicals, and mineral medicines. They administered them according to the rules of sympathy and antipathy, and judged the disease by the afflicting planet and its aspects.[503]

The intrigue to treat disease with some sort of mineral, herb, or concoction has been present throughout time and has continued to our present day. There are many proven valuable pharmaceutical therapies in use, but the need for their use often could be greatly reduced by following a different lifestyle of exercise and diet. Is it feasible that by depending upon a medicinal rather than lifestyle changes thus eliminating or reducing the need for therapy could fall under the definition of sorcery? Pharmaceuticals are heavily used in the mind therapy sciences, from anxiety, attention deficit disorder, depression, to psychosis. There are times when nothing short of a specific medicine will be of value in treatment; however, for many problems there are other solutions. It is man's preoccupation with the belief that for every symptom and distress there is a medicinal therapy that could be thought of as a deception or sorcery.

Wednesday Feb. 9, 2011 *The Oregonian* a Portland, Oregon newspaper carried and article entitled "Take two pills and call me in 2000 years." Underwater archeologists had found a ship wreck (age— 2000+ years) in the Mediterranean Sea 40 years ago, but just recently the Smithsonian Institute had analyzed the pills found in a container in the ship. These were medicinal tablets. DNA revealed them to be a variety of herbs—celery, alfalfa, wild onion, radish, cabbage, wild carrot, yarrow, jack bean and hibiscus, willow, aster, common bean and nasturtium. This same article tells that *The Hippocratic Collection* is a series of ancient Greek texts attributed to Hippocrates which refers to 380 medicinal herbs used for a variety of ailments. Records show that Greek physicians used 45 different herbs in the pharmaceutical approach to health and healing.

One of the leading causes of death is an adverse reaction from drugs even when given properly by the practitioner. When we combine the accidental wrong medicine, or overdose etc., we recognize there is a major problem with use of medicinal therapies. These problems not only occur from physicians, but from patients as well. It would be a wise choice to seek ways of dealing with illness and disorders with as few medicines as possible.

---

503   Hall, Manley, *The Story of Healing,* Citadel Press, NY, (1928), p. 162.

In the writings of E.G. White, the words "sorcery," "sorcerer," and "sorceries" are found many times. She equates the word "sorcery" with spiritualism, witchcraft, magic, hypnosis, magnetic healers, false healers, earthly enchantments, divination, love of wealth, and fame. Whatever form of deceit the devil uses to confuse and deceive men comes under her definition. There is a movement with some physicians across this country to blend conventional medicine with alternative and complementary methods; this blending is referred to as *integrative medicine.* There has been a rapid increase in the number of clinics adopting this *mix* of the scientific with the non-scientific. This blending is most deceptive for people who are unaware of the devil's sorceries.

> Andrew Weil M.D. has devoted the past 40 years to developing, teaching and educating others on the principles of integrative medicine. Weil is an internationally recognized expert on integrative medicine, medicinal herbs, and mind-body inter-actions.... He is a clinical professor of internal medicine and the founder and director of the Program of Integrative Medicine (PIM) at the College of Medicine, University of Arizona in Tucson. Weil received both his medical degree and his undergraduate AB degree in biology (botany) from Harvard University.[504]

Dr. Weil is the author of many books. A review of the titles of these books reveals his interest in meditation, deep breathing, guided imagery, sound, and music therapy. He also has vast influence with the public. He trains other doctors in converting to the integrative method of practice. The following quotation will give some insight to the direction of his beliefs and teachings and their orientation. Dr. Weil wrote about his *fire walking*:

> I once did a forty-foot walk over an extremely hot bed of coals without experiencing any burns or even any sensation of heat. (The coals just felt crunch.) This was in a large group with Tony Robins, where everyone got very charged dancing to African drums, chanting, and engaging in other rituals. On another occasion I got burned attempting a mere six-foot walk over cooler coals. On that occasion, there were no exciting rituals, no charismatic leader, and only a small group of not-very bonded individuals.[505]

Upon reading the above comment from Dr. Weil I thought again of the verse in Deuteronomy 18:9-12:

---

504 http://www.webmd.com/andrew-weil
505 http://www.drweil.com/drw/u/id/QAA221693#_ga=1.182122402.481573435.1465163041
     http://www.maslow.com/

When thou art come into the land which the Lord thy God giveth thee, thou shalt not learn to do after the abominations of those nations. There shall not be found among you anyone that maketh his son or his daughter *to pass through the fire*, or that useth divination, or an observer of times, or an enchanter, or a witch. Or a charmer, or a consulter with familiar spirits, or a wizard, or a necromancer. *For all that do those things are an abomination unto the Lord;* and because of these abominations the Lord thy God doth drive them out from before you.

What is it that attracts and motivates people to fire-walk? What is to be gained from it? What prevents burns to the feet? It is an act performed in many places of the world. I lived for a short time in Phuket, Thailand, where once a year a festival was held for worshiping Satan. It was my understanding that fire-walking was a part of this festival. I have been in *pagan provinces* of Russia where similar festivals are held. Revelation 13:13, 14 (NIV) gives an answer to the above question:

And he performed great and miraculous signs, even causing fire to come down from heaven to earth in full view of men. *Because of the signs he was given power to do on behalf of the first beast, he deceived the inhabitants of the earth.*

Satan will use fire to cause men to believe that man is God. God sent fire from heaven to ignite the sacrifice of Abel; at Solomon's dedication of the temple; at the sacrifice Elijah offered on Mount Carmel, and He sent fire to consume the soldiers of Ahaziah, king of Israel, when they went to arrest Elijah. In the days of Daniel God preserved the three Hebrews in the fiery furnace.

Just because God has allowed Satan to have power over fire, we need not be deceived if all miracles are tested by the scriptures.

By sending fire down from heaven at the end of time and protecting those who walk in fire, does not Satan hold himself out to be God? Does he not deceive by these miracles he performs? Should we not carefully consider the teachings of those people who are led by his power? They may be highly trained in the science of conventional medicine, yet the deception comes as they blend in Satan's method of healing with God's methods. Let the followers of Christ beware.

Another popular physician and author, Gabriel Cousens M.D. , also leads the march toward integrative medicine. His orientation is revealed by his quotation found in chapter 7 (Ayurveda) in this book. Dr. Cousens has a popular following in regard to his dietary writings. He writes of foods being held over chakra areas of the body to establish which colored foods, when eaten, would most enhance the power of the chakras. His books strongly reflect Ayurvedic and Hindu concepts.

Another powerful influence enticing interest in New Age/New Spirituality exists in the USA, Canada, and in areas of the world where the television show of Oprah Winfrey penetrates. She has featured many individuals on a repeated basis who by their appearances on her show and their books, promoted by Oprah, have given great exposure and the potential of acceptance of New Age/Neo-Pagan/New Spirituality concepts by vast millions of people. Marianne Williamson famous for her promotion of A Course on Miracles which originally had been channeled by a spirit to Helen Shucman; Gary Zukov and his book, *Seat of a Soul,* espouses the divinity of man; Oprah's endorsement of the book *The Secret,* by Rhonda Byrne which teaches that we are all *God*; Echart Tolle and his book published in 2008 entitled *A New Earth Awakening To Your Life's Purpose,* teaching a shift in consciousness with an indwelling of divinity referred to as *Christ*; promotion of the popular Mehemet Oz M.D., a Muslim and Sufi (mystical order in Islam), intertwines the occult with his knowledge of nutrition and lifestyle; all recipients of powerful promotion by Oprah's show. Dr. Oz now has his own TV show wherein he mingles the good with the bad. His wife is a Reiki Master also a follower of the late world renowned spiritualist Emmanuel Swedenborg; Dr. Oz is a strong promoter of her spirit powered healing technique.

Rick Warren, *America's pastor*, author of *The purpose Driven Church* and *The Purpose Driven Life,* launched January 15, 2011 a 52 week course from his Saddleback Church on wellness. This program is titled *The Daniel Cha*llenge and was a weekly program guided by Mehemet Oz M.D., Daniel Amen M.D., and Mark Hyman M.D., all well trained specialists and versed in health and nutrition but also heavily engaged in promoting New Age/Neo-Pagan concepts. They bring up-to-date nutrition and healthful living information, but blend in Eastern meditation techniques as an important component of health.

Rick Warren has far reaching influence, his organization is extended to and has communication with more than 160 nation network, and 400,000 ministers and priests have attended his teaching seminars.[506]

From the pen of Ellen White we find:

> The God of heaven came to Paul, and through the Spirit of God miracles were wrought. But there were some men there, who tried to imitate the miracles, and the evil spirit fell upon them, and they were beaten and bruised because they

---

506 Smith, Warren, *A Wonderful Deception,* Lighthouse Trails Publishing, Silverton, OR, (2009), p.ix.

took the name of Jesus to use in their sorcery. *They cannot mix; they cannot mix at all.*[507]

God's design for health and healing is not to be mixed with that of Satan's. Let us review the basics of what has been presented in this book. The devil desires to draw men's minds away from recognizing God the Creator. He devised a counterfeit story of creation based upon the blending of two opposing divisions of a supposed universal energy, which is considered god. This energy, when blended in the right proportions, brought about the creation of the universe (cosmos), earth, and man. This universal energy (god) is said to be in all substances of the universe, including man. Man need only to bring the god within himself to a higher level to obtain immortality.

Man's journey on earth, according to the pagan, is to escape from the cycle of reincarnation, and to progress upward to become an ascended master or god himself. This may take many lifetimes. Many ways are promoted to shorten the journey to godhood, often called *higher consciousness.* Yoga meditation, yoga exercises, qi gong exercises, and psychedelic drugs used to connect with spirit entities are some of the ways believed to shorten the pathway to Nirvana or god-hood. Another way to hasten this progression toward godhood is to be a follower of a guru. I invite the reader to pause and reflect upon the contrast between the theory and variety of modalities presented by *energy or vibrational medicine,* and the instructions God gave through E.G. White in 1863 and 1865 as to how the Health Reform Institute was to be operated. Our Creator was to be upheld as the Source of healing and His physical and spiritual laws were to be followed. The plan of operation was simple: no coffee, tea, alcohol, or tobacco; plant-food diet with only small amounts of milk, cream and eggs, if at all; exercise; rest; regularity of meals with no eating between, abundant use of water for bathing and drinking, and placing our trust in God for healing.

There is a power in the universe and it is the power of God. It is not inherent in the planets. It is not hidden away in the mind of man waiting for some gimmick to release it. It is not accessed by pendulums or radionic machines, or by mindless meditation. The power of God is accessed by prayer and Bible study, and obedience to His physical and spiritual laws.

Like the Samaritans who were deceived by Simon Magus, the multitudes, from the least to the greatest, give heed to these *sorceries,* saying: 'this is the great

507   White, E.G., *Sermons and Talks Volume* II, Chapter 8 – Heaven's Part in Life's Conßict, manuscript 1, (1890), p. 61.

power of God.'[508] But the people of God will not be misled. The teachings of this false Christ are not in accordance with the Scriptures.[509]

Take each verse of this chapter (Revelation 18), and read it carefully, especially the last two: 'And the light of a candle shall shine no more at all in thee; and the voice of the bridegroom and of the bride shall be heard no more at all in thee: for thy merchants were the great men of the earth; for by thy *sorceries (magic arts)* were all nations deceived. And in her was found the blood of prophets, and of saints, and of all that were slain upon the earth.'[510]

...It is fondly supposed that heathen superstitions have disappeared before the civilization of the twentieth century. But the word of God and the stern testimony of facts declare that sorcery is practiced in this age as verily as in the days of the old time magicians. The ancient system of magic is, in reality, the same as what is now known as modern spiritualism.[511]

Those who give themselves up to the sorcery of Satan may boast of great benefit received; but does this prove their course to be wise or safe? What if life should be prolonged? What if temporal gain should be secured? Will it pay in the end to have disregarded the will of God? All such apparent gain will prove at last an irrecoverable loss. We cannot with impunity break down a single barrier which God has erected to guard His people from Satan's power.[512]

---

508 White, E. G., *The Great controversy*, Pacific Press, Nampa Idaho, (1888), pp. 624,625, Acts 8:10.

509 White, op. cit., p. 625.21.

510 White, E.G., 16 *Manuscript Releases*, The Ellen G. White Estate Inc., Washington, DC, p. 270.2.

511 White, E.G., *Acts of the Apostles*, Pacific Press Publishing Assn., Mountain View, CA, (1911), p.289.

512 White, E.G., *Evangelism*, Review and Herald Publishing Association, Washington D.C., (1946) p. 219.

CHAPTER 18
HYPNOSIS

I once received a call from the hospital to come quickly to care for a lady who had been water skiing. She had fallen into the water and had been run over by a boat, sustaining severe injury to one leg. Upon reaching the emergency room, I saw the patient had several huge lacerations across her thigh, inflicted by the propeller of the boat. She had lost much blood and looked pale. The bleeding had stopped so there was time to give her blood and fluids intravenously before taking her to the operating room. The injuries were so large and destructive to her leg that I decided to ask a plastic surgeon to join me in caring for her in the operating room.

We were able to save the leg and expected proper healing and the return to normal use. Three days later, I scheduled a change of the bandages on the leg. By that time the bandages had crusted and dried, sticking to the wounds. Changing the dressings was going to be painful.

The plastic surgeon arrived in her room before I did and proceeded to change the dressings. When I entered the room, the patient had her eyes closed; she was not showing any tension or any sign that she was in distress. When I spoke to her, the doctor said that she was sleeping but he would awaken her soon. He finished with the new dressings then told her that he was going to count backward from 5 and when he got to zero she would awake.

He counted five, four, three, two–she began to move, one and zero–she awoke and was happy and smiling, as well as delighted that the dressings were changed and she knew nothing of the ordeal. It seemed wonderful. Who could object to such a pleasant method of dealing with injuries? I was surprised to learn that the surgeon used hypnosis. I had known him for several years and operated with him many times. I was opposed to the use of hypnosis and never suggested it to my patients. I was embarrassed to have had this happen to one of my patients without first being able to share with her my concerns about its use.

Why should I object? Was it not wonderful to relieve someone from a painful procedure? Why would I oppose this humane approach?

Was it not better than giving a pain medication an hour prior and then removing the bandages? She was wide-awake and pain free and did not remember the procedure.

Some doctors in medical practice have used hypnosis for many years and it is considered an acceptable method of treatment in the medical field. It has been used as an anesthetic in operative procedures, as well as in treatment of psychological ailments. Yet many physicians choose not to use it in their practices.

What is hypnosis? How does it work? Where does it come from? Why does not every doctor use it? These are important questions that deserve answers. Let us first look at a dictionary definition. "Hypnosis" is:

> An induced state of mind in which the subject is responsive to the suggestions of the hypnotist. This state may be to the degree of resembling sleep, called a hypnotic trance.[513]

This suggests that there are degrees of hypnosis that are below the hypnotic trance. What of its origin? Let us consider the comments made in the *New Age Encyclopedia*:

> What is now called hypnosis has existed in almost all societies in the past, though its nature was only rarely understood or appreciated. Hypnotic phenomena began to be studied in Europe in the sixteenth century, when these occurrences were attributed to magnetism, which was understood to be a subtle influence exerted by every object in the universe on every other object.[514]

The Bible tells of the serpent (in a tree) that spoke to Eve and "beguiled," or deceived her.[515]

> Satan tempted the first Adam in Eden, and Adam reasoned with the enemy, thus giving him the advantage. Satan exercised his power of *hypnotism* over Adam and Eve, and this power he strove to exercise over Christ. But after the word of Scripture was quoted, Satan knew that he had no chance of triumphing.[516]

Medical history texts record hypnotic phenomena being studied by physicians, such as Paracelsus, in Europe in the mid-16th century. Its power source was explained as a magnetic fluid which connected all substances in the universe and which could not be seen, demonstrated, or measured. In the seventeenth century it again appeared in the writings of several notorious

---

513 *Miriam Webster Advanced Dictionary.*
514 *New Age Encyclopedia,* Gale Research, Detroit, MI, (1990), p. 28.
515 Genesis 3:13; 2 Corinthians 11:3.
516 White, E.G.; Letter 159, 1903, (5BC 1081).

physicians.[517] The power of suggestion, or hypnosis, was used by these physicians to treat medical conditions.

In the eighteenth century, Emanuel Swedenburg (1688–1772) studied this *magnetism* credited to hypnotism and tied it in with his interest in the spiritual world. This, in turn, laid the grounds for spiritualism.[518] Swedenburg and his ideas of spiritualism influenced the world of the occult for nearly two centuries.

If you were to consult an encyclopedia on the word *hypnosis*, you would most likely find that a physician, Franz Anton Mesmer, is referred to as the father of modern hypnosis. He is not truly the father of hypnosis, but he did make it so well known that for nearly a century this phenomenon was known as *Mesmerism*. Let us review Dr. Mesmer's history.

He graduated from medical school in Vienna in 1766. That same year he published a book, *On the Influence of the Planets*, in which he proposed stroking diseased patients with magnets to affect a cure. In 1773, he claimed his first cure by the use of magnets. Mesmer was a believer in astrology and felt the body of man was a microcosm of the macrocosm (universe). He felt that man, earth, and the universe were tied together with a universal magnetic fluid. Mesmer continued his medical practice using magnets to cure disease.[519]

Mesmer heard of a Swabian priest, John Gassner, who was simply passing his hands across diseased bodies and effecting "cures:

> Mesmer observed Gassner and thought it was done by the power of the same magnetic fluid that he felt explained his activities with magnets. He then dispensed with the magnets and achieved equal results by use of his hands. Eventually he dispensed with the hand technique and used the mind only as the modality of influencing animal magnetism (power believed to effect hypnotism).[520]

In 1784, a book written by French doctor and spiritualist, Jean Philippe Francois Deleuze, referred to these same phenomena (hypnotism) as *animal magnetism*. Deleuze seemed to want to separate the name *Mesmer* from the method.[521]

> For much of the nineteenth century, the term '*animal magnetism*' also encompassed clairvoyance, empathy, mediumistic trances, and many other

---

517   *New Age Encyclopedia,* op. cit., (1990), p. 28.
518   *Ibid.*, p. 28.
519   *Ibid.*, pp. 28, 58.
520   *Ibid.*
521   *Ibid.*, pp. 28–29, 58.

psychic abilities and psychological phenomena, the relationships between which were far from clear.[522]

Let us briefly review the influence of Dr. Mesmer and the different methods he used in his medical therapy. First, he started by passing magnets across the bodies of his patients. He would make large tubs and fill them with chemicals to produce an electrical charge, placed on the tubs were iron knobs. People would stand around the tubs holding on to the iron knobs in order to receive *magnetic* therapy. His treatments progressed to simply passing of hands over the body.

Eventually, he used only the mind to accomplish the desired effect. The hypnotic state could be so deep that surgical procedures could be performed during the trance. To accomplish this involved not only an expert *mesmerist,* but also a willing, submissive person. A British surgeon, James Esdaile (1805–1859), practiced in India and used the trance state for anesthesia during surgery. He performed 261 painless operations with mesmerism as the only anesthetic. When he returned to Scotland, he found that mesmerism used as an anesthetic did not work well there.[523]

The inducement of the hypnotic state by suggestion was used in many ways by the various practitioners who became skilled in its use.[524] The British Medical Society, in 1893, concluded that hypnosis was a true science even though they were not able to perfectly explain it. There could be no doubt that it was much more than a sham or fake act. Great influence and results did indeed occur with its use and it appeared as though its action was only positive with little to no adverse side effects.

The American Medical Association was much slower in embracing this form of treatment. Physicians at large were not fully convinced of its value, though there was no denying that it had great power to affect a person. There was no real lasting effect on disease. It seemed to be more related to the treatment of the mind and so has not been widely used by all physicians. Hypnosis was given official sanction by the American Medical Association in 1958.

We are warned that it will be in the area of *science* that Satan will exert such deceptive practices in the last days. In the days of Paul and Timothy, there also existed false sciences and Paul gives us warnings concerning them:

> O Timothy, keep that which is committed to thy trust, avoiding profane and vain babblings, and oppositions of science falsely so called. (I Timothy 6:20).

522 *Ibid.,* p. 58.
523 Garrison, Fielding H. M.D., *History of Medicine,* W.B. Saunders & Co., Philadelphia, PA, (1929), p. 428.
524 *Ibid.,* p. 369; *New Age Encyclopedia,* (2003), p. 58.

Dr. Franz Joseph Gall (1757-1828) was an anatomy instructor. He was the first to show that different parts of the brain had specific functions.[525] He carried this too far, however, and felt that the character and personality could be recognized by observing the bumps and ridges on the skull. This idea he carried even further, suggesting that the mind, character, and personality could be altered by massage to the head, or pressure applied to specific areas of the skull. This concept was named *phrenology.*

Phrenology was a pseudo-science and was adopted by those practicing mesmerism and other occult therapies. The spiritualist movement was attracted to phrenology and mesmerism. E.G. White had much to say concerning the practice.

> Satan uses these very things to destroy virtue and lay the foundation for spiritualism.[526]

> The sciences of phrenology, psychology and mesmerism have been the channel through which Satan has come more directly to this generation, and wrought with that power which was to characterize his work near the close of probation.[527]

In a private letter to someone in 1901, Ellen White made it clear that the false sciences of phrenology and mesmerism (hypnotism) are *Satan's own science.* (Letter 130, 1901). 2 SM 349-50)

> A perilous Science: We do not ask you to place yourself under the control of any man's mind. The *mind cure* is the most awful science which has ever been advocated. Every wicked being can use it in carrying through his own evil designs. We have no business with any such science. We should be afraid of it. Never should the first principles of it be brought into any institution.[528] (Written in 1901) (Emphasis added)

> The theory of mind controlling mind was originated by Satan to introduce himself as the chief worker, to put human philosophy where divine philosophy should be. Of all the errors that are finding acceptance among professedly Christian people, none is a more dangerous deception, none more certain to separate man from God, than is this. Innocent though it may appear, if exercised upon patients, it will tend to their destruction, not to their restoration. It opens a

525 Garrison, op. cit., p. 539.
526 White, E.G., *Testimonies Vol.* 1, Pacific Press Publishing Assn., Mountain View CA, (Now Nampa, ID) (1867), pp. 296–297.
527 White E.G., *Messages to Young People, Review and Herald,* Southern Publishing Assn., Nashville, TN, (1930), p. 57.
528 White, E.G., *Medical Ministry,* Pacific Press Pub. Assn., Mountain. View, CA, (1932), p. 116.

door through which Satan will enter to take possession both of the mind that is given up to be controlled by another and of the mind that controls.[529]

The business world is offered commercial mind-training courses by a variety of teachers. Some of these courses teach hypnotism even though the title of the course will not suggest so. Course titles such as *Conditioning, Programming, Brain-wave* Training, *Alpha Training*, etc., may actually be hypnosis. There can be consequential adverse effects to the student taking part in such a course. Elmer and Alyce Green (researchers in psychology), in their book, *Beyond Biofeedback*, state that thousands of students in these courses will sooner or later experience serious mental changes such as neurosis or even psychosis. They warn that the greatest danger, however, is obtaining psychic advisers who are assistants in the course. The Greens warn that there is the possibility of mediumistic "possession" via the influence of the advisers.[530]

The point brought out by the Greens that there is great danger in allowing another individual to control or even strongly influence us in the science of *mind control,* brings to mind advice given long ago on the same point.

In April 2011, I received a copy of an article that appeared in a Colorado town's newspaper, *Highlands Ranch Herald,* April 4, 2011. This article was lauding and promoting the value of using hypnotism in childbirth. I share with you some comments found in this article.

> HypnoBirthing, which is a registered trademark, has been found to significantly reduce stress and improve the well-being of newborns, and classes are now being offered at Westridge Recreation Center. *Even the family education center at Littleton Adventist Hospital is planning on training nurses and physicians on how to assist mothers who use HypnoBirthing,* ...HynoBirthing classes teach expecting parents how to wipe away anxiety through positive thoughts and reassurance. Hypnosis CDs containing messages directed at *imaging* a healthy birth; *visualization* of good outcomes and pain-free childbirth are also part of the 2 1/2 hour class sessions. (Emphasis added)

Reading this article brought to me a feeling of sadness as I remembered the many warnings given through the years by the author E.G. White regarding Christians using hypnotism as individuals or of its practice being brought into Adventist hospitals. Note these quotations:

Warning to a Physician Who Favored Hypnosis. -- I am so weighed down in your case that I must continue to write to you, lest in your blindness you

---

529 White, E.G., *Mind, Character, and Personality* Vol. 2, Southern Publishing Assn., Nashville, TN, (1977), p.712.

530 Green, Elmer and Alyce, *Beyond Biofeedback,* Knoll Publishing Co., (1977), pp. 319-323.

will not see where you need to reform. I am instructed that you are entertaining ideas with which God has forbidden you to deal. I will name these as a species of *mind cure*. You suppose that you can use this *mind cure* in your professional work as a physician. In tones of earnest warning the words were spoken: Beware, beware where your feet are placed and your mind is carried. God has not appointed you this work. The theory of mind controlling mind is originated by Satan to introduce himself as the chief worker, *to put human philosophy where divine philosophy should be.*

No man or woman should exercise his or her will to control the senses or reason of another so that the mind of the person is rendered passively subject to the will of the one who is exercising the control. This science may appear to be something beautiful, but it is a science which you are in no case to handle.... There is something better for you to engage in than the control of human nature over human nature.

I lift the danger signal. *The only safe and true mind cure covers much. The physician must educate the people to look from the human to the divine. He who has made man's mind knows precisely what the mind needs.* (Emphasis added)[531]

A great danger occurs when we seek counseling from professional or lay counselors. The education and source of knowledge of so many of these individuals is from the cistern of modern psychology. (See Chapter 20 *Psychology—Science of the Soul*). The counselor may be a Christian, but if his education and mind are fixed in the philosophy of modern world psychological principles, his very influence on you to accept his advice has danger. The principles of counseling must come from the scriptures; our Creator is the Great Counselor.

>**Appears Valuable and Wonderful.**--In taking up the science you have begun to advocate, you are giving an education which is not safe for you or for those you teach. It is dangerous to tinge minds with the science of *mind cure*. {2MCP 714.2}

>This science may appear to you to be very valuable, but to you and to others it is a fallacy prepared by Satan. It is the charm of the serpent which stings to spiritual death. It covers much that seems wonderful, but it is foreign to the nature and spirit of Christ. *This science does not lead to Him who is life and salvation...*[532] (2MCP 714.3)

---

531   White, E.G., op. cit., p. 713-714.
532   *Ibid.*

An experienced mesmerist attempted to hypnotize Mrs. White sometime around 1845. He had proclaimed that he could do so and cause her to have a vision. She allowed him to try for 30 minutes and yet he could in no way influence her state of mind.

> I told him that the Lord had shown me in vision that mesmerism was from the devil, from the bottomless pit, and that it would soon go there, with those who continued to use it.[533]

The methods used today by Satan started in the courts of heaven and were taken to the Garden in Eden. They worked in heaven, in the garden, and they work now. We have been warned.

> There are doctors and ministers who have been influenced by the hypnotism exercised by the father of lies. Notwithstanding the warnings given, Satan's sophistries are being accepted now just as they were accepted in the heavenly courts. The science by which our first parents were deceived is deceiving men today. Ministers and physicians are being drawn into the snare.[534]

There are people who feel they are wise enough to take parts of these false sciences and use them to their advantage; but the warning is given to have nothing to do with them. Even to investigate the theories can expose us to Satan's power. Our duty is to direct the mind of man to God, the true mind therapist.

---

533   *Ibid.*, p. 719.
534   *Ibid.*, p. 719.1.

CHAPTER 19
BIOFEEDBACK

A common medical complaint with which doctors are challenged is headaches. When a patient complained of such to me I would place my hand on the back of their neck and feel for tight muscles and tender points at the base of the skull where the neck muscles attach. When there was tenderness on the skull I could be reasonably sure that that person had excess tension of the neck muscles, and the pain was a result of the chronic contraction of these muscles. The point on the skull where the muscles attach becomes sore and contributes to the headache. I would advise the patient to practice relaxing these muscles several times a day, to massage the neck muscles, apply moist heat, and to attempt to discover initiating stress factors that led to the tenseness.

In the 1960's, I read in medical journals of another method of treating people with stress headaches. This method was called *biofeedback*. Simply stated, it was a procedure where electrodes were attached to the muscles of the neck, which in turn would be attached to an oscilloscope showing electrical nerve impulses stimulating the neck muscles. With conscious effort, an individual could learn to reduce the excess nerve impulses and tension in the muscles, and the headaches would cease. Biofeedback sounded harmless and possibly might work better than the method I used. The procedure was not done by physical therapists in my area and so I never prescribed this treatment method.

Migraine headaches usually occur from a different physiological dysfunction than tension headaches. They occur on one side of the head, and usually are preceded by symptoms of dimming vision on one side and strange sensations at various locations. Sometimes apparent weakness of certain muscles will be manifest. These symptoms occur, it is believed by physicians, as a result of artery constriction over one side of the brain; after a few minutes, the same vessels will dilate resulting in pain. Many factors, including mental stress, can trigger such a headache. Present-day therapy involves using medicines to cause constriction of the dilated artery with varying degrees of relief.

This type of headache may last from a few hours to days. It is often incapacitating, affecting the ability to attend school or work. Migraine headaches are notoriously difficult to treat.

Medical literature has featured articles telling of the use of *biofeedback* as treatment for migraine headaches. These articles reported that up to 80% of patients with migraines received great relief by using biofeedback treatments. It sounded like good, safe therapy, and I never had any adverse thoughts against such a method. Over time, it was shown that many other physical ailments, such as high blood pressure, some gastrointestinal disorders, asthma, neuromuscular disorders such as post-stroke rehabilitation, cerebral palsy, spinal cord injuries, anxiety states, Reynaud's phenomena, etc., have been helped with the use of biofeedback.

In the 1980's, I began to be aware of different types of medical treatments referred to as alternative or complementary medicine. I had concerns about those treatments as it appeared to me that hypnotism— spiritualism was probably the source of their power. When reading articles and books written by Christian authors explaining the nature of certain alternative therapies, I would notice that biofeedback was included in the list of treatment methods those books advised against.

In 1987, the Biblical Research Committee of the General Conference of Seventh-day Adventists presented a report of a study entitled *The New Age Movement and Seventh-day Adventists*. In this paper is a section dealing with various medical treatment methods that were believed to be *spiritualistic* in nature. Three times the word *biofeedback* is mentioned as one such method. I found that this same labeling of biofeedback occurred in several other books written to expose spiritualism in alternative medicine methods. I was surprised and questioned this label against biofeedback. It occurred to me that I needed to do some in-depth study of biofeedback and to arrive at my own conclusion on this issue. I will share with you my discoveries.

Before proceeding with biofeedback investigation I wish to establish the definition as to the word biofeedback. It is possible in this discussion for confusion to occur between the word *monitoring* and biofeedback. Monitoring refers to some mechanical or electrical device, such as an electroencephalogram, electrocardiogram, or electromyography, which reveals electrical biological functioning. Applying electrodes to neck muscles and to an oscilloscope, wearing any type of apparatus to reveal physiological functioning such as a blood pressure monitor, is using a monitor. When I use the word *biofeedback,* I am speaking specifically to a method that uses a combination of monitoring and adding a mental act to facilitate an altered state of consciousness. This is usually achieved by use of any one or combination of the following: *muscle relaxation, deep breathing exercises*, use of a *mantra* or repetitive sentences/ phrases, and by use of *visualization*.

The special paper prepared by the Biblical Research Committee listed several sets of questions that need to be answered as a person studies medical treatment methods to determine if they are *spiritually* safe. The committee took these questions from Dr. Warren Peters' book, *Mystical Medicine*. They are excellent questions. No single question should determine the issue, but several questions, when answered, should give evidence of a spiritualistic relationship before you finalize judgment.

The first set of questions was Where did the method come from; what is its source? Does it have mystical roots? With what other therapies is it often associated? What did the founder believe? What is the life story of the founder or founders?

A renowned German brain physiologist, Oscar Vogt of the Berlin Institute, during the 1890's was using hypnosis in guided sessions. Some of the people in the sessions learned to put themselves, for a self-determined time, into a state similar to the hypnotic state they achieved with the doctor's guidance.[535],[536] Vogt found he could have these people, in their auto-hypnotic practices, treat and alleviate many different stress-like medical disorders with which they were afflicted. In the early 1900's, Johannes Schultz, a psychiatrist and neurologist in Berlin, continued the work that Vogt started. This state of self-hypnosis was called "autohypnosis."

Schultz wanted to perfect autohypnosis because it would eliminate the tendency of the participant to develop dependence on the hypnotist. It was recognized that the state of self-hypnosis could be induced by 1) using certain basic verbal formulas repeated over and over by the individual desiring autohypnosis; repeating these phrases contributed to developing a state of pronounced 2) *relaxation* of the muscular and vascular systems, as did practicing 3) *deep, slow breathing*; 4) *visualizing* colors, objects, and abstract concepts.

> This is followed by meditating on one's own feelings or on the image of another person, and finally, at the deepest level, *one may interrogate and get "answers from the unconscious"* levels of one's own nature, as Schultz put it.[537]

Dr. Wolfgang Luthe had been a student of Schultz, and continued the work after Schultz's death. Luthe called autohypnosis *autogenic training* in a book authored by Schultz and Luthe (1959). In the early 1960's, Dr. Joe Kamiya of San Francisco attached an electroencephalograph to college students' heads

535 Green, Elmer Ph.D., and Alyce M.A. , *Beyond Biofeedback,* Knoll Publishing Co., (1989), p. 26.
536 Hill, Ann, *A Visual Encyclopedia of Unconventional Medicine,* Crown Publishing Inc. NY, (1978), p. 190
537 Green, op. cit., p. 27.

to see if they could, at will, change their brain wave patterns. He found they could. He came up with the word *biofeedback.*

> He studied the brain waves of Zen meditators and proposed that it might be possible to develop a 'psychophysiology of consciousness.'[538]

Dr. Kamiya presented a lecture at the Psychophysiological Research Society meeting in 1965, which was attended by one, Elmer Green, Ph.D., a physicist and psychologist. It was the first time Dr. Green had heard of biofeedback. He was inspired to investigate this ability to self-control brainwave patterns.[539]

There were many therapists who dabbled in the use of autogenic training, but one outstanding investigative group led the way to what we now call *biofeedback.* Dr. Green, along with Alyce Green, M.A., a psychologist, and Dale Walters Ph.D., a colleague, were investigators at the Menninger Foundation, a psychiatric institute in Topeka, Kansas. In 1965, they began to explore the autogenic techniques in their research. Dr. Green developed electronic devices to monitor physiological changes while people were in autogenic training. They could see changes in the rate of nerve impulses, muscular tension and relaxation, temperature of the skin in specific locations, and brain wave amplitude and rates.

From these studies of autohypnosis or biofeedback, brain wave monitoring studies were done. By *muscle relaxation, deep slow breathing,* and use of *mantra* phrases along with *visualization,* a certain brain wave rate called *theta* could be achieved. It is at this level of brain activity that the autohypnosis takes place. Dr. Green stated the following:

> In my view theta training is a form of accelerated meditation– and the benefits to students are incalculable. They range from better physical functioning, to improved emotional balance, to sharpened intellect, to true creativity–to the solution of insoluble problems in unpredictable ways, coming into mind as from another dimension.[540]

With the addition of electronic monitors, a person could see evidence of changes in his physiology as he practiced the *autohypnosis* or *autogenic training,* or as it is now called, *biofeedback.* The Greens' work and writing for scientific journals has made biofeedback well known, and has rapidly increased belief in, and use of, this technique.

---

538 *Ibid.,* pp. 44, 118, 119.
539 *Ibid.*
540 *Ibid.,* preface xiv–xv.

At this point in our discussion of biofeedback the difference should be made clear again between *monitoring* some physiologic function of the body versus *biofeedback*. Monitoring of blood pressure, skin temperature, brain wave, or heart by appropriate mechanisms is not biofeedback. Biofeedback is a procedure wherein monitoring various physiologic activities of the body is done, but the critical difference is the added emphasis of combined use of *muscle relaxation, deep slow breathing, visualization and repeating a mantra word or phrase.* These practices together can bring about an altered state of consciousness, bringing the mind to a neutral or stilled state, opening it for spirit control.

Dr. Elmer and Alyce Green refer to biofeedback as *Western Yoga.*[541] In their book, *Beyond Biofeedback,* both Elmer and Alyce express their belief in the *universal energy* concept of the cosmos and its relationship to man. They have, from youth, studied and practiced the astrological concepts of the East. In their book preface (p. xix) they state:

> From our viewpoint, the development of full human potential starts most easily with mastery of *body* energies (through internal control of images, emotions, and volition), and the process can be extended to energies which influence the outside world.[542]

The book tells the story of their life, which is deeply entrenched in the Eastern teachings. I quote again from their book *Beyond Biofeedback*:

> During those years Alyce and I read continuously in the fields of metaphysics, parapsychology, and theosophy, searching for and constructing a framework of ideas that would correspond with our own experiences and at the same time be reasonable in terms of a possible science in which mind and matter were not forever separate.[543]

The practice of using *mantras, muscle relaxation, rhythmic deep breathing,* and *visualization* to induce changes in brain wave patterns and induce physiological function change is of concern. The use of mantras (repetitive phrases), relaxation, deep breathing, and visualization is an integral part of Eastern religions and has long since found its way into Christianity with the use of prayer beads, and more recently, in various styles of prayer, often referred to as *contemplative prayer.* Even Bible verses can be used as mantras. The Eastern religions use mantras to alter consciousness; actually, they eliminate thinking. Body and/or muscle relaxation practices are integral

---

541   *Ibid.,* p. 16.
542   *Ibid.,* Preface xix.
543   *Ibid.,* p. 13.

to hypnosis techniques. *The Indian gurus have warned that rhythmic deep breathing is a time-honored method for entering altered states of consciousness and for developing psychic power. Visualization* (forming a mind picture) is a method of attempting to change and manipulate the physical reality by mental pictures. Dave Hunt, in his book, *Seduction of Christianity, Spiritual Discernment in the Last Days,* states:

> Shamanistic visualization is an attempt to create or manipulate the physical world by the practice of 'mental alchemy.' It is based upon the ancient sorcerer's belief that the entire universe is an illusion (called *maya* in Hinduism) created by the mind.[544]

One leading proponent of visualization, Adekaide Bry, says that it can be used to create whatever you want. Visualization, as practiced in this pagan philosophy, is an attempt to mimic God's power of creation—by the breath of His mouth." (Psalms 33: 6).

The ancient roots of this type of thinking can be found in Greek mythology. Dave Hunt tells in *The Seduction of Christianity* that the Egyptian god, Thoth, (to the Greeks, Hermes), taught that the physical world could be transformed through *mental imagery*.[545] Also of bygone times has been the use of *visualization* in yoga to create reality with the mind and achieve union with the supreme Hindu god, Brahman. Also mentioned is the comment that visualization is a widely used technique in psychic healing.[546] It is a regular practice in training psychic healers. Do not confuse visualization, (which is an attempt to bring something into reality, or into materialization by the thought itself) with our creative ideas, plans, and mental activities that we use to work, design and function by every day. That is not what is referred to by the word *visualization*.

Chapter 47 of Isaiah warns us of the end result of trusting in sorceries and enchantments. Evil and desolation and final destruction by fire will be our lot. The astrologers, stargazers, and sorcerers will not be able to save us. It is very clear that the most prominent investigators and authors on the subject of biofeedback are deep believers in, and practitioners of, Eastern mysticism.

Second set of questions What company does this technique keep? Who uses it and what other therapies accompany its use? From the above information we see that biofeedback developed out of hypnosis, actually is hypnosis under a different name. In the book, *The Illustrated Encyclopedia of Body-Mind*

---

544 Hunt, David, McMahon T.A., *Seduction of Christianity, Spiritual Discernment in the Last Days,* Harvest House Publishing, Eugene, OR, (1985), p.138.
545 *Ibid.,* p. 140.
546 *Ibid.,* p. 141.

Disciplines by Nancy Allison, chapter 4 titled, 'Mind/Body Medicine,' lists the names of therapeutic techniques that are associated. They are Biofeedback Training*, Guided Imagery*, Hypnotherapy*, Interactive Guided imagery*, Psycho-neuroimmunology*.[547]

Chapter 4 of *The Illustrated Encyclopedia of Mind-Body* opens with the following paragraph:

> Mind/body medicine is a contemporary term used to describe a number of disciplines that study or approach, healing the physical body, transforming human behavior, by engaging the conscious or unconscious powers of the mind. While: 'mind/body medicine' is a term used in this section of the encyclopedia to describe a growing field of study and practice in contemporary Western medicine, it is also used by others to describe ancient Eastern disciplines such as yoga, meditation, traditional Chinese medicine, and subtle energy therapies. The variety of disciplines that comprise mind/body medicine in this encyclopedia combine a theory of the relationship between body and mind that has much in common with these ancient Eastern disciplines with Western scientific models of biology and chemistry....[548]

The use of biofeedback started with therapists employing hypnosis-type therapies, and its use has extended into many health disciplines.

Third set of questions: What is the ultimate direction that the therapy is headed? Am I led toward Jesus Christ or away from Him? Do I still need Him as a Savior, or have I become my own savior?

Biofeedback is considered to be the yoga of the West.[549] It is based on the same principles as *yoga* of the East. The basic principle is that within SELF lies all the wisdom of the universe. The body has all the intelligence and power to heal itself and also to grow into a higher consciousness called the *Supreme Self*. The following quotation is from a letter from Dr. Elmer Green to Mr. Ihori, a Japanese businessman who wrote enquiring about the theory of biofeedback, and if it would be applicable to his employees. The reply to Mr. Ihori is summarized as follows: Deep within the unconscious mind of each person is hidden the *Source of Creativity*, which has the solution to all human problems. It is known by various names such as *Tao* (the way) in China, *True Self* in Zen, Jiva in India and in Tibet *Lotus*.

How does one bring out this hidden Source of Creativity? By putting the *body at complete rest*, the *emotions at peace*, and the *mind stilled* while

---

547 Allison, Nancy, *The Illustrated Encyclopedia of Mind/Body Disciplines,* Rosen Pub. Group Inc. NY, (1999), p. 64.

548 *Ibid.*, p. 64.

549 Green, op. cit., p. 76.

conscious and ready to receive impressions from the creative center of the subconscious mind.

Biofeedback is an efficient, effective manner of bringing out this *Source* by having the person place him/herself in the theta brain-wave status. This demonstrates through the electroencephalographic (EEG) feedback wherein an electrode is applied to the left occipital area of the scalp, over the visual part of the brain. The final remark in Dr. Green's letter to Mr. Ihori states:

> In my view theta training is a form of *accelerated meditation*– and the benefits to students are incalculable...[550]

Richard Willis, in his book *Holistic Health Holistic Hoax?* tells of the experience that Drs. Malcolm and Vera Carruthers had in their autogenic training classes conducted in England. They reported that everyone that became completely relaxed wanted to "go further." The doctors realized that the western approach, such as autogenic training or biofeedback, brought a level of treatment that meshed with the traditional spiritual practices of the East, similar to Eastern meditation. They then moved from autogenic training to the practice of yoga and meditation. The Carruthers felt that autogenic training is the best way to develop inner awareness, and this led them to seek the best Eastern meditation practices.[551] Willis tells us that:

> The most popular form of Eastern meditation practiced by millions in the West is Transcendental Meditation (TM) which originated with Maharishi Mahesh Yogi.[552]

In this form of meditation, a mantra word or phrase is given to the student by the instructor. This *secret mantra* is repeated over and over in the mind as one rests in a comfortable position. The mantra is to facilitate bringing the mind into a *passive* attitude. The student is advised to meditate twice a day for 20 minutes. By using this style of meditation, physiologic changes occur. Herbert Benson M.D. writes in his book, *The Relaxation Response,* that a hypo-metabolic state would occur within three minutes of starting transcendental meditation and the oxygen consumption of the mediator would be reduced by 20%, signifying a profound relaxation response.

The words given to be repeated, the mantra, are actually names of Hindu gods and one is calling on those gods to possess oneself. I made mention of

---

550   *Ibid.,* preface xiv.
551   Willis, Richard J.B., *Holistic Health Holistic Hoax?,* Pensive Publications, 10 Holland Gardens, Watford Hertfordshire, England WD2 6JW, (1997), p. 223.
552   *Ibid.,* p. 223.

this fact at a seminar I was conducting on the subjects of this book in the state of Massachusetts where there is a large ashram for training people in transcendental meditation. A young gentleman came to me afterward with a puzzled expression on his face. He asked me:

> How did you know that the names given in the secret mantra were names of Hindu Gods? I worked at the transcendental ashram and became a member. When I was initiated, I knelt before an alter with idols of pagan gods and was given their names for my mantra.

In this belief system for health and healing, there is no room for a Creator God. There is no room for understanding the forces of darkness–of Satan and his angels, no place to understand that Satan has been allowed great power to influence man, and no room to understand that Satan has been allowed power over electrical forces. E.G. White wrote of the result of this type of teaching as follows:

> None are in greater danger from the influence of evil spirits than those who, notwithstanding the direct and ample testimony of the scriptures, deny the existence and agency of the devil and his angels. So long as we are ignorant of their wiles, they have almost inconceivable advantage; many give heed to their suggestions while they suppose themselves to be following the dictates of their own wisdom...There is nothing the great deceiver fears so much as that we shall be acquainted with his devices.[553]

Fourth set of questions: Does the treatment method follow known laws of physiology? Does it teach and direct the patient to seek to know and follow God's laws of health?

Hypnosis, autogenic training, or biofeedback, do not operate by any known laws of physiology. However, there are physiological changes that do occur through the autonomic nervous system in an individual. The explanation is that the body knows how to heal itself when it is told to do so. The practitioner's use of these modalities seldom gives appropriate attention to the underlining causes of disease.

The treatment methods spoken of in this book, and many more that have not been mentioned, have no basis in known laws of physics or chemistry. All have come about as a result of a theory based on pagan religious beliefs, and a false understanding of the origin of the universe and man. For 100 years, proponents of these methods have tried their best to reconcile these methods

553   White, E.G. The Great Controversy, Pacific Press Publishing Assn., MT. View, CA, (1950). P. 516.

with known science. They have failed. Dr. Green mentions in his book that he took postgraduate studies in physics at UCLA so as to be able to demonstrate a scientific connection between his beliefs and experiences in Eastern mysticism and the physical laws that modern science recognizes.[554]

Eastern mysticism's declares that all substance of the cosmos, earth, and man originate from universal energy, and is said to be divided into seven levels (frequencies), or densities of energy. The question arises, why is it not possible for science, with its delicate instruments, to detect this energy force? These energy levels are labeled by author Green, E–1 through E–7. E–1 refers to the transformation of energy into the physical universe, including the human body. The higher levels (frequencies) of energy that are written about have to do with the mind and consciousness that is *higher consciousness*. Science has no instruments to detect these supposed higher levels of energy and Green tells us why they are not measurable by science:

> Humans have all the parts and can therefore detect a greater spectrum of energies. Instruments are made of minerals, and lack the transducer components needed for detection of E–2 through E–7 energies. In other words, living beings are coupled to the cosmos better than scientific devices, which are, after all, quite limited tools.[555]

In contrast to the above is God's way. We follow His spiritual and physical laws to maintain health. We look to God for the power to heal. He is our Creator and Sustainer and Redeemer.

> Thousands, I was shown, have been spoiled through the philosophy of phrenology and animal magnetism, (*hypnotism, autogenic training, biofeedback*) and have been driven into infidelity. If the mind commences to run in this channel, it is almost sure to lose its balance and be controlled by a demon.[556]

> Some will be tempted to receive these wonders as from God. The sick will be healed before us. Miracles will be performed in our sight. Are we prepared for the trial which awaits us when the lying wonders of Satan shall be more fully exhibited? ...We must all now seek to arm ourselves for the contest in which we must soon engage. Faith in God's Word, prayerfully studied and practically applied, will be our shield from Satan's power and will bring us off conquerors through the blood of Christ.[557]

---

554   Green, op. cit., p. 296.
555   *Ibid.*, p. 304.
556   White, E.G., *Testimonies* Vol. I; Pacific Press Publishing Assn., Mt. View, CA, (1948), p. 297.
557   *Ibid.*, p. 302.

Fifth set of questions: Who receives the credit for healing, God the Creator or Satan the created? Dr. Green states the following:

> Why did biofeedback prove helpful in the treatment of so many and varied disorders? Suddenly I realized that it isn't biofeedback that is the 'panacea'– *it is the power within the human being to self-regulate, self-heal, re-balance.* Biofeedback does nothing to the person; it is a tool for releasing that potential.[558]

Contrast this statement with the following comment:

> Jesus has not taught them this philosophy. Nothing of the kind can be found in His teachings. He did not direct the minds of poor mortals to themselves, to a power which they possessed. *He was ever directing their minds to God, the Creator of the universe, as the source of their strength and wisdom.*[559]

Five sets of questions show positive answers for identifying spiritualism in biofeedback. I no longer wonder why it has been listed as such in Christian books that have been written to expose the devil's wiles. The special report by the Biblical Research Committee included biofeedback as a procedure that we should shun. You will have to decide for yourself if biofeedback is a procedure you would choose to use. My goal is to present enough documented information in order for you to make an intelligent decision.

You may have noticed that the testimonies of people, as to the value of different treatment methods, or the personal experience of individuals who experienced relief and apparent healing from use of various alternative healing modalities, have not been included as testing criteria. This book does not present the idea that these methods do not give apparent benefit. The purpose of the book is to help us in answering the question, *who makes it work, what power is behind it?*

E.G. White in Selected Messages book II page 52-53 gives testimony supporting the statement in the above paragraph. Apparent healing or miracles are not proper tests as to the source of power.

> The man who makes the working of miracles the test of his faith will find that Satan can, through a species of deceptions, perform wonders that will appear to be genuine miracles. It was this he hoped to make a test question with the Israelites at the time of their deliverance from Egypt.—Manuscript 43, 1907.

> ...we may be among the number who will see the miracles wrought by Satan in these last days, and believe them. Many strange things will appear as wonderful

558   Green, op. cit., p. 116.
559   White, op. cit., p. 297.

miracles, which should be regarded as deceptions manufactured by the father of lies. — Letter 136, 1906

We need not be deceived. Wonderful scenes, with which Satan will be closely connected, will soon take place. God's Word declares that Satan will work miracles. He will make people sick, and then will suddenly remove from them his satanic power. They will then be regarded as healed. These Works of apparent healing will bring Seventh-day Adventists to the test. Many who have had great light will fail to walk in the light, because they have not become one with Christ.—Letter 57, 1904 (emphasis added)

I would like to present one additional bit of information to help you in making your decision about whether biofeedback is good, rational treatment, or if it falls into the domain of the mystical. Dr. Green, in his book *Beyond Biofeedback*, has an entire chapter on the use of *volition* in biofeedback therapy. Synonyms for volition are *the will* or *to choose*. A person must first *choose* to participate in biofeedback, for without this willingness, the treatment will be ineffective. The following is from the book, *Beyond Biofeedback*.

Fundamental among (man's) inner powers, and the one to which priority should be given, is the *will's* central position in man's personality and its intimate connection with the core of his being–his very self....[560]

Dr. Green also states:

Volition (will) is at the heart of the mind-body problem.[561]

Attitude is a critical feature in biofeedback training, because volition (will) is influenced by what one believes.[562]

Elmer and Alyce Green are correct in their assessment of the power of the will. It is vital in deciding which power will control us.

Through the right exercise of the will an entire change may be made in the life. By yielding up the will to Christ, we ally ourselves with divine power. We receive strength from above to hold us steadfast. A pure and noble life, a life of victory over appetite and lust, is possible to everyone who will unite his weak, wavering human will to the omnipotent, unwavering will of God.[563]

---

560 *Ibid.*, p. 58.
561 *Ibid.*, p. 59.
562 *Ibid.*, p. 66.
563 White, E.G., *Counsels on Health,* Pacific Press Pub. Assn., Mt. View, CA, (1923), p. 440.2

The will is the governing power in the nature of man, bringing all the other faculties under its sway. The will is not the taste or the inclination, but it is the deciding power, which works in the children of men unto obedience to God, or unto disobedience.[564]

Every human being possessed of reason has power to choose the right. In every experience of life God's word to us is, "Choose ye this day whom ye will serve," (Joshua 24:15). Every one may place his will on the side of the will of God, may choose to obey Him, and by thus linking himself with divine agencies, he may stand where nothing can force him to do evil.[565]

564 White, E.G., *Child Guidance;* Pacific Press Pub. Assn., Mt. View, CA, (1954), p. 209.1.
565 *Ibid.,* p. 209.3.

CHAPTER 20

SECULAR PSYCHOLOGY"SCIENCE OF THE SOUL?"PART I

Near the time I was writing the finishing pages of the book *Spiritualistic Deceptions in Health and Healing* I realized there was need for a chapter on spiritualism's influence on the medical discipline of psychology. In the years since that book was published I have had repeated requests to include such a chapter in any future book. Those requests have come from people who have either attended a seminar that I have conducted exposing spiritualism in health and healing, or have read the book *Spiritualistic Deceptions in Health and Healing*.

Those requests have been far more than just suggestions; they are urgent pleas even to the point of sending to me valuable text relevant to the subject. These individuals shared with me what they had seen and experienced firsthand in therapy that they now recognized as having spiritualistic overtones.

In an earlier chapter the subjects of phrenology and mesmerism (hypnotism) were presented. Quotations, from E. G. White, relevant to phrenology and mesmerism as laying the foundation for spiritualism had also included the word *psychology* as being of the same nature. Let us review one of those statements:

> I have been shown that we must be guarded on every side and perseveringly resist the insinuations and devices of Satan. He has transformed himself into an angel of light and is deceiving thousands and leading them captive. *The advantage he takes of the science of the human mind is tremendous*. The sciences of *phrenology*, *psychology*, and *mesmerism* (hypnotism) are the channels through which he comes more directly to this generation and works with that power which is to characterize his efforts near the close of probation.[566] (Emphasis added)

I found it difficult to accept that modern psychology continued to fit the definition as categorized by the above quote and from other similar statements by the author, E.G. White. I did not doubt that the definition fit at the time it was written but felt that over time psychology had risen above and out of

566   White, E.G., *Counsels for the Church*, (1991), p. 329.4.

that definition to a status based upon science. As I have pursued the study of modern psychology, I have at times not only been surprised by what I learned, but even *stunned.* As

I further researched comments of *mind—cure, mind—therapy,* I read a quotation that raised high my interest in pursuing the answer for a question lingering in my mind. Why was *psychology* included in the mind—cure comments that E.G. White referred to as laying the foundation for spiritualism? I quote:

> **The true principles of psychology are found in the Holy Scriptures**. Man knows not his own value. He acts according to his unconverted temperament of character because he does not look unto Jesus, the Author and Finisher of his faith. He who comes to Jesus, he who believes on Him and makes Him his Example, realizes the meaning of the words "To them gave He power to become the sons of God."[567] . . . (Emphasis author's)

> **Laws of the Mind Ordained by God**.--He who created the mind and ordained its laws, provided for its development in accordance with them.[568]

A small book *Christians Beware* by Magna Parks, Ph.D. came into circulation in 2007 and at the same time as did *Spiritualistic Deceptions in Health and Healing* by Edwin A. Noyes M.D. Magna Parks, a practicing psychologist for twenty years had encountered a written sermon that had been delivered prior to a church body. As she read, she found she was at odds with the content of the sermon and proceeded to study to determine whether she was wrong in her understanding or the pastor was mistaken. What she learned shocked her and changed the way she practices psychology and counsels. No longer does she rely upon the standard principles of counseling that she learned in her training, she found that scripture contains answers to problems of the mind that she often encounters in her patients. Her book is a recommended read for anyone interested in mind—cure therapy.

Magna Parks has with consummate skill condensed an immense subject into 78 pages of simple clear and concise phrases that all can understand. She has brought to focus three theories in psychology which she feels create the greatest influence today, *psychoanalytic*, *behaviorist*, and *humanistic perspectives*. She also states that the two theories with the most influence on Christianity are psychoanalytic and humanistic.[569]

567 White, E.G., 1. *Mind/ Character/Personality,* Southern Publishing Association, Nashville Tennessee, (1977), p. 10.
568 *Ibid.*
569 Parks, Magna Ph.D., *Christians Beware! The Dangers of Christian Psychology*, Teach Services, Inc., Brushton, New York, (2007), p. 5.

She also identifies several of the leading personalities that have over the last 100 plus years most influenced the present day disciplines of psychiatry and psychology. The central theme to be found in secular psychology according to Parks is the fixation on "Self." That within "Self" is the elements for mind therapy.

At this point in our discussion I think a definition of psychology would be appropriate as the explanation of the original meaning of the word goes a long way toward establishing common ground for understanding forthcoming comments. From *Webster's New World Dictionary, the Third Edition* (1988) the Greek word psyche, has as one of its definitions "*soul,*" and is stated to be the origin of the English word *psychology,* which refers to the science of the *mind* or *soul;* also one of the definitions is the "science of animal and human behavior." An 1828 Noah Webster's Dictionary defines *psychology* as follows:

> PSYCHOLOGY, n. [Gr. soul, and discourse.] A discourse or treatise on the human soul; or the doctrine of the nature and properties of the soul.

From *Young's Analytical Concordance to the Bible* the Hebrew word *nephesh* is translated in English to *soul.* The Bible speaks of the soul nearly five hundred times, referring to *mortal* animal and man.

This chapter has as its purpose to share with the reader what I learned as I sought to understand why psychology, as pointed out by E.G. White, would be used by Satan to increase his power of deception near the close of probation. This chapter is focused on the quote that psychology can lay a foundation for spiritualism.

WHAT IS SPIRITUALISM?

The lie told in the Garden of Eden "you will not die" is the foundation of spiritualism, that there is life after death and that the *soul* is separate from the body. Belief in this false doctrine as well as the deification of the dead can lead to communion with the dead which actually is communion with demons, fallen angels. Part of the lie at Eden was that man would progress to become wise like God and know good and evil. These two lies are the foundation of pantheism.

> It is fondly supposed that heathen superstitions have disappeared before the civilization of the twentieth century. But the word of God and the stern testimony of facts declare that sorcery is practiced in this age as verily as in the days of the old-time magicians. The ancient system of magic is, in reality, the same as what is now known as modern **spiritualism**. Satan is finding access to thousands of minds by presenting himself under the guise of departed friends. . . .

> The magicians of heathen times have their counterpart in the spiritualistic mediums, the clairvoyants, and the fortunetellers of today. . . . Could the veil be lifted from before our eyes, we should see evil angels employing all their arts to deceive and to destroy. Wherever an influence is exerted to cause men to forget God, there Satan is exercising his bewitching power. . . . The apostle's admonition to the Ephesian church should be heeded by the people of God today: "*Have no fellowship with the unfruitful works of darkness, but rather reprove them.*"[570] (Emphasis added)

At this point in our discussion a review of the principles of Satan's counterfeit pagan religion— nature worship that originated in Babylon, and was known as part of the Babylonian Mysteries is helpful for understanding the following discourse.

Primordial evolution theory replaced the Biblical account of the creation of the world—"by the breath of His mouth," by Jesus Christ the Divine Son of God. In the pagan false story of creation, God is removed from His creative power and set aside. The *creative power* is divided into two parts, good— evil, positive—negative, or yin—yang, and this power is considered as *god.* With evolutionary time the two parts of energy were supposedly blended harmoniously to the point that all material substance was created, the cosmos, world, and man. All material substance is said to be made of this same *creative power, or energy,* so each substance is out of the same original universal source (energy) and has all the attributes of, and is a part of, everything. Synonyms of this creative power are *consciousness, collective consciousness, Self, subliminal Self,* and a hundred other names, even the blasphemous use of the name that God called Himself, the *I AM.* The entire theory has a name— *pantheism.*

A refinement of pantheism wherein God is left in the equation of creation but that he in turn left a *spark* of Himself in everything he created so that innately each of us has latent divinity within. This false concept is given the name *panentheism.* This branch of pantheism claims that the soul is immortal and that we are gods. The belief that the soul has immortality is still prevalent today, even throughout Christendom. The God *within* concept leads to the glorification and infatuation of *Self.* Humanistic psychology has utilized this theme, further demonstrated by the term *Self-esteem.*

To identify spiritualism in psychology one or both of two teachings will need to be demonstrated to be a component of this discipline, namely 1) life continues after death—immortality of the soul; and 2) teaching of progression to the godhood of man—divinity within. That would not apply to every precept under the name of psychology but only to those teachings wherein

---

570   White, E.G., *Conflict and Courage,* (1970), p. 343.

such concepts are found. So we need to look at the teachings of psychology in the 1800's, early 1900's and forward until today. First we need to investigate the history of those who developed and influenced the establishment of the teachings and philosophy of this branch of medicine. Were they believers in such doctrines as the immortality of the soul, and or divinity within man.

SOCRATES—PLATO—ARISTOTLE

Therapeutic psychology arose out of philosophy. Philosophy is the science (so called) of estimating values and the superiority of any belief, situation, action, condition, or substance over another as determined by the mind of man. In this world's history the Greeks were known for having great philosophers. The *psyche* (soul) was a subject of much discussion by these Greek philosophers. The belief in the *immortality* of the psyche or soul had its start in this world in the Garden of Eden, and was carried down to Babylon and spread to the world with the language dispersion from Babylon.

I recently read with interest some translated writings of Socrates, Plato and Aristotle from the text *History of Psychology, Fundamental Questions,*[571] wherein those philosophers discussed their concept of the soul. The ancient religions of India, Egypt, and China all have the doctrine of the immortality of the soul as revealed by *The Book of the Dead* from Egypt and the *Tibetan Book of the Dead*. St. Thomas Aquinas (1224-1274A.D.) writes of the immortality of the soul and about the soul after death.[572] In *History of Psychology* the great philosophers from Socrates up to the modern times are reviewed and some of their writings that have been translated into English are included. The belief in the separation of the soul from the body and immortality of the soul seems to be a dominant concept of these philosophers. In the late 1700's and early 1800's the term psychology began to be used when referring to the study of the mind and gradually the discipline of mind therapy was considered under this term. Psychiatry is the term used for a medical doctor who specializes in diagnosis and treatments of neurosis and psychosis. Many of the 19th and 20th century thought leaders in the field of psychology believed in the immortality of the soul. This fact will be more clearly recognized as we look at leading psychologists and psychiatrists of the modern area. Remember, the definition of *spiritualism* is the belief of life after death and communication between the living and the dead can occur, which practice is strongly prohibited in the Bible. E.G. White adhered to an enlarged definition of the term *spiritualism*

---

571 Munger, Margaret P., *The History of Psychology, Fundamental Questions,* Oxford University Press, Oxford, England, (2003).

572 *Ibid.*, pp. 46-65.

as illustrated in the following snippets taken from *The Great Controversy* pp. 551-562.

> That man is the creature of progression; that it is his destiny from his birth to progress, even to eternity, toward the Godhead; each mind will judge itself and not another; the judgment will be right because it is the judgment of self; any just and perfect being is Christ; true knowledge places man above all law; whatever is right is right; all sins committed are innocent; denies the origin of the Bible; the Bible is a mere fiction; Love is dwelt upon as the chief attribute of God.

The doctrine of life after death and divinity within mankind had its origin from the lie told in the Garden of Eden, and is the foundation of Eastern thought and Western occultism. It is the doctrinal principles of principles of pagan religions and or nature worship. *To* recognize seeds of spiritualism within psychology we need an understanding of the Eastern explanation of man. 1) The soul separates from the body of man, continues in life after death and is immortal. 2) This soul is composed of a conscious mind and has subconscious and super conscious components, which in turn are a part of a *universal mind,* referred to as *Universal Consciousness, Self, Subliminal Self, Higher Self, god.* As man's mind is believed to be a part of a *universal mind—god,* man therefore has divinity within and the pursuit of life is to bring this divinity into full bloom, escape reincarnation, and join the spirit world of nirvana, and to enjoy an eternal life of bliss.

There are a number of practices which are applied in the field of mind therapy whose working power is explained by their proponents as an extension of the unconscious mind as spoken of in the preceding paragraph. These are hypnotism, clairvoyance, visualization, telepathy, channeling, meditation, yoga, transcendental meditation, Extra Sensory Perception, and others. There is the ever present belief and teaching that within *Self* resides all the wisdom of the universe, and the power of all healing. A myriad of techniques are designed to access that presumed power from within. There are a large number of theories related to the function of the mind and mind therapy which are promoted in the field of psychology.

> According to Alan E. Bergin and Sol L. Garfield, editors of the *Handbook of Psychotherapy and Behavior Change,* 1994, p. 6, tell us that there are more than

400 differing psychotherapeutic methods offered to the public and by 10,000 varying techniques.[573]

Why so many? Answer: proof by scientific testing of its theories, diagnosis, and therapies is difficult to come by. Undoubtedly there are many principles adhered to in psychology that do have value and are free of spiritistic influence.

In my study for evidence of spiritualistic influence in psychology I have repeatedly come across certain names that are referred to by various authors, as being *thought* leaders and theorists in the field of psychology, such as James, Freud, Jung, Rogers, and Maslow. These men have set general theories during the past 100 plus years in the field of mind science. We will look at the history of each of these individual practitioners and teachers in our search for *seeds* of spiritualism that may have entered into secular psychology as may be practiced.

In the latter half of the nineteenth century including the early years of the twentieth century, *Mesmerism,* also known as *hypnotism* and *suggestion*, was commonly used in dealing with mind—cure therapy in the United States and Europe.[574]

> By 1885 the 'psychotherapeutic movement' that had begun in Europe in the middle 1860's with Liebault and developed rapidly in the next decade was making headway in the United States, principally through the efforts of psychologists William James, G. Stanley Hall, Joseph Jastrow, and James Mark Baldwin, and of a few physicians.[575]

WILLIAM JAMES M.D. (1842-1910)

In 1890 William James, an illustrious Harvard professor of psychiatry, wrote an article carried in Scribner's Magazine entitled the *Hidden Self.* He wrote that science had ignored mysticism, the occult, spiritualism, faith healing, and hypnotism because it could not be well understood and classified. James called for more study and research in this area. James was first hired to teach at Harvard, his academic home for virtually his entire career. He explored the occult and took forays into psychical research, séances, and, of

---

573   Gabbert, Dan, *Biblical Response Therap®, Healing God's Way,* Gabbert Family Resources, Aardvaark Global Publishing Co., LLC, (2008); p. iv; Available at Black Hills Health and Education Center, PO Box 19, Hermosa, SD 57744, www.bhhec.org

574   Hale, Nathan G., *Freud and the Americans, The Beginnings of Psychoanalysis in the United States,* Oxford University Press, (1971), pp. 229, 230.

575   *Ibid.*, p. 229.

course, several varieties of religious experience, authoring the book, *Varieties of Religious Experience*.

The medical professionals and public at large were interested in and utilized hypnosis, suggestion, mental healing, multiple personalities, automatic writing, psychic research, etc., and it peaked in the 1890's to decline slightly and then surge again between 1905 and1910.

A high point, prior to the present time, in American history for use of hypnosis and suggestion for mental therapy was in the first decade of the twentieth century.[576] Adelbert Albrecht, editor of the Journal of Criminal Law and Criminology, stated in 1913 that:

> Several psychotherapeutists in America claimed to have cured hundreds of cases of alcoholism and its consequences by hypnotism[577]

In America at this same time, movements referred to as the *Emmanuel Movement* and *Christian Science* were popular. To combat the nervousness and evils of the day the Reverend Elwood Worcester started a crusade combining *liberal Christianity, Subliminal Self,* and the other methods used in that day for psychotherapy; this was called the Emmanuel Movement because they first started their meetings Nov. 11, 1906 in the Emmanuel Church building. This movement did not necessarily utilize professionals for administering therapy and soon spread across the country among different protestant organizations, Baptist, Congregationalist, Unitarian, and Presbyterian, etc. These movements aroused interest in *Subliminal Self* and hidden powers with possible connection with the *Great Beyond*; this was the beginning of public awareness of the *Unconscious*. Ellen White mentioned these movements in her comments regarding mind—cure therapy.

> There are many who shrink with horror from the thought of consulting spirit mediums, but who are attracted by more pleasing forms of spiritism, such as the *Emmanuel movement*. Still others are led astray by the teachings of *Christian Science*, and by the mysticism of *theosophy* and *other Oriental religions*.[578]

SIGMUND FREUD M.D. 1856-1939:

At the time of the above mentioned peak use of hypnotism in Europe and the United States, a neurologist psychiatrist Sigmund Freud, from Vienna, Austria came to the United States in 1909 to present a series of lectures on

576 *Ibid.*, p. 230.
577 *Ibid.*, p. 227.
578 White, E.G., Evangelism, Review and Herald Publishing Association. Hagerstown, MD, (1946), p. 606.

mind—cure that he had developed, he called it *psychoanalysis*. Freud tells us that he had used hypnotism but:

> I have given up the *suggestive* technique and with it *hypnotism* because I despaired of making the suggestion strong and durable enough to effect a permanent cure. In all severe cases I saw the *suggestion* crumble away and the disease again made its appearance.[579]

Freud was a practitioner of psychiatry, and a researcher in neurology. He presented in 1909 to a group of psychiatrists in the United States the concept of psychopathology (deranged mental activity) as originating from the subconscious mind" and he introduced a technique of *mind— cure* he called *psychoanalysis*. He had dropped the use of hypnotism and simply explored with the patient the history of their childhood and youth. Freud was an atheist, did not believe in spirits and explained occult happenings as an extension of the subconscious. His central pillar of doctrine was the *subconscious* and tied in most mental dysfunction with some sort of sexual relationship. Freud had also used cocaine as therapy for mental dysfunction. He eventually discarded cocaine for therapy as he did hypnosis. Freud was an interpreter of dreams and also used this technique in the psychoanalysis process.

Freud did change the direction of psychotherapy in the U.S. and there was a decline in use of many of the occult techniques. However he added fuel to the fire in the concept of *subconscious*. The subconscious was the source of subliminal Self, instincts, man's memory, reserve energies, etc. The subconscious was believed to be more sensitive to good and evil than our conscious mind; it was a connection to the *Universal Mind* or *Spirit*.

> Its roots were the *Infinite*, it was closer to the Universal Spirit. The subconscious then was uncanny: it healed; it remembered everything; it solved problems; it could impart glorious, undreamed-of resources.[580]

Another movement in the first two decades of the 20th century in the U.S. was the *New Thought Movement* originated by a professional hypnotist Phineas Parkhurst Quimby (1802-66), "philosopher- mesmerist-healer-scientist." He taught that many diseases could be cured by suggestion and thus were therefore illusionary. Another mesmerist and spiritualist, Mary Baker Eddy carried the New Thought Movement on into *Christian Science*. A New Thought Sanitarium on the Hudson River in 1909 was offering treatments of:

---

579   Hale, op. cit., p. 227.
580   *Ibid.*, p. 241.

...psychic experiments, non-church religion, admonitions to conquer the world with sheer sentiments of optimism, electric shocks delivered through a serrated gold crown, hypnotism, and suggestion.[581]

The New Thought and Christian Scientists treatments for the mind were the most popular. From 1882 to 1908 the number of Christian scientists had grown from less than one hundred to 85,000. These movements claimed to be effective on all ailments.[582] It was into this mixture of hypotheses that Freud introduced his own hypothesis of psychoanalysis:

> Psychoanalysis is concerned with the discovery of events in the past life of the individual and with their consequences for him, and neither the events nor the consequences can ever be exactly the same for two people.[583]

Freud had a great impact on psychology in the United States in the early 1900's. He used dream analysis, confession, and looking to the past as the source of mental problems. This approach tended to blame parents for the patients mental disorders. The philosophy was expanded by others until supposedly returning to the womb and to previous lives via hypnotism became part of the psychologist's modus operandi.

It was out of this hypothesis of past life experiences, including intrauterine development and birth experience, that is portrayed as deciding the stability or instability of the future mental health of an individual. This is the basis for the concept of *re-birthing*, and finding the *inner child, divine within* (*divine child* by Jung) in psychotherapy.

Although Freud was not known as a spiritualist and tried to explain psychic phenomena as arising out of the subconscious he still took decided interest in such as he was a member of the Society (S.P.R.) that attempted to investigate on a scientific basis psychic happenings. Freud was elected as a Corresponding Member of the British Society for Psychical Research in 1911, and in 1915 he became an Honorary Fellow of the American Society for Psychical Research. In December, 1923, the Greek Society for Psychical Research honored him similarly. Matthew Raphael, author of *Bill W. and Mr. Wilson*, a book about the cofounders of Alcoholics Anonymous, shares with us on page 161 Freud's dabbling in spiritism. A comment from Raphael:

---

581   *Ibid.*, p. 246.
582   *Ibid.*, p. 245.
583   Bettelheim, Bruno, *Freud and Man's Soul,* First Vintage books Edition, (1984); Random House Inc., New York p. 42.

...As we have seen, Sigmund Freud, whose highest ambition was to put psycho-analysis on a scientific footing, nonetheless took notice of psychical (occult) phenomena—much to the chagrin of his closest disciples, who felt a need to bury the offending facts or else to explain them away. An entire chapter of Ernest Jones' monumental biography (of Freud) is dedicated to Freud's *open-mindedness* about *occultism* (he was a member of the Society for Psychical Research) and his publication, over Jones's protestations, of his papers on telepathy.

Ernest Jones MD, Freud's biographer and coworker stated that it was generally held that Freud's greatest contribution to science was his *interpretation of Dreams* and the concept of *the unconscious mind.*

C.G. JUNG M.D. , 1875-1961:

Probably the best know name in the field of psychiatry and psychology is that of Carl Gustav Jung M.D., a Swiss psychiatrist. His name is recognized the world over and is associated also with the discipline of psychology. He was born in Kesswil, Switzerland by Lake Constance July 26, 1875 to Paul and Emilie (Preiswerk) Jung. His father Paul, was a Parson in the Swiss Reform Church; his mother came from a family of many Parsons, her father and eight uncles.

Carl's maternal grandfather, Parson Samuel Preiswerks' first wife died, thereafter he held weekly intimate conversations with her spirit, to the irritation of his second wife.[584] Samuel's second wife Agusta, Carl's maternal grandmother was gifted with the ability to see *spirits.*[585]

Emilie, daughter of Samuel and Agusta, too had the gift of seeing spirits. Her father would have her stand behind him as he prepared his sermons so as to keep the ghosts from annoying him as he studied.[586] Emilie, Carl's mother kept a diary which listed all of the strange experiences she encountered. She spoke of it as "spookish" phenomena and strange occurrences.[587] Carl once saw the following come from his mother's bedroom door.

> I slept in my father's room. From the door to my mother's room came frightening influences. At night Mother was strange and mysterious. One night I saw coming from her door a faintly luminous, indefinite figure whose head detached itself from the neck and floated along in front of it, in the air, like a

---

584   Jaffe', Aniela, *From the Life and Work of C.G. Jung,* Harper and Row, Publishers, N. Y., NY, (1971), p. 2.
585   *Ibid.,* p. 2.
586   *Ibid.*
587   *Ibid.*

little moon. Immediately another head was produced and again detached itself. This process was repeated six or seven times.[588]

Carl, as do all people, had dreams, however, he had a life-long fascination with interpretation of dreams. The first dream he remembers came to him when he was between three and four years of age. He tells us in his book *Memories, Dreams, and Reflections*, that this dream was to "preoccupy me all my life."[589] The dream consisted of a phallic symbol 15 feet high and one and one half to two feet diameter seated on a golden throne in a room deep into the subterranean parts of the earth. He heard in the dream his mother's voice saying "Yes, just look at him that is the man eater!" The symbol he later determined to represent "the dark Lord Jesus, and a Jesuit priest." He tells us that the dream haunted him for years and he never shared it with anyone.

> At all events, the phallus of this dream seems to be a subterranean God 'not to be named,' and such it remained throughout my youth, reappearing whenever anyone spoke too emphatically about Lord Jesus. Lord Jesus never became quite real for me, never quite acceptable, never quite lovable, for again and again I would think of his underground counterpart, a frightful revelation which had been accorded me without my seeking it. The Jesuit's 'disguise' cast its shadow over the Christian doctrine I had been taught. ...Lord Jesus seemed to me in some ways a god of death, helpful, it is true, in that he scared away the terror of the night, but himself uncanny, crucified and bloody corpse....[590]

Before Carl could read, his mother had read to him *Orbis Pictus*, and old, illustrated children's book, containing an account of exotic religions, primarily Hinduism . Illustrations of the chief God's of the Hindus were portrayed; Brahman, Vishnu, and Shiva which he had an "inexhaustible source of interest in."[591] He felt an affinity with these illustrations with his *original revelation— his earliest dream.*

> If there arise among you a prophet, or a dreamer of dreams, and giveth thee a sign or a wonder, And the sign or the wonder come to pass, whereof he spake unto thee, saying, Let us go after other gods, which thou hast not known, and let us serve them; Thou shalt not hearken unto the words of that prophet, or that dreamer of dreams: for the LORD your God proveth you, to know whether ye love the LORD your God with all your heart and with all your soul. Ye shall

588   Jung, C.G. , *Memories, Dreams, and Reflections,* recorded and edited by Aniela Jaffe'; translated from the German by Richard and Clara Winston, Random House, Inc. (1989), p. 18.
589   *Ibid.,* p. 11.
590   *Ibid.,* p. 13.
591   *Ibid.,* p. 17.

walk after the LORD your God, and fear him, and keep his commandments, and obey his voice, and ye shall serve him, and cleave unto him. And that prophet, or that dreamer of dreams, shall be put to death; because he hath spoken to turn (you) away from the LORD your God, which brought you out of the land of Egypt, and redeemed you out of the house of bondage, to thrust thee out of the way which the LORD thy God commanded thee to walk in. So shalt thou put the evil away from the midst of thee. Deut. 13: 1-5

In the spring of 1895 Carl began his studies at the University of Basel in the study of medicine. His father died in 1896. Six weeks after his father's death he dreamed of his father returning and standing before him. In the dream his father had recovered and was coming home. The dream repeated itself a few days later; it seemed real and forced Carl to think about life after death.

At the end of the second semester of his studies at the University Carl discovered in a library of a classmate's father, a book on spiritualistic phenomena, dating from the 1870's. It was the history of the beginning of spiritualism of that day. Questions concerning this subject plagued him and he read extensively of occultic author's writings, Zollner, Crooks, Kant's *Dreams of a Spirit Seer*, several other authors, and seven volumes of Swedenborg, a renowned spiritualist.

In 1897 C.G. Jung lectured to a club at the University setting forth his views that the soul exists, is intelligent, immortal, and he believed in the reality of spirits and spiritualism by evidence of occult activities, believed in hypnotism, clairvoyance , telepathy, telekinesis, second sight, prophetic dreams, messages of dying people, horoscope calculations, observed levitation. (Found in the Foreword for C.G. Jung, *Psychology and the Occult*)

During the summer recess of 1898 an event happened that Carl records in Memories, p. 104, 105 that would "influence him profoundly." He was sitting in one room studying and in the next room his mother was sitting and knitting and with the door open between rooms. Suddenly a noise like a pistol shot rang out. Carl found that a large walnut table top had split suddenly right through solid wood, even in a climate with plenty of moisture so the table was not excessively dried out. Two weeks later he arrived home to find his mother, sister, and maid in a state of agitation. Again a loud crack like noise had occurred, however, no new split could be found in the table. The noise had come from the sideboard, an old piece of furniture which contained bread and culinary tools. Carl found the bread knife broken into many pieces. He had the knife examined by an expert in steel and was told the steel had no defects in it.[592]

---

592 *Ibid.*, p. 105,6.

He shortly became aware of relatives who were engaged in *table turning* and enjoying séances conducted by a fifteen year old cousin medium. He joined these relatives at the table for séances on Saturday nights for two and one half years. There was communication in the form of tapping noises from the walls and the table. Movements of the table apart from the medium were hard to determine and so he accepted the association between the tapping noises and communications in the séance. He wrote his doctrinal thesis on these experiences and communications received in the séances.[593] He states in *Memories* the following:

> All in all, this was the one great experience which wiped out all my earlier philosophy and made it possible for me to achieve a psychological point of view.[594]

This contributed to Jung's choice of psychiatry as a specialty in spite of it being held in contempt by most physicians and non-physicians of his day. The doctors knew little more than laymen about psychiatric diseases and mental illness was a hopeless and fatal situation casting its shadow over a psychiatrist's reputation. December 10, 1900 found Carl Jung working as an assistant at Burgholzli Mental Hospital, Zurich, so began a life and practice of psychiatry that was to influence the world, for better or for worse.

Jung tells us in *Memories* that he used hypnosis in the early part of his work but soon gave it up because he felt it added to working with the unknown causes of mental disorders and the apparent beneficial results often did not continue. He chose to analyze all aspects of the patient's life and thereby arrive at a probable source for cause and effect in psychiatric disorders. So Jung began developing his *psychological point of view* to affect therapy to the mentally afflicted. The treatment for mental disorders in the early 20th century was very limited; more effort was placed on diagnosis than on therapy as almost nothing was known as to the etiology of mental abnormalities, or what could be done to improve the condition. Hypnosis was widely used as therapy in the latter part of nineteenth century and early twentieth.

Throughout *Memories, Dreams, and Reflections* Jung tells of different dreams and his attempt to interpret them. In 1914 he had three dreams he writes about in his chapter of *Confrontation with the Unconscious* and speaks of being under so much stress he practiced *Yoga* exercises in order to hold his emotions under control.[595]

---

593   *Ibid.*, p. 107.
594   *Ibid.*
595   *Ibid.*, p. 177.

Jung speaks of some fantasies he developed such as The Biblical figures *Elijah* and *Salome* as well as a large black snake. Then came another *fantasy figure* which Jung says came out of the unconscious, that of *Philemon*. Philemon in this story was a pagan and carried an influence of old Egypt and Gnosticism. Jung states that these were entities in his psyche which he did not produce by imagination or by any method. Philemon was one of these; Philemon represented a force which was not of his self. Jung said that in his fantasies he held conversation with Philemon.

> Psychologically, Philemon represented superior insight. He was a mysterious figure to me. At times he seemed to me quite real, as if he were a living personality. I went walking up and down the garden with him, and to me he was what the Indians call a guru.[596]

Fifteen years from the first appearance of Philemon in Jung's life he had a conversation with a friend of Gandhi that told him his guru (Gandhi's friend's guru) was an ancient Hindu master; Jung asked him if he were referring to a *spirit*? He replied to the positive and Jung states that at that moment he thought of Philemon. Gandhi's Hindu friend stated that there are live gurus and ghost gurus as well.[597]

Jung tells us in *Memories* that around 1916 an inner change began within him, he felt an urge to give shape to something. He was compelled from within to express what his spirit guide Philemon might have said, and he wrote in three nights *The Seven Sermons to the Dead.*[598] Before he started writing he had the feeling that the air was filled with ghostly entities. His house seemed to be haunted as his daughter saw a white figure passing through the room. His second daughter, stated that twice in the night her blanket had been snatched away; and his nine year-old son had an anxiety dream involving the devil. The next day at five P.M. the doorbell began to ring without anyone to ring it.

> The house was "crammed full of spirits," Jung cried out "For God's Sake, what in the world is this?" "Then the spirits answered back, "We have come back from Jerusalem where we found not what we sought."
>
> ...They were packed deep right up to the door, and air was so thick it was scarcely possible to breathe.[33]...Then it began to flow out of me, and in the course of three evenings the thing was written. As soon as I took up the pen,

596   *Ibid.,* p. 183
597   *Ibid.,* p. 184.
598   Jung, op. cit., p. 190.

the whole ghostly assemblage evaporated. The room quieted and atmosphere cleared. The haunting was over. [599]

The Seven Sermons to the Dead was one of the key works of Jung. It was the spirits answer to the "*nature of God*," the *universe*, and *man*, and contained the *seeds* for his future writings in psychology. Jung had the fantasy of being a *Parson to the Dead*. In *Memories* he explained this strange concept by saying that the soul establishes a relationship to the unconscious which corresponds to the mythic land of the dead. This would give the dead a chance to manifest themselves through a medium.

C.G. Jung explained as did Freud, those ghosts, spirits, and loud noises (poltergeist), and dreams all, as coming out of an unconsciousness, which each person possessed within themselves. He did not accept influences and power coming from fallen angels (demons). He rejected the great controversy between Satan and Jesus Christ as nonexistent and sought to explain the occult on the unconsciousness of the mind. This concept grew into the doctrine of "Self" that is so prevalent in the field of psychology today.

Jung had studied Gnostic writers during the years between 1918 and 1926, they too, according to Jung, had the concept of the unconscious. He stated that he began to understand in the years between 1918-20 that the goal of psychic development is the SELF. He, while being commandant of a prison camp in Switzerland during the First World War began to draw mandalas. These symbols are of a round design and with the entire symbol directing attention to the center of the mandala. The center represented the *Self*-concept mentioned above. He had a dream in 1927 which brought to conclusion his forming doctrine of *Self*. He stated that through the dream he understood that the *Self* is the principle, orientation, and meaning in the process of development of consciousness. Symbols of the Zodiac are related to the archetypes which Jung's spirit guide Philemon encouraged him to believe haunted the collective unconscious. Consequently Jung had great respect for astrology and used it in his analysis. "In cases of difficult diagnosis I usually get a horoscope," wrote Jung.[600]

It took the first forty-five years of his life with all of the dreams, occultic phenomena, spirit guides, (Philemon), inner symbols, levitation happenings, Seven Sermons to the Dead etc., to form his theory of the *unconsciousness*.[601] *Analytical psychology* is the product of all of Jung's efforts to puncture the empty shell of psychological therapy during his life time. He felt need of strengthening and shoring up this theory of consciousness, unconsciousness,

---

599   *Ibid.*, pp. 190, 191.
600   Hunt, op. cit.., p. 76.
601   Jung, Memories, op. cit. 199

and the collective consciousness he postulated. He felt he found that added strength when he studied Gnosticism and then became fascinated by the study of *alchemy*. He felt that alchemy's addition to the knowledge of Gnosticism gave him historical basis to bolster the theory of the unconscious. It added a historical connection to the past and a bridge to the future, to the modern psychology of the unconscious.

> As I worked with my fantasies, I became aware that the unconscious undergoes or produces change. Only after I had familiarized myself with alchemy did I realize that the unconscious is a *process,* and the psyche is transformed or developed by the relationship of the ego to the contents of the unconscious. In individual cases that transformation can be read from dreams and fantasies. In collective life it has left its deposit principally in the various religious systems and their changing symbols. Through the study of these collective transformation processes and through understanding of alchemical symbolism I arrived at the central concept of my psychology: *the process of individuation.*[602]

Jung wrote many articles on occult phenomena, the little book *Psychology and the Occult* is a booklet containing three essays by Jung. Essay 1) *On Spiritualistic Phenomena,* 2) *The Psychological Foundations of Belief in Spirits,* 3) *The Soul and death.*

Psychology and the East is a book composed of works by Doctor Jung. He was asked to review certain ancient writings of the Oriental religions and those written commentaries constitute this volume. These commentaries are taken from his Collected Works and translated to English. A comment at the beginning of the book *Psychology and the East, The Collected Works of C.G. Jung* is given by Alfred Plaut, M.D. states the following:

> By temperament, Jung is nearer to the Eastern attitude of introversion and hence to the "God inside." This enables him to understand the Eastern emphasis on detachment and inner vision and to compare the latter with the imagery of the collective unconscious, with which Eastern man appears to be in direct and almost constant contact.[603]

He writes commentaries on *Alchemical Studies* and *The Secret of the Golden Flower,* and from these commentaries, one realizes that alchemy is another counterfeit story of redemption by emphasizing the transformation of physical matter such as base metal into gold and in so doing one can attain immortality. He also wrote "*Psychological Commentary on The Tibetan Book*

---

602 *Ibid.,* p. 209.
603 Jung, C.G. , *Psychology and the East,* Princeton University Press, (1978). Jacket cover back side.

of the Dead. Author Nandor Fordor in his book, *Freud, Jung and Occultism* remarks that many of Jung's beliefs were derived from *The Tibetan Book of the Dead.* Jung stated that it had been his constant companion since its publication in 1927.[604]

> The book gives instructions to the dead and the dying and serves as a guide to the dead during the heavenly and hellish journey of forty-nine days between death and rebirth.[605]

Jung's work, *Psychological Commentary on the Book of the Dead,* contains some revealing concepts commented on and found in his Collected Works:
1. The psyche (soul) has divine creative power within itself.
2. The creative ground of all metaphysical assertion is *consciousness,* the invisible, intangible manifestation of the *soul.* 3) The soul is assuredly not small, but the radiant *Godhead* itself. 4) Thus far the Bardo Thodol (Book of the Dead) is,… an initiation process whose purpose it is to restore to the soul the *divinity* it lost at birth.[606]

Jung tells us that the application of this spiritualistic theory was the basis of Freud's psychoanalysis. Also that when the European passes through this *Freudian domain* his unconscious contents are brought to view by analysis and he then journeys back through the world of infantile-sexual fantasy to the womb.[607] Jung continues:

> Originally, this therapy took the form of Freudian psychoanalysis and was mainly concerned with sexual fantasies. This is the realm that corresponds to the last and lowest region of the Bardo, known as the *Sidpa Bardo,* where the dead man, unable to profit by the teachings of the *Chikhai* and *Chonyid Bardo,* begins to fall a prey to sexual fantasies and is attracted by the vision of mating couples. Eventually he is caught by a womb and born into the earthly world again. The European passes through this specifically Freudian domain when his unconscious contents are brought to light under analysis, but he goes in the reverse direction. He journeys back through the world of infantile-sexual fantasy to the womb. It has even been suggested in psychoanalytical circles that the

604   Fodor, Nandor, *Freud, Jung, and Occultism,* University Books, Inc., New Hyde Park, New York, (1971) p. 157.
605   *Ibid.*
606   Jung, C.G. , *Psychology and the East, from The collected Works of C.G.Jung,* Volumes 10,11,13,18, Princeton University Press, (1978) pp. 62, 63, 64.
607   *Ibid.,* p. 65.

trauma par excellence is the birth-experience itself—nay more, psychoanalysts even claim to have probed back to memories of intra-uterine origin.[608]

...Freud's psychoanalysis leads the conscious mind of the patient back to the inner world of childhood reminiscences on one side and on the other to wishes and drives which have been repressed from consciousness. The latter technique is a logical development of *confession*. It aims at an artificial introversion for the purpose of making conscious the unconscious components of the subject.[609] (Emphasis added)

Today we have "pop psychologists" that purport to take one back into the womb by a process of deep breathing, and in so doing release the hypothetical psychological cramps of the original birthing experience, that is said to have allowed formation of anxieties, frustrations, etc., that man experiences. Below are some snippet explanations as to what today is referred to as "rebirthing."

(...) **Rebirthing** is an American form of prana yoga that is closest to Kriya Yoga. It may be called scientific breathing rhythm or spiritual breathing. Simply described, it is a relaxed, intuitive, connected breathing rhythm, in which the inhale is connected to the exhale, and the inner breath is merged with the outer breath. This merging of pure life energy with air sends vibrations through the nervous system and circulatory system cleaning the body, the human aura, and nourishes and balances the human mind and body. Rebirthing - Maha Yoga: Spiritual Breathing, by Leonard Orr

...**Rebirthing** is called rebirthing because many times the suppression that comes up and is released is related to birth trauma. When a rebirthee has released enough suppression (usually in 10 to 20 sessions) they have mastered the breath and feel safe enough with the process to rebirth themselves whenever they want. What is Rebirthing? By Russell J. Miesemer

(http://www.apologeticsindex.org/r08.html)

Contrast the above philosophy—psychology with scriptural reference to a rebirth.

The Savior said, "Except a man be born from above," unless he shall receive a new heart, new desires, purposes, and motives, leading to a new life, "he cannot see the kingdom of God." John 3:3, "Marvel not that I said unto thee, ye must be born again." I Corinthians 2:14; John 3:7.

---

608 *Ibid.*
609 *Ibid.*, p. 84.

But how can one receive this rebirth? The book *Steps to Christ by E.G. White,* p. 8 gives the answer:

> It is impossible for us, of ourselves, to escape from the pit of sin in which we are sunken. Our hearts are evil, and we cannot change them. "Who can bring a clean think out of an unclean? Not one." "The carnal mind is enmity against God: for it is not subject to the law of God, neither indeed can be." Job 14:4; Romans 8:7. Education, culture, the exercise of the will, human effort, all have their proper sphere, but here they are powerless. They may produce an outward correctness of behavior but they cannot change the heart; they cannot purify the springs of life. There must be a power working from within, a new life from above, before men can be changed from sin to holiness. That power is Christ. His grace alone can quicken the lifeless faculties of the soul, and attract it to God, to holiness.

I find very interesting a comment by C.G. Jung in relationship to, the *autogenic training* (later referred to as *biofeedback*) of the German physician, Johannes Schultz M.D., which Jung says consistently *links with yoga.* Schultz's chief aim, Jung says, is to break down the "conscious cramp" and the repression of the unconscious caused by it. Jung tells us his (Jung's) method is built upon *confession* similar to Freud's and he also uses *dream analysis* but on the *unconscious mind* philosophy they differ. He sees the unconscious as a *collective psychic disposition,* characterized by creativity in nature.[610]

Additional Bible texts reveal to us God's warnings in use of dream interpretation.

> Behold, I (am) against them that prophesy false dreams, saith the LORD, and do tell them, and a cause my people to err by their lies, and by their lightness; yet I sent them not, nor commanded them: therefore they shall not profit this people at all, saith the LORD. Jeremiah 23:32

> For thus saith the LORD of hosts, the God of Israel; Let not your prophets and your diviners, that (be) in the midst of you, deceive you, neither hearken to your dreams which ye cause to be dreamed. For they prophesy falsely unto you in my name: I have not sent them, saith the LORD. Jerimiah 28: 8, 9

> For the idols have spoken vanity, and the diviners have seen a lie, and have told false dreams; they comfort in vain: therefore they went their way as a flock, they were troubled, because (there was) no shepherd. Jeremiah 10: 2

---

610   *Ibid.*, p. 85.

Specific to yoga, kundalini yoga, tantric yoga, Lamaism, and Taoistic yoga of China, Jung sees *parallels* for interpreting his "collective unconscious." He intends for everything possible to be done which will *switch off* the conscious mind so as to allow the unconscious mind to emerge. He accomplishes this by using active imagination, imagery, and visualization in a special training technique for switching off consciousness.[611]

The final article in *Psychology and the East* from the works of Jung that I wish to refer to is "The Psychology of Eastern Meditation." To better understand the East Indian's spirituality a vision of his understanding of the *soul* is presented. Jung explains it by telling us that to the Indian the world is a mirage, a façade, and his reality is closer to what we say is a myth or a dream. The Christian looks upward and outward to a divine power from a Creator God, while the Eastern man looks down and inward, into *self-immersion through meditation*. God is understood to be in all things including man so to access God; the Hindu will sink the altar in his temple down into a deep depression or hole rather than have it raised up above the worshiper as we do in the West.[612]

For the Indian *true reality*—the soul, is quite different than what the Christian understands as the soul. The Biblical *soul* encompasses the body, mind, and spirit of a living being. It is all one, and with death, the soul ceases to exist. The body returns to dust, there is no thought and the life which God gave to the body returns to God for his keeping. Notice the following Bible verses which present this understanding.

> And the LORD God formed man (of) the dust of the ground, and breathed into his nostrils the breath of life; and man became a living soul. Genisis 2:7 and so it is written, the first man Adam, was made a living soul.... I Corinthians 15:45 For the living know that they shall die: but the dead know not anything, neither have they any more a reward; for the memory of them is forgotten. Also their love, and their hatred, and their envy, is now perished; neither have they any more a portion forever in any (thing) that is done under the sun. Ecclesiatics 9:5, 6 And the second angel poured out his vial upon the sea; and it became as the blood of a dead *man*; and every living soul died in the sea. Revelation 16:3 Behold, all souls are mine; as the soul of the father, so also the soul of the son is mine: the soul that sinneth, it shall die. Ezekiel 18:20

In Eastern thought *true reality—soul—*spirit, is considered a component of universal energy, prana, chi, etc., and the physical body is said to contain the *divine within*, the soul does not cease to exist at death of the body but passes on to *nirvana* or continues by passing into another body—reincarnation. The

611   *Ibid.*, pp. 85.
612   *Ibid.*, p. 170.

practice and exercise of *yoga* is also a way to reach the inner depths of this divine within—Self. Yoga is much older than Buddhism; "Buddhism itself was born of the spirit of yoga."[613]

Yoga is an act of worship in Eastern religions; it is a sacred act, similar to gathering together in song, praise, sermon, and prayer for the Christian. To refer to *Christian yoga* or utilizing it as a recreational physical activity (yoga exercises) is repugnant and sacrilegious to the Eastern mind. Jung attempts to build a bridge which he hopes to lead the European to an understanding of yoga, to do this he uses a series of symbols.

The *sun*, our source of heat and light, is a central point in the visible world. As the source of heat and energy upon which our world depends, it or its image has been accepted by many the world over as divine and worshiped as such. Special meditations and yoga exercises to the sun exist in every Eastern culture. In the Bible the *sun* has been used as a reference to Jesus Christ, as in an allegory. The Eastern mind turns to the sun in meditation attempting to "descend into the fountainhead of the psyche, into the unconscious itself." The Indian likes to enter into the maternal depths of Nature while the European desires to rise above the world.

Yoga exercises to the sun begin with concentration on the setting or rising sun, the sun is gazed upon until an after image is seen when the eyes are closed. Jung mentions that a method of hypnosis is facilitated by gazing at a bright object and he feels that the viewing of the sun as explained is meant to produce a similar hypnotic effect. Meditation of the *round* sun must accompany the fixation upon it. Eventually the meditator experiences himself as the only thing that exists, taking the highest form of consciousness. To reach this goal it is necessary to go through the above exercises of mental discipline to be free of the illusions of this world, and to reach the place where the psyche (soul) is one with the universe.

In the following quotation Jung compares these Eastern ways with the *spiritual exercises of Ignatius Loyola*:

> The *exercitia spiritualia* pursue the same goal. In fact both methods seek to attain success by providing the meditator with an object to contemplate and showing him the image he has to concentrate on in order to shut out the allegedly worthless fantasies. Both methods, Eastern and Western, try to reach the goal by a direct path....[614]

C.G. Jung continues in his attempt to bring understanding of yoga to the Western mind. *He is doing this because in this article under review,*

---

613   *Ibid.,* p. 168.
614   *Ibid.,* p. 171.

he concludes that the theory of "psychology of the unconsciousness", first initiated by Freud, and further developed by himself in the "psychology of the collective unconsciousness" is to the West what yoga is to the East. More simply stated: *they are of the same origin.*[615] This conclusion is further enunciated by remarks of Jung in his book *Man in Search of a Soul*. He says that Western Theosophy is just an amateur's imitation of the East. That the use of astrology is again taken up, which is daily bread to the Oriental. The study of the sexual life is surpassed by the Hindu. Richard Wilhelm showed Jung that certain complicated processes discovered by analytical psychology are described in ancient Chinese texts. We mention again the parallel between Yoga of the East and psychoanalysis as pointed out by Oskar A.H. Schmitz.[616]

Jung in ending his essay, *The Psychology of Eastern Meditation* makes the all-important contrast of meditation, yoga and Eastern thought, the parallel of Freud's and his, Jung's, theory of the *psychology of the unconscious* in contrast to the Christian thought grounded in the Bible. The Christian reaches his goal of salvation through faith in the merits of the shed blood of Jesus Christ the Divine Son of God, while *nirvana, being one with the universe—Samadhi*, is reached by the Eastern mind by going deep into SELF to join with the spirit world of Brahman.

In the Freudian and Jungian concept of the unconscious we find the origin of the inner child, inner self, inner healing, divine child—(Jung), etc. J. Beard points out that inner healing is an off shoot of Freudian and Jungian theories rooted in the occult. They have moved from the field of psychology into the church.

> A variety of "memory-healing" psychotherapies are masquerading under Christian terminology and turning Christians from God to self. Among the most deadly are 'regressive' therapies designed to probe the 'unconscious' for buried memories which are allegedly causing everything from depression to fits of anger and sexual misconduct, and must, therefore, be uncovered and 'healed.'[617]

In the first half of the 20th century that aspect of spiritualism "Self—the divine within" is seen to have been fostered and promoted by the philosophy and writings of these personalities presented. In the following chapter exposure is made of the subtle and imperceptible progression of the subject of "Self" in psychology through the latter half of the 20th century.

---

615 *Ibid.*, pp. 172-5.
616 Jung,C.G. , Modern Man I Search Of A soul, A Harvest Book-Harcourt, Inc., Orlando, Florida, (1933), p. 216.
617 Beard, J., *Inner Healing/Healing of Memories: Christian or Occult?* http://www.rapidnet. com/jbeard/bdm/Psychology/inheal.htm

CHAPTER 21
SECULAR PSYCHOLOGY "SCIENCE OF THE SOUL"? PART II SECOND HALF OF 20TH CENTURY

CARL ROGERS 1902-1987:

One of the most influential minds in the field of psychology in the last half of the 20 century is that of Carl Rogers. He is one of the founding fathers of Humanistic Psychology and also had great influence in establishing research in this field. He started his advanced education training in a theological seminary, but after two years he transferred to Teachers College, Columbia University, receiving a MA degree and then in 1931, a PhD in Psychology. He was on the faculty of Ohio State University, University of Chicago, University of Wisconsin—Madison, Western Behavioral Sciences Institute, and Center for Studies of the Person. He was known for originating *the person centered approach* for counseling and psychotherapy.

Carl Rogers's theory of the *Self* is considered to be *humanistic* and phenomenological.[618] His theory is based directly on the *phenomenal field* personality theory of Combs and Snygg.[619] An encyclopedia tells us that he wrote 16 books and many journal articles defending his theory.

In his book, *Client-centered Therapy* (1951), Rogers divides his theory into nineteen *propositions*. We will consider those propositions that pertain to the theme of this chapter, searching for and identifying seeds of *spiritualism* in psychology. Propositions numbers four and five relate to how the *Self*, the *I* or the *Me* is formed in man's development. Numbers eleven and twelve tell us that man's ways of behaving which have been adopted by his organism are formulated within the concept of S*elf*. The remaining propositions continue to elaborate on the theme of S*elf*. In his propositions outlining man's development of his personality, the main issue is the development of a *Self-concept* and the progress from an undifferentiated *Self* to being fully differentiated. A *Self Concept* definition:

---

618   Pescitelli, Dagmar, *An Analysis of Carl Rodgers' Theory of Personality,* Listed in Wikipedia/ Carl Rodgers. (1996).

619   Combs, Arthur W. and Snygg, Donald (1949), *Individual Behavior: A New Frame of Reference for Psychology,* New York, Harper & Brothers, Article on Snygg and Combs' "Phenomenal Field" Theory.

Self-Concept...the organized consistent conceptual gestalt composed of perceptions, of the characteristics of 'I' or 'me' and the perceptions of the relationships of the 'I' or 'me' to others and to various aspects of life, together with the values attached to these perceptions. It is a gestalt which is available to awareness though not necessarily in awareness. It is a fluid and changing gestalt, a process, but at any given moment it is a specific entity. (Rogers, 1959)[620]

If you find yourself confused by this definition of *Self*, you are not alone. Perhaps it will clear some as we progress in this study.

First we need to understand more of what *Humanism* is and then attempt to decipher the meaning of *humanistic psychology*. If a person reviews encyclopedias, or goes to the Internet and reviews the various web sites on the subject of *humanism* a voluminous number of articles are available. They cover the history of this thought and terminology going back to ancient Greek philosophers, ancient Asian and Renaissance humanism, and tracing its influence forward to our present time. Humanism is a *world view and moral philosophy* that places humans above their Creator God. In fact it does not accept the idea of a God, never mind a Creator God. It sees man as the center of the universe. In the ancient pagan concepts expounded on earlier in this book we spoke of the belief that man was the *microcosm* of the *macrocosm* (the universe). We presented a figure of a man standing within a circle, within another circle. This figure represented man as the center of the universe and under this symbol in the book *Magic and the Supernatural* by Maurice Bessy, figure 220, is written:

Man, as conceived in astrology, reflects the rhythms and structure of the universe in the same way as the universe mirrors the rhythms and structure of Man himself, everything is part of everything.

In the pagan belief man has a *super consciousness, True Self, Self,* which is the connecting link (divine within) to the wisdom of the universe and when man connects "all is One, One is all", "as above so below," immortality or godhood is achieved. In Freud's and Jung's philosophy and psychology this access to universal wisdom is through the *subconscious* and/or *collective consciousness* respectively, which is synonymous, as I understand it, with the expression *Self* used by humanists.

620 Rodgers, Carl (1959). *A Theory of Therapy, Personality and Interpersonal Relationships as Developed in the Client-centered Framework.* In (ed.) S. Koch, Psychology: *A study of Science.* Vol. 3: *Formulations of the person and the social context,* New York: McGraw Hill.

Humanist Manifesto I of 1933, declared the followers to be religious humanists and in their view traditional religions were failing to meet the needs of their day. They claimed to form a religion that would meet the needs of their day.[621]

Human Manifesto II of 1973, states that a faith and knowledge are required for hope for the future and that traditional religion renders a disservice to humanity. Manifesto II recognizes the following groups to be part of their naturalistic philosophy: *scientific, ethical, democratic, religious*, and *Marxist* humanism.[622]

Human Manifesto III of 2003, secular humanists consider all forms of religion, including religious Humanism to be superseded by *secular* Humanism, a religion that does not believe in God. Their view is compatible with atheism and agnosticism. They do not consider metaphysical issues, or the existence of immortal beings (spirits).[623]

Rogers is not known for being involved in paranormal psychology during most of his career, denies having any type of mystical experiences, or drug induced altered state of consciousness. XE "altered state of consciousness" Yet as he aged he gradually began to accept that there was really something to the experiences so many wrote about. He stated that the most convincing statements he encountered in the reporting of the paranormal were from Carlos Castaneda, and this man's encounter with the mystical through a Yaqui Indian medicine man—shaman.[624] He also gradually changed his concepts of what happens at death, from a total end of a person to the probability of life after death. He expands further on this subject as he relates the circumstances in his wife's final illness and eventual death.

Helen Rogers and Carl visited a medium in the later days of the illness that lead to her death. Helen experienced contact with a deceased sister and facts were shared by the sister that were totally convincing to both Helen and Carl.

> The messages were extraordinarily convincing, and all came through the tipping of a sturdy table, tapping out letters. Later, when the medium came to our home and my own table tapped out messages in our living room, I could only be open to an incredible and certainly non-fraudulent experience.[625]

621 http://www.americanhumanist.org/Who_We_Are/About_Humanism/Humanist_Manifesto_I

622 http://www.americanhumanist.org/Who_We_Are/About_Humanism/Humanist_Manifesto_II

623 Kurtz, Paul, *Living Without Religion: Eupraxophy,* Prometheus Books, Amherst, NY, (1995), p. 8.

624 Rogers, Carl R., *A Way of Being,* Houghton Mifß in Company, New York, New York, (1995), pp. 253, 254.

625 *Ibid.*, p. 90.

He tells of Helen having dreams and visions of a family member telling her she would be welcomed "on the other side." She experienced the sight of evil figures and the devil by her hospital bed. She eventually dismissed the devil and he left for good. She had a vision of a white light that came close, and lifted her from the bed and then put her back upon the bed. The evening of her death, friends of Carl who had a long scheduled appointment with the medium, held a séance session. Contact was made with Helen and she answered their questions. She told them she heard everything that was said while she was in a coma the night of death and again she experienced the white light and spirits came for her. She had taken the form of a young woman; dying had been without stress.[626]

Carl said that these events gave him a lot of interest in all types of paranormal phenomena. He accepted spirit life and reincarnation.[627] He found quite appealing the view that the individual *consciousness is but a fragment of a cosmic consciousness* and the fragment would be absorbed back into the cosmic consciousness upon the death of the individual, essentially the Eastern view of life after death.[628] Rogers had developed an interest in the exploits of Carlos Castaneda and his initiation into the sorcerer's world "Where the man of knowledge has a spirit ally, where the impossible is experienced." Rogers comments further:

> These and other accounts cannot simply be dismissed with contempt or ridicule. The witnesses are too honest, their experiences too real.

> All these accounts indicate that a vast and mysterious universe— perhaps an inner reality, or perhaps a spirit world of which we are all unknowingly a part— seems to exist.[629]

William Kilpatrick writes that he was present when Rogers related the following. After Helen's death Carl Rogers was ridden with guilt because he had formed a *new relationship* during his wife's illness, so after her death he with a group of people consulted an Ouija board, in spite of no previous use of the board, suddenly letters began to form...:

> It is Helen, and her message is one of complete absolution: "Enjoy, Carl, enjoy! Be free! Be Free!"

---

626 *Ibid.*, p. 91.
627 *Ibid.*, p. 92.
628 *Ibid.*, p. 88.
629 *Ibid.*, p 99-102.

"Well by gosh!" says Rogers, and he wipes his hand upward across his brow. "What a wave of relief swept over me when I heard that."

From the group, exclamation of awe can be heard: "That's incredible!" "Fantastic!"

And now it seems everyone in the group has had their mystical and quasi-mystical experiences:...premonitional dreams, poltergeists, and encounters with something known as "the white light." Whenever the latter is mentioned there are nods of familiarity, as though the white light were an old friend or a new G.E. product.[630]

Rogers, in *A Way of Being,* expresses his acceptance of and belief in the use of altered states of consciousness. He comments on the feeling of transcending experience of unity, where the individual self is a part of the whole area of higher values, such as beauty, harmony, and love. There is that feeling of being *one* with the universe. He shares the belief that the mystic's experience of union with the cosmos is confirmed by solid science. He shares with the reader his experience of when being closest to his *inner intuitive self;* he comes in touch with the unknown in himself. When he is in an altered state of consciousness he is full of healing and energy, just to be near the patient transmits healing. He speaks of the *life force* that is in each patient and therapist, which he tells us is like a meditative experience wherein he feels himself as a center of consciousness, "very much a part of the broader, universal consciousness."[631] (Emphasis added)

On the front cover of his book, Carl R. Rogers has written "The Founder of the Human Potential Movement Looks Back on a Distinguished Career." It appears to me that Rogers' influence upon the field of psychology is based upon the same foundation as Freud, Jung, and of the Eastern pagan doctrines, i.e., the lie told in the Garden of Eden, "you will become wise like God." That you have within *Self* access to the wisdom of the universe; it lies latent and must be developed. These teachings have indoctrinated the world through the influence of Eastern thought and similarly in the Western world in a disguised form, at times, under the banner of *psychology*—the science of the soul.

I have chosen to present the work of psychologists Abraham Maslow next, to illustrate progression in the development of *Self* in psychology toward more open spiritualistic concepts and practices.

---

630   Kilpatrick, William Kirk, *The Emperor's New Clothes* (Crossway Books, (1985), pp. 176,7.
631   Rogers, op. cit., pp. 128-130.

Abraham Maslow 1908-1970:

Maslow is considered one of the founders of Humanistic Psychology along with Carl Rodgers. Maslow considered humanistic psychology a *third force* in the field of psychology, the first field was of *Freudian*, the second *behaviorism*. Maslow added to the theories of Rodgers with the concept of *Self-actualization*, that of reaching the point of highest possible attainment for an individual. Humanistic psychology ushered in several different therapies; all guided by the idea that people possess *inner resources* for full attainment and therapy is designed to help clear away those things which tend to block this fulfillment.

Self-actualization of Maslow could be compared with the *self-realization* of yoga, both look to the inner Self to secure the ultimate growth and refinement of the soul. The inner-Self is the sub-consciousness of Freud, the collective consciousness of Jung, the Self- Concept of Rodgers and the Super-consciousness of the Eastern religions—*the god within.*

Maslow had a lot to do with the establishment of Transpersonal Psychology discipline. In 1969 Maslow, Grof and Sutich initiated publication of the *Journal of Transpersonal Psychology.* The Association for Transpersonal Psychology was founded in 1972. Transpersonal Psychology focuses on the *spiritual* aspects of life while parapsychology focuses on *psychic* phenomena. *Transpersonal psychology attempts to describe and integrate the experience of mysticism within modern psychological theory*. Transpersonal psychology is associated with New Age dogma.[632] This variant of psychology is often regarded as a *fourth* force of psychology, which in Maslow's judgments summarized in Wikipedia "*Transpersonal Psychology*":

> Transcends Self-actualization of Humanistic psychology.[633] Unlike the other first three schools of psychology i.e., psychoanalysis, behaviorism, and humanistic psychology which more or less deny the transcended part of soul, transpersonal psychology integrates the whole spectrum of human development from prepersonality to transpersonality.[634] Hence transpersonal psychology can be considered the most integrated complete psychology, a positive psychology par excellence.[635] From personality to transpersonality, mind to meditation, neuroscience to Nirvana, it is a complete wholesome science for all round development and treatment.[636]

---

632 http://Wikipedia.org/wiki/Transpersonal_Psychology p. 3.
633 http://www.maslow.com/
634 http://www.transpersonalcentre.co.uk
635 http://www.britanica.com/bps/additionalcontent/18/36678143/ Complementary-Research-Methods-in-Humanistic-and-Transpersonal-Psy-chologty-A-
636 http://www.psychotherapyuk.com/psychotherapy-london/psychotherapylondon.htm

In more understandable terms we could say that Transpersonal Psychology is more openly connected with the tenets of the neo-pagan—New Age mysticism than are the other disciplines of psychology. Now we trace the progression of the Self-concept onward into more open New Age theosophy through *Psychosynthesis* of Roberto Assagioli, M.D.

Roberto Assagioli 1888-1974:

Dr. Assagioli was an Italian Jewish neurologist and psychiatrist, having trained at the same mental hospital as did C.G. Jung in Switzerland. He learned psychoanalysis but was not satisfied with this discipline as he felt it was not complete and proceeded to develop what he called psychosynthesis. He was influenced by both Freud and Jung and felt that Jung was the closest to his theory. Psychosynthesis is broadly defined as a spiritual and holistic application of psychology having been developed out of psychoanalysis. It is an attempt to develop the "higher psychic functions, the spiritual dimension."

In 1938 he was imprisoned in Italy by Mussolini for one month due to his humanistic teachings and he used that month to investigate his inner-Self.[637] Assagioli sees the *will—the power of choice* in a central position of *Self-consciousness*. He combines the Eastern approach to mental health with Western psychology in a stronger way than most other psychologists have done. His writings are frequently quoted in the field of holistic health as well as mental health.

Will Parfitt, a practitioner of psychosynthesis for 40 years, in an article on the Internet titled *Roberto Assagioli The Kabballist,* presents what is known about Assagioli's connection to the Jewish secret society *Kabbalah.* Assagioli's library contained many books of mystical nature, writings of Gershom Scholem (the founder of modern Jewish mysticism), works of Alice Bailey and Theosophy, the works of Plato, etc. Most striking were psychospiritual articles written by Assagioli describing the psyche identical to the Kabbalah's description of the psyche. The psyche is divided into three divisions: the lower unconscious, the middle unconscious, and the upper unconscious which is the Soul—Self.

Assagioli was careful in his writings to avoid mention of the Kabbalah or its doctrines, yet it is apparent that he subscribed to its tenets. The Kaballah is pantheistic in its doctrines; it is mystical. Parfitt tells us that:

> Psychosynthesis easily interfaces with the *Kabbalistic Tree of Life* to create a model that can be effectively applied in many areas, particularly in the fields of healing, counseling and psychotherapy. Indeed, an understanding of the Kabbalistic Tree of Life is useful for practitioners of all types of therapeutic

---

637   http://en.wikipedia.org/wiki/Roberto_Assagioli

work. The larger, synthesizing context of the Kabbalah enables different models to be included without any subsequent loss of the integrity of each system.[638]

The Psychosynthesis psychology of Assagioli goes beyond transpersonal psychology in that it is quite open to the Eastern spiritualistic—pantheistic teachings. It can be seen that the pantheistic *Self* can be found in Freud's, Jung's, Rodger's, Maslow's, and Assagioli's psychologies, and that over time the progression to openness of a pantheistic tone is recognized.

Herbert Benson M.D.:

An author and researcher who is not a psychologist, but has become well known in the medical world; a cardiologist, and founder of Mind/Body Medical Institute at Massachusetts General Hospital in Boston, MA. He is a graduate and associate professor of Harvard Medical School. He is author or co-author of many scientific publications and authored a number of books which have sold more than 4 million copies in several languages. He was an early promoter of spirituality in medical practice. His work has been a bridge, joining medicine with religion, East with the West, mind with the body, and belief with science. His research and writings have had a significant influence in the field of medicine.

Dr. Benson and his work were included in the chapter *Ayurveda*, Meditation section. I wish to review its role in mind—therapy; its contribution to the field of psychology.

A discipline known as *The Relaxation Response* brought forth by Herbert Benson M.D. has had considerable influence upon the medical community. Dr. Benson conducted quality medical research, studied the physiological changes in the autonomic nervous system in followers of *Maharishi Mahesh Yogi* while they practiced *Transcendental Meditation*, and then he named those physiological effects of transcendental meditation *The Relaxation Response.* *R*emember, it took *meditation* to produce the relaxation response. He studied the effects of this relaxation technique upon various medical disorders in his Harvard research lab. He was able to show beneficial effects upon high blood pressure, help in reducing illicit drug use, benefit for migraine headaches, lower cholesterol levels, overcome insomnia, stimulate creativity, relieve various pain syndromes, and various anxiety disorders.

Dr. Benson is also Chief of the Division of Behavioral Medicine, New England Deaconess Hospital in Boston. His book, *The Relaxation Response,* has sold millions. It gained wide acceptance by the medical community because it showed benefits under controlled trials that met with the medical

---

638 http://www.willparfitt.com/

standards of research. The methods presented by Benson are easy and without cost. This method he considered as harmless to the physical body. However, it was not evaluated as to its effect upon the long term spiritual health. William A. Nolen M.D. wrote an endorsement to the relaxation response as follows:

> I am delighted that someone has finally taken the nonsense out of meditation... Without the need to waste hundreds of dollars on so-called "Courses," the reader knows how to meditate—and how to adopt a technique that best suits him or herself. This is a book any rational person—whether a product of Eastern or Western culture—can whole heartedly accept.[639]

Not only medical professionals but also the mental health establishment has accepted Dr. Benson's *Relaxation Response* as quality science and many therapists have utilized his technique. In 1975 it was introduced to the armed forces, "the *meditative* technique, cleansed of ideology," and made a smashing hit with the Admirals and chief of naval education. It became a standard in indoctrination of new recruits throughout the armed forces. All basic training programs use it because of its effect *as an alternative to drug use.*[640]

What is this Relaxation Response that the doctor has made so popular? Benson reviewed the past and present religions of the world, including practices of *shaman* of primitive tribes throughout the world, looking for and selecting a particular practice used in healing that tended to be common to all. He found that meditation similar to transcendental meditation contained the principles that were found in the healing practices he had reviewed in his study of the various ancient religions as well as certain present religions.

All non-Christian and mystical Christian systems have some form of Eastern type *meditation* in their religious practices. Apostolic style Christianity does not, it has the practice of what we refer to as study and prayer as its particular method of communion with God. However, within the Christian movement there has been a mystical branch as traced by Benson. It started with St. Augustine (354-430), and then continued through monastics of the desert (desert fathers) during the early Middle Ages, using the mantra as a form of prayer tool.

> The meditation practices and rules for living of these earliest Christian monks bear strong similarity to those of their Hindu and Buddhist renunciate brethren several kingdoms to the East... the meditative techniques they

---

639   Benson, Herbert M.D., Klipper, Miraiam Z., *The Relaxation Response,* Wings Books, a Random House Company, New Jersey, (1975), cover of book.
640   Ferguson, Marilyn, *The Aquarian Conspiracy,* J.P. Tarcher, Inc., Los Angeles, Distributed by St. Martin's Press, New York, (1980), p. 237.

adopted for finding their God suggest either a borrowing from the East or a spontaneous rediscovery.[641]

A book by an unknown author with the title of *A Cloud of Unknowing* written possibly in the fourteenth century promoted the use of a *passive mind* to achieve a contemplative mind (meditation). There are records of people in the Christian faith known as *Christian mystics* who practiced some form of meditation down through the centuries. We have continuation of this movement in the Christian community today teaching a similar practice, referred to as contemplative prayer.

The Relaxation Response is composed of four elements, previously listed in the chapter on Ayurveda but important to review at this point: 1) A *quiet environment*; 2) an *object* to dwell upon, *word* or *sound in repetition* (mantra) or to gaze upon some *object or symbol*; 3) *passive attitude*, an empting of all thoughts from one's mind; facilitated by deep rhythmic breathing; 4) a *comfortable position* allowing the same position for at least 20 minutes.

Medical research has substantiated that there are very definite effects upon our nervous system and endocrine system by use of these methods. The involuntary nervous system reacts to many methods of relaxation and stress reduction. The rate of metabolism will be slowed within minutes by 20% or more as revealed by the reduced utilization of oxygen. Blood lactate levels drop revealing that the muscles are in a more relaxed state, blood pressures will become lower, heart rate slows, breathing rate slows, and the brain wave changes from the beta rhythm to alpha rhythm which is a slower rate of electrical brain waves. All these changes result in improvement of various medical conditions as mentioned in the first paragraph of this section.

If the Relaxation Response is so easy, cheap, safe, accessible, and effective for problems that are not always responsive to medicines, why has this section on Relaxation Response been placed in this chapter which is exposing Satan's deceptions that are infiltrating the mental health field? Because it is insidious, deceptive, and *spiritualistic*. Dr. Benson has proposed the technique as a neutral method between science and religion by changing the word *meditation* to *Relaxation Response* and suggests use of Christian terms in the mantra. Many health professionals have accepted it. Some spiritual leaders believe they would not be partaking of its spiritualistic pagan tenets if they choose to use this method.

Meditation and yoga are worship acts and practices made to pagan gods. Transcendental meditation is a particular method of yoga wherein a secret

---

641   Goleman, Daniel, *The Meditative Mind* (Los Angeles, CA: Tarcher/Putman Inc. 1988), p. 53; Reported in Youngen, Ray, *A Time of Departing,* Lighthouse Trails Publishing, Silverton, Oregon, (2002), p. 42.

mantra is given that is never to be shared with anyone. This manta is in fact a name of a Hindu god and when the mantra is used the meditator in turn is calling upon that Hindu god to possess him or herself.

Some may doubt the above statement. I will share with the reader a recent experience that makes clear to me this is so. I was conducting a seminar on the subjects of this book in Massachusetts March 2010 and I had shared the above statement with those in attendance. Following the lecture a young man came to me with a question—how did I know this fact that the mantra given in transcendental meditation is the name of a Hindu god and that to repeat it is to call on that god to *possess* the meditator? I could not recall at that moment where I learned such, however, he told me I was correct, that it was a secret not to be revealed. He had once worked for the great Transcendental Meditation Ashram near Lancaster, Massachusetts and had been initiated into transcendental meditation; he had received the secret name of a Hindu god and bowed before two altars to Hindu gods in this initiation. One and one half years later he had surrendered his life to Jesus Christ and became a baptized Christian.

The Relaxation Response is a name given by Dr. Benson to the physiologic changes measured on transcendental meditators he used in his research. This *meditation* that he measured had the same response on the nervous system that occurs from meditation of Eastern religions, of Shamanism, of Christian mystics, Western occultism, of yoga, etc. For certain there are real effects, hundreds of experiments and studies substantiate that it is not a sham; *there is a power* in these practices. How does hypnotism bring changes to our nervous system to the degree that painless surgery has been done while under its influence, or painless surgery with patient awake with acupuncture? Men are able to walk or run through white hot coals of fire without burning flesh or clothing. Is this the answer?

> These Satanic agents claim to cure disease. They attribute their power to electricity, magnetism, or the so-called "sympathetic remedies," while in truth they are but channels for Satan's electric currents. By this means he casts his spell over the bodies and souls of men.--Signs of the Times, March 24, 1887.

In the Appendix H (*Satan's Ground*), there is a list of more than thirty different conditions or situations that are considered *Satan's ground* by Ellen White. Is it possible that a thirty-five hundred plus year old worship procedure, designed to worship and connect the worshiper to Satan's spirit world could be considered as *Satan's ground,* and an act that the worshiper of the Creator God would choose to avoid?

What has made The Relaxation Response so deceptive is *a name change*. Most of the medical profession at the time Dr. Benson was doing his research rejected practices coming from Eastern thought. By demonstrating physiologic changes from meditation and changing the name, prejudice was overcome. One of Dr. Benson's investigators, Dharma Singh Khalsa, M.D. shares with us his confirmation of the way that Dr. Benson was able to gain the medical professions acceptance of his relaxation response therapy.

> ...Transcendental Meditation, popularized by the Beatles, and the relaxation response, was popularized by Harvard's Dr. Herbert Benson. Dr. Benson, who directed a postgraduate course I took at Harvard Medical School, was chiefly concerned with isolating the most obvious healing aspect of meditation, and therefore focused his research almost solely upon simple, worry-free relaxation. *In so doing, he made meditation palatable to the medical community.*[642] (Emphasis added)

Dr. Khalsa is author of the book *Meditation as Medicine*, wherein he compares the relaxation response and Transcendental Meditation with his method—*Meditation as Medicine*. He makes the comment that *visualization, guided imagery, progressive relaxation*, and *affirmation are forms of meditation* but lack the value and full effects he sees from his method—*Meditation as Medicine*. He refers to Relaxation Response as the *kindergarten version* of *Medical Meditation.*[643] Khalsa points out that *Medical Meditation* has unique attributes wherein specific breathing patterns are utilized; postures are specific even to the position of the hands and fingers; specific mantras that give selected sounds; and a special mental focus are used. What makes the difference between a *kindergarten* level practice and one of superior effectiveness? Answer: the *spiritual sensitivity of the operator*, or said another way, the operator's close connection to the powers of the occult.

Dr. Benson followed his book, *The Relaxation Response,* with a second book, *Beyond Relaxation Response,* which brings out additional areas of interest not mentioned in the first book, *The Relaxation Response.* In this second book he emphasizes the *faith factor.* He speaks of two powerful spiritual vehicles: 1) meditation 2) personal religious convictions. The statement is made in his book that the use of Relaxation Response is to form a bridge between two disciplines, the practice and art of *meditation* and your *traditional faith.*[644] How does one connect an ancient practice designed to alter one's level of consciousness and to connect man with the spirit world and blend it with the Christian faith?

---

642   Khalsa, Dharma Singh M.D., *Meditation as Medicine*, Stauth, Cameron, New York, NY, (2001), p. 7.
643   *Ibid.*, p. 10.
644   Benson, Herbert M.D., *Beyond Relaxation Response,* A Berkeley Book, Times Books edition , 1984, Berkley edition ,(1985), New York, NY, p. 6.

As I read through this small book it soon became clear that the book is written to persuade one, of the beliefs of the Eastern thought, i.e.,, the origin of man coming from a theorized *energy* and not from a Holy Being—Creator God. Buddhism's doctrines are cautiously introduced throughout the book in a masterful way suggesting a blending of these principles with other religions including Christianity by use of the technique (Eastern style meditation) spoken of as the Relaxation Response.

A third book by Benson, *Your Maximum Mind*, moves the reader one more step further toward changing one's world view of reality. In this text Benson recommends his *Relaxation Response* technique as a means of:

> ...Our research has shown that to pass into the so called *hypnotic state*, the Relaxation Response is first elicited. Then, the hypnotist may suggest various actions to the individual being hypnotized.[645] (Emphasis added)

This above quotation is telling us that all that is needed after the Relaxation Response is reached is to have a hypnotist make suggestions and the meditator will respond accordingly. Is that not fully *hypnosis* when the Relaxation Response has been reached? Another question comes to my mind: what is the difference between a *hypnotist* and any other person that might give suggestions to the meditator that has achieved the Relaxation Response? I suggest this answer: the hypnotist has placed him or herself under the control of occult powers. What about the person who attained the *Relaxation Response*?

If I choose to use the Relaxation Response for stress or other reasons, how do I know when I have reached the full response? Dr. Benson gives the answer in *The Maximum Mind*, pages 38, 39:

> It's interesting that many people who have elicited the Relaxation Response— and experienced increased communication between the two sides of the brain—express the experience as a sort of "wholeness." They use such terms as "unboundedness," "infinite correlation," "well-being," and "intense wakefulness." Also, those in this state tend to have much greater awareness of the richness of details which surround them in their environment.
>
> Often people just say that the state is inexpressible; it's beyond words and language and can only be felt, not described. In its most intense form, this type of experience is known as a "peak experience"—whether you're talking about a spiritual insight, a winning sports effort or some personal intellectual break through.

---

645   Benson, Herbert M.D., *Your Maximum Mind*, Times Books, Division of Random House, Inc., New York, (1987), p. 38.

Benson in the same chapter as above refers to a Dr. Stanley R. Dean, professor of psychiatry at the Universities of Miami and Florida, who makes the following comment on this *peak experience*. As one that:

> ...produces a superhuman transmutation of consciousness that defies description. The mind, divinely intoxicated, literally reels and trips over itself, groping and struggling for words of sufficient exaltation and grandeur to portray the transcendental vision. As yet, we have no adequate words.

In the research laboratory when this state of full Relaxation Response has been reached, monitoring of brain waves reveals alpha and theta brain waves in both hemispheres. These are the wave lengths of a slowed brain activity which results from a passive mind, and theta is specifically the rate demonstrated in biofeedback and hypnotic trance.

The book, *Your Maximum Mind,* by Benson has as its purpose to share with the reader Dr. Benson's belief that by use of the Relaxation Response the brain can be tuned to bring forth its full potential. He presents the story of research that his laboratory from Harvard University did in Tibet, monitoring Tibetan monks as they meditated. One group of monks came into a room at 40 degrees Fahrenheit and took wet cloths, wrapped them over their bodies. Meditation style (*gTummo Yoga*), was entered into. The wet cold clothes within three to five minutes began to steam and in thirty to forty minutes the clothes were dry. They repeated this act several times.

Another group of monks living at 17,000 feet elevation walked in the early evening up to an elevation of 19,000 feet and dressed in sandals, loin cloth and a thin cotton cloth over the body. They took off their sandals squatted down with their heads resting on the ground in front of them and entered into *gTummo Yoga*. The temperature was zero degrees Fahrenheit. Thus they spent the night without even a shiver, in the morning they arose shaking off snow that had settled on them during the night and walked back to their monastery.

Dr. Benson shares with us his belief that the monk's ability to do these acts is a result of the *Relaxation Response—meditation* and relying profoundly upon their Buddhist faith. Might it not be the same power that prevents burns to clothing and skin for those who walk forty feet through white hot coals of fire?

In the book, *Your Maximum Mind,* Herbert Benson reveals how by use of the Relaxation Response we can increase our abilities in academic activities, music, health, creativity, spirituality, etc. We do this by bringing ourselves into the fullness of the Relaxation Response then exposing ourselves to any of those endeavors we wish to excel in. The level of achievement in that art will be much higher than we are able to achieve without using this technique. Why not take advantage of it?

Can I find in the Bible any suggestion that this is the way to enrich my spiritual life? Is there any hint of such in the books written by E.G. White? I have not found any suggestion of such. I do find the advice to seek wisdom from God. Solomon asked wisdom from God and was blessed with such. We cannot serve two masters at one time, it is always only one. Is it spiritually safe? The Christian will find his growth in abilities and wisdom coming from the Creator God of the universe, not hidden within his consciousness to be brought forth through an occult power.

> That their hearts might be comforted, being knit together in love, and unto all riches of the full assurance of understanding, to the acknowledgement of the mystery of God, and the Father, and of Christ; *In whom are hid all the treasures of wisdom and knowledge.* Colossians 2: 2, 3 (emphasis added)

Herbert Benson comments further:

> So when you are in this state of enhanced left-right hemispheric communication, it's easier to process information and view situations in a new and innovative way. In other words, a *cognitive receptivity* or *plasticity of cognition* occurs, in which you actually *change the way you view the world.*[646] (Emphasis added)

Benson told the *L.A. Times*:

> ...in his clinical experience, about 60-70% of those who begin a meditation-type practice primarily for medical reasons (often at the recommendation of their doctor) adopt the teachings. (Buddhism). L.A. Times *Quiet the Mind, Heal the Body*, 1/12/03

False Science of Mind Cure:

Philosophy since the time of Socrates and Plato considered the workings of the mind and expounded upon man's understanding of its workings. Man added to man's ideas; the scriptures were not consulted in an attempt to explain the mind, psychology became a discipline of its own. Scriptures were not accepted and an anti-Creator—God attitude was present through the ages. The *tradition of men* helped to devise many of the concepts and dogma that went into forming modern mind sciences. Undoubtedly there also has been worthwhile advancement in knowledge in the mind sciences that is valuable and not connected with spiritistic influences. It is important to make clear that there are psychologists and psychiatrists that do not use techniques that are related to the methods exposed in this chapter. However, it is important that we

---

646 *Ibid.*

understand these principles so if we choose professional aid in mental health that we are intelligent in those practices that are tainted.

> Says Paul, "Beware lest any man spoil you through philosophy and vain deceit, after the tradition of men, after the rudiments of the world, and not after Christ." (Colossians. 2:8) This scripture is especially applicable as a warning against modern Spiritualism. If the mind commences to run in the channel of phrenology and animal magnetism, it is almost sure to lose its balance. "Vain deceit" takes possession of the imagination. Many think there is such *power in themselves* that they do not realize their need of help from a higher power. Their principles and faith are "after the traditions of men, after the rudiments of the world, and not after Christ." Jesus has not taught them this. He does not direct the minds of men to themselves, but to God, the Creator of the universe, as the source of strength and wisdom.[647]

> For thousands of years Satan has been experimenting upon the properties of the human mind, and he has learned to know it well. By his subtle workings in these last days he is linking the human mind with his own, imbuing it with his thoughts; and he is doing this work in so deceptive a manner that those who accept his guidance know not that they are being led by him at his will. The great deceiver hopes so to confuse the minds of men and women that none but his voice will be heard.[648]

True Science Mind Cure:

At the beginning of the previous chapter this quote from book 1 *Mind, Character, and Personality* by E.G. White, p. 10 was presented. I desire to draw attention to it once again. Many pages in this chapter have been written exposing a false science of mind—cure that looks to Self—the divine within, as the power and means for restoration of mental health.

> **Laws of the Mind Ordained by God.**--He who created the mind and ordained its laws, provided for its development in accordance with them.

To have mental health it is first necessary to exercise the *power of the will*—to choose:

> No servant can serve two masters: for either he will hate the one, and love the other; or else he will hold to the one, and despise the other. Ye cannot serve God and mammon. Luke 16:13

---

647   White, E.G., ST, November 13, (1884), par. 1.
648   White, E.G., Letter 244, (1907). {MM 111.2.}

Satan cannot touch the mind or intellect unless we yield it to him[649]

> Christ can do nothing for those who are *yoked* up with the enemy. His invitation to us is, "*Come unto Me*, all ye that labor and are heavy-laden, and I will give you rest. Take **My yoke** upon you, and learn of Me; for I am meek and lowly in heart: and ye shall find rest unto your souls. For *My yoke* is easy, and My burden is light." When in our daily experience we learn His meekness and lowliness, we find rest. There is then no necessity to search for some mysterious science to soothe the sick. We already have the science which gives them real rest--the science of salvation, science of restoration, the science of a living faith in a living Savior.[650]

Within the scriptures are to be found the principles for safe and effective therapy for the mind. Those that may be looking for help and guidance for mental wellbeing, choose not only a Christian health professional but also one who finds in the scriptures his guidance for assisting patients in securing mental health. I have become acquainted with books written by authors that are guided by scriptures in their professional endeavors. Undoubtedly there are many more such professionals. I wish to share some names of authors and books so written.

First: A book entitled *Christians, Beware! The Dangers of Secular Psychology* by Magna Parks, Ph.D., a previously practicing psychologist. Her book is written, about an oftentimes confusing subject. With simplicity and clarity she tells her story of twenty years of psychological counseling following the secular methods taught by the schools she attended.

She once read a sermon that challenged the usual principles of therapy in psychology counseling and found it in opposition to her way of treatment. She studied to expose the error of understanding of psychology by this pastor as revealed in his sermon.

Her pursuit in this study led her to the conviction that he was right and thereafter she turned to the scriptures for her source of wisdom in bringing mental health to her patients. The conclusion Dr. Parks came to in her search for the *guiding principle* used in secular psychology is summarized in the following quotation.

> It is my prayer that what you have read in this book will provoke you to re-examine your perspective on secular psychology as it relates to your life as a

---

649   White, E.G., *2 Mind, Character, and Personality,* Southern Publishing Association, Nashville, TN, (1977), p. 710.

650   White, E.G., *Medical Ministry,* Pacific Press, Nampa Idaho, (1932), p. 117.

Christian. The teachings of secular psychology point us to one object—self. This is completely contrary to God's desire for us to be focused on Him.[651]

Second: *Depression The Way Out* by, Neil Nedley, M.D. , is another book that approaches mental health utilizing the physical, mental, and spiritual approach. It is especially directed at mental depression. Dr. Nedley is an internal medicine practitioner and during his specialty training he became interested in the mental affliction of depression. This disorder is extremely widespread in our country. He recognized that the results of the usual therapy were not very beneficial. The customary medical approach has been treatment of depression largely by medication. In his book Dr. Nedley places great emphasis upon lifestyle and changing our patterns of thinking, avoiding negative thoughts and carrying an attitude of gratitude. The value of helping people see themselves as having *true value* because they were bought with a price, the life of the Son of God, and avoiding the pursuit of *self-esteem* is emphasized.[652]

Third: Daniel L. Gabbert with 25 years of full time Christian ministry of which 13 have been in church pastoral ministry, six as a mental and spiritual health coach at Black Hills Health and Education Center, in Hermosa, South Dakota. There he conducts training seminars for those wishing to learn and share with others God's method of healing the mind. He has written a special training manual entitled, *Biblical Response Therapy®, Healing God's Way.* He too, has recognized the infatuation of *Self* by the mental health field. He exposes in great detail this false focus; tracing its origin from Satan in his rebellion—sin against God and to its infection and spread in man, therein identified as *Self.* In the preface of his manual the following words reveal the focus:

> The purpose of this manual is to provide sincere Christians the basic principles for leading hurting people along the incredible path of spiritual and mental healing and restoration **found in God's word.** These principles are based solely upon the precepts of healing the thought life (the habits of thinking and feeling) as found in God's word....[653]

The information prepared for the training course and contained in Gabbert's syllabus recognizes the influences of our physical health upon the function of the mind and thought life, the effects of diet, exercise, and even our world view. The syllabus material is based on scripture and occasionally selections from the author E.G. White as follows:

---

651   Parks, Magna, *Christians, Beware! The Dangers of Secular Psychology,* Teach services, Brush New York, (2007), p. 77.

652   Nedley, Neil M.D. , *Depression the Way Out,* Nedley Publishing, Ardmore, Oklahoma, (2001), chapter 5.

653   Gabbert, Ibid., p. i.

Man was originally endowed with noble powers and a well-balanced mind. He was perfect in his being, and in harmony with God. His thoughts were pure, his aims holy. But through disobedience, his powers were perverted, and *selfishness* (self) took the place of love. His nature became so weakened through transgression (sin) that it was impossible for him in his own strength, to resist *the power of evil* (Satan).[654]

IN CONCLUSION:

The purpose and goal of this chapter has been to search for seeds of spiritualism in the field of psychology/mind cure. This study was initiated because of statements by the author E.G. White naming phrenology, mesmerism (hypnotism), and psychology as laying the foundation for *spiritualism.* This statement is made several times in her writings. This search proceeded guided by definitions of spiritualism as understood by Ellen White, which are: man's consciousness in death, (*immortality*); spirits of dead return to minister to the living; no difference between righteousness and sin; man will judge himself; men are unfallen demigods (*divine within, pantheism*); Theosophy principles, theory of *animal magnetism* (which includes universal energy, universal mind, divine mind, *Self* and or *Divine Self*, consciousness, unconscious, and all synonyms).

> Spiritualism declares that there is no death, no sin, no judgment, no retribution; that men are unfallen demigods; that desire is the highest law; and that man is accountable only to himself....[655]

Thousands of men and women have been involved in the field of psychiatry and psychology and different forms of mind—cures but this discourse has presented only a few names that are more prominent in the literature of psychology as having formulated theory concepts which have influenced the field of psychology/mind-cure over the past 120 or so years. Within this book the foundational precepts of Eastern religions and mysticisms as well as Western occultism (Theosophy) have been presented. These in brief are: man's origin is from a blending of a universal divine energy, therefore man has divinity within—Self, man by his works progresses toward godhood, belief in reincarnation and that man eventually reaches *nirvana* (spirit's paradise).

Did we find any of the above defined aspects of spiritualism in psychology? Let us review: the concept of life after death (immortality) was found in philosophy writings down through the ages; the theories of the subconscious

---

654   White, E.G., *Steps to Christ,* Review and Herald Publishing Association, Hagerstown, MD, p. 17.
655   White, E.G., *Evangelism*, Review and Herald publishing Association, Hagerstown, MD, (1940) p. 608.

of Freud; collective consciousness of Jung; *self* of most other psychologists; are in reality synonymous with the doctrine of Eastern mysticisms and Western occultism. They are presented as apart from religion, but in reality I believe they constitute a near-religion with the same core dogma of Eastern religions, that is—*the divine within*.

This conclusion is illustrated by tracing the gradual change in the concepts of psychology during the past century. Freud was anti-religion and denied there were spirits until his later years; however, he promoted the doctrine of *intelligence in the unconscious*. Jung's life was filled with contact with the spirit world and by his own words this influence helped him formulate his theories of psychology, that of the collective unconscious which is the same as the Eastern consciousness. Rogers and Maslow were leaders in humanistic psychology which places man as possessing the *divine within*, Maslow moved farther than Rogers toward Eastern mysticism as seen in his interest in what is called *transpersonal psychology* which is an emphasis on *spirituality,* but not Biblical directed spirituality. Assagioli was oriented in psychology but also accepted parapsychology (occult manifestations) into the discipline of trans-psychology. Herbert Benson, the scientist, has taken the Eastern practice of meditation, repackaging it as relaxation, bridged it to religion for treating stress, anxieties, and various medical disorders.

Satan has not only controlled pagan man's loyalty by his *counterfeit teachings* of salvation by works, but also great parts of the Christian civilization by the greatest deceptive doctrine found in secular psychology, *Self.* I do not believe that all psychologists or psychiatrist are directed by this false doctrine in their therapy. There are undoubtedly practitioners who do follow the Biblical model of "True Science Mind—Cure."

The *law of the universe* is: God gives all things to the Son, who gives to the created, who in turn returns love to the Son, and the son to God, completing the great circle of beneficence. Satan introduced *Self* as a substitute for the love of God.

Eating of the fruit of the *Tree of Knowledge of Good and Evil* was proclaimed by Satan to make *man wise like God—man possessing within self all healing and wisdom of the universe. T*his is the theme of Satan's counterfeit story of God's creation and salvation.

In Paul's second Epistle to the Thessalonians, he exhorts to be on guard and not depart from the faith. He speaks of Christ's coming as an event to immediately follow the work of Satan in *spiritualism* in these words: "Even him, whose coming is after the working of Satan with all power and signs and lying wonders, and with all deceivableness of unrighteousness in them that perish; because they received not the love of the truth, that they might be saved. And for this cause God shall send them strong delusion, that they should believe a lie: that they all might be damned who believed not the truth, but had pleasure in unrighteousness.[656]

The warnings of the word of God regarding the perils surrounding the Christian church belong to us today. As in the days of the apostles men tried by tradition and philosophy to destroy faith in the Scriptures, so today, by the pleasing sentiments of higher criticism, evolution, spiritualism, theosophy, and pantheism, the enemy of righteousness is seeking to lead souls into forbidden paths. To many the Bible is as a lamp without oil, because they have turned their minds into channels of speculative belief that bring misunderstanding and confusion. The work of higher criticism, in dissecting, conjecturing, reconstructing, is destroying faith in the Bible as a divine revelation. It is robbing God's word of power to control, uplift, and inspire human lives. By *spiritualism*, multitudes are taught to believe that desire is the highest law, that license is liberty, and that man is accountable only to himself.[657]

The follower of Christ will meet with the "enticing words" against which the apostle warned the Colossian believers. He will meet with spiritualistic interpretations of the Scriptures, but he is not to accept them. His voice is to be heard in clear affirmation of the eternal truths of the Scriptures. Keeping his eyes fixed on Christ, he is to move steadily forward in the path marked out, discarding all ideas that are not in harmony with His teaching. The truth of God is to be the subject for his contemplation and meditation. He is to regard the Bible as the voice of God speaking directly to him. Thus he will find the wisdom which is divine.[658]

In these days when skepticism and infidelity so often appear in a scientific garb, we need to be guarded on every hand. Through this means our great adversary is deceiving thousands and leading them captive according to his will. The advantage he takes of the sciences, *sciences which pertain to the human mind*, is tremendous. Here, serpent-like, he imperceptibly creeps in to corrupt the work of God.[659]

---

656 White, E.G., *Confrontation*, (1971), pp. 91, 92.
657 White, E.G., *Acts of the Apostles*, Pacific Press Publishing Association, Nampa Idaho, (1911), p. 474.
658 *Ibid.*
659 White, E.G., *op. cit.*, 1MCP p. 19.1.

CHAPTER 22

MINDFULNESS—MEDITATION— BUDDHISM

Mindfulness meditation has captured the interest of the world in the   field of psychology and stress management the past few years. Interest in it has swept across America like a tidal wave and there seems to be no end in sight. We have been exposed and grown accustomed to Hindu type meditation and yoga over the past 50 or more years. But, what is this *mindfulness* you speak about? You say it has grown and spread everywhere, yet I have not heard of it and what's more I do not understand the word *mindfulness*.

Courses of mindfulness meditation are offered in many businesses, universities, government agencies, counseling centers, schools, hospital, religious groups, law firms, prisons, military, and other organizations. The business world, has taken a strong interest in the technique evidenced by articles in the business press, in books on leadership, and on the Internet. A book with the title of, *Resonant Leadership Renewing Yourself and Connecting with Others Through Mindfulness, Hope, and Compassion,* by Boyatzis and Mckee[660] along with many other books have added force to this popular subject.

The University of Massachusetts Medical School Center for Mindfulness in Medicine, Health Care, and Society, as well as Carroll's book, *The Mindful Leader,*[661] published in 2007 amplifies the widespread utilization of this style of meditation. Many fortune 500 companies utilize mindfulness for training programs as well as the CEOs of some companies practice such.[662] This University center has promoted the integration of mindfulness meditation in mainstream medicine and health care through patient care, research, academic medical and professional education. These activities have been directed by Saki f. Santorelli, EdD, MA, and with the founding of the center by Jon Dabat-Zinn, Ph.D. 18,000 people have completed an 8 week mindfulness-based stress

---

660   Boyatzis, R.E., McKee, a., *Resonant Leadership: renewing yourself and connecting with others through mindfulness, hope and compassion,* Boston: Harvard Business School Press, (2005).

661   Carroll, M. *The Mindful Leader: Ten principles for bringing out the best in ourselves and others,* (first edition) Boston, (2007): Trumpeter.

662   *Ibid.*

reduction program offered by this center.[663] Mindfulness meditation has and is making itself felt throughout the discipline of psychology.

What is mindfulness? How does it differ from other meditative techniques? What is the advantage? What is its origin? Is it spiritually safe? The term *mindfulness* is a translation of *Sati* of the Pali language into the Sanskrit word *smrti*, meaning "that which is remembered." David explains:

> Sati is literally "memory" but is used with reference to the constantly repeated phrase "mindful and thoughtful"; and means that activity of mind and constant presence of mind which is one of the duties most frequently inculcated on the good Buddhist.[664]

Shambhala Publications Presents, *A Guide to Buddhism,* and lists the basics of Buddhism:

> Four Noble Truths; The Eightfold Path; 1. Karma; 2. Attachment; 3. The Three Marks of existence; 4. Koans: *Mindfulness*; 5. Bardo; 6. Heart Sutra; 7. Loving-Kindness; 8. Pure perception.[665] (Numbers added by author)

This article on the Internet on Buddhism continues in attempting to define mindfulness.

> Mindfulness is the English translation of the Pali word sati. Sati is an activity. What exactly is that? There can be no precise answer, at least not in words. Words are devised by the symbolic levels of the mind, and they describe those realities with which symbolic thinking deals. Mindfulness is pre-symbolic. It is not shackled to logic. Nevertheless, mindfulness can be experienced—rather easily—and it can be described, as long as you keep in mind that the words are only fingers pointing at the moon. They are not the thing itself. The actual experience lies beyond the words and above the symbols. Mindfulness could be described in completely different terms than will be used here, and each description could still be correct.[666]

This meditation technique referred to as "mindfulness" was introduced by the Buddha about 25 centuries ago and is a set of mental activities aimed at experiencing a state of *uninterrupted mindfulness*. The article elaborates further with a comment that when this mindfulness meditation is prolonged,

---

663 http://www.umassmed.edu/content.aspx?id=41252. Center for Mindfulness in Medicine, Health Care, and Society, University of Massachusetts Director Saki F. Santorelli, EdD, MA
664 Rhys Davids, tr. T.W., *Buddhist Suttas,* Clarendon Press, (1881), p. 107.
665 http://www.shambhala.com/
666 http://www.shambhala.com/

using proper techniques, that the experience is profound and *it changes ones entire view of the universe*. This article is spread over three pages with additional paragraphs attempting to describe what mindfulness is. I will share the first sentence in several different paragraphs describing mindfulness to illustrate the difficulty in understanding what mindfulness meditation is.

> Mindfulness is a subtle process that you are using at this very moment. 2) Mindfulness is mirror-thought. 3) Mindfulness is non-judgmental observation. 4) Mindfulness is an impartial watchfulness. 5) Mindfulness is non-conceptual awareness. 6) Mindfulness is present-time awareness. 7) Mindfulness in non-egotistic alertness.[667]

I finally found a paragraph that had a sentence that made sense to me. *Mindfulness is not thinking.* Just reading this article and others like it in the attempt to explain this technique brings about feelings of mental confusion. Are you with me? Are you beginning to sense what "mindfulness" is? It is simply the Buddhist's word for bringing the mind into the silence, passive mode, an altered state of consciousness—Eastern style meditation. Then this altered state of consciousness opens to the possibility for the mind to be influenced and/or controlled by satanic agencies.

> In these days when skepticism and infidelity so often appear in a scientific grab, we need to be guarded on every hand. Through this means our great adversary is deceiving thousands, and leading them captive according to his will. The advantage he takes of the sciences, sciences which pertain to the human mind, is tremendous. Here, serpent like, he imperceptibly creeps in to corrupt the work of God.

> This entering in of Satan through the *sciences* is well devised. Through the channel of phrenology, psychology, and mesmerism, he comes more directly to the people of this generation, and works with that power which is to characterize his efforts near the close of probation. The minds of thousands have thus been poisoned, and led into infidelity. While it is believed that one human mind so wonderfully affects another, Satan, who is ready to press every advantage, insinuates himself, and works on the right hand and on the left. And while those who are devoted to these sciences laud them to the heavens because of the great and good works which they affirm are wrought by them, they little know what a power for evil they are cherishing; but it is a power which will yet work with all signs and lying wonders--with all deceivableness of unrighteousness. Mark

---

667 *Ibid*

the influence of these sciences, dear reader, for the conflict between Christ and Satan is not yet ended. . . .[668] (Emphasis added)

This 2500 year old Buddhist style meditation has been *secularized* for use in coping with stress, chronic pain control, immune disorders, anger, fear, greed, thoughts, feelings, attention, emotions, skills, addictions, performance, creativity, and changing the structure of our brains. It is proclaimed to change our relationship to life. It involves "inward investigation," to promote well-being. It is partaking of an ancient Eastern practice to inform, affect, and compliment life. It is said to now be based in science but was once in the realm of mystics and philosophers.[669]

Ron Kurtz a psychologist, a Buddhist for more than 35 years, and author of the online text *Hakomi Method of Mindfulness Based Body Psychotherapy*. Hakomi is a name he gives to his psychotherapy which, in turn, utilizes mindfulness as a principle component of therapy. We connect to Ron Kurtz's online book *Hakomi Method of Mindfulness Based Body Psychotherapy*.

1. Mindfulness is undefended consciousness. It has been defined as "the clear and single-minded awareness of what actually happens to us and in us at the successive moments of perception."
2. It is a skill; it improves with practice. *It is a traditional form of meditation*, especially for beginners, It is a traditional method of self-study.
3. In mindfulness, there is no intention to control what happens next. It is a deliberate *relinquishing of control*. That is why the first focus in traditional practice is often on the breath. To pay attention to the breath and not control it is more difficult than one might imagine, especially when we think about how little attention we ordinarily pay to breath and how well it works outside of our conscious control. Mindfulness is a way of *surrendering*.
4. In mindfulness, one attempts to calm the mind, to *silence thoughts*.
5. One focuses inward on the flow of one's experience.
6. In Hakomi, we use it in small doses (30 seconds to a minute).[670] (emphasis added)

668	White, E.G., *2 Selected Messages,* Review and Herald Publishing Association, Washington D.C., (1958), p. 351.
669	*Smalley, Suan, Winston, Diana, Fully Present: the Science, Art, and Practice of Mindfulness,* DaCapo Lifelong, Cambridge, MA, (2010), pp. xvii, xviii.
670	http://www.scribd.com/doc/6673762/HAKOMI-Methode p.4 (on line book) by Ron Kurtz (Now deleted from scibd.com)

In literature espousing Hakomi style psychotherapy, there is claim made by its practitioners that unconscious *core beliefs* of an individual can be made conscious through use of the *mindfulness* technique and that, in turn, this offers the opportunity to alter and change those fundamental core beliefs. A person's world view—"where did we come from", "why are we here", and" where are we going", are as a result of being placed in *mindfulness* subject to change.[671] "Mindfulness practice is a spiritual discipline."[672]

Ron Kurtz in his book tells us that when a person has attained a state of mindfulness the person becomes very still and **the eyelids flutter up and down over closed eyes**. This movement of the eyelids is almost always an accurate sign that the client is in mindfulness. Kurtz states that he uses this sign "all of the time."[673]

Psychologist Kurtz elaborates further in his use of mindfulness in his practice. He tells of when a person makes a change in their state of consciousness that their voice may become childlike, and vocabulary and speech are as a child. Past emotions and emotional memories from childhood may present, the face may express past childhood emotions. When this happens Ron Kurtz says the psychologist needs to contact that *inner child* by directly speaking to it, such as "you are feeling your youth again," etc. He further comments:

> When the child appears, you want to contact it....This childlike state is a very fruitful state to work with. The client is, in a sense, innocent and open, ready to be helped by an adult. I like to engage a client's adult self in the process of working with the child.

> I want the adult to help me understand what's going on with the child. I want to help the client self -engage with her child in a nourishing way, more nourishing than the child experienced in her formative relationships.[674]

This dialogue is wherein the patient communes with *another voice*, her or his *own youthful voice*. Is this a disguised spirit—demon contact?

> In dealing with the science of mind cure (hypnosis), you have been eating of the tree of the knowledge of good and evil, which God has forbidden you to touch.... Cut away from yourselves everything that savors of hypnotism, the science by which satanic agencies work.[675] E. G. White, Letter 20, 1902 (2SM, p. 350).

---

671   *Kurtz*, op. cit., p. 67.
672   *Ibid.*, p.36.
673   *Ibid.*, p. 124.
674   *Ibid.*, p. 23.
675   White, E.G., Letter 20, 1902 (*2 Selected Messages,* (1958), p. 350).

There are varying stages of entering into hypnosis. The first stage is entered by focusing on something, anything such as a light, sound, flame, or breathing. This is done until fatigue occurs and the awareness of outside activities wanes. Relaxation follows next, etc. The Bynum Scale of Hypnotic Susceptibility lists the following first five of 30 levels of hypnotism:

1. No Objective Change
2. Relaxation
3. *Fluttering of Eyelids*
4. Closed Eyes
5. Complete physical relaxation.[676]

To summarize the issue of *mindfulness*, I believe it to be, Buddhist meditation with the possibility of progressing to higher levels of hypnotism and at times channeling of spirit entities— demons. Let us now reflect upon this quotation:

> ...The mind cure is one of the most dangerous deceptions which can be practiced upon any individual. Temporary relief may be felt, but the mind of the one thus controlled is never again so strong and reliable....[677]

A comment in the book *The Great Controversy* comes to mind at this time as I struggle to clear the confusion created in my mind in attempting to understand and describe the great variety of definitions and explanations for this word *mindfulness*:

> Spiritualism teaches "that man is the creature of progression; that it is his destiny from his birth to progress, even to eternity, toward the God-head.". "The throne is within you."...Satan has substituted the sinful, erring nature of man himself as the only object of adoration, the only rule of judgment, or standard of character. This is progress, not upward, but downward.[678]

676　www.hypnosisforyou.com (now off Line)
677　White, E.G., *2 Mind, Character, and Personality,* Southern Publishing As sociation, (1977), p. 706.
678　White, E.G., *The Great Controversy,* Paciþ c Press Publishing Association, Nampa Idaho, (1888) pp. 554, 555.

CHAPTER 23

12 Steps — To Where? Part I

I was asked: what is your stand on 12 Step programs? My response was: what about 12 Steps? The answer came back to me: well, your seminars and book *Spiritualistic Deception in Health and Healing,*

expose spiritualism in health care, but you have said nothing about 12 step programs and we have personally taken programs where 12 steps were used and have concern. This comment surprised me. First, I knew only a little about the 12 step doctrine and in past years had felt no hesitancy to recommend participation in Alcoholics Anonymous 12 step program. Second, I was not as informed as I might have been that the 12 step approach had expanded as a framework for recovery therapy in so many different avenues.

There were several individuals encouraging me to study this issue and if a second book exposing spiritualism in health care was to be written, I was urged to include a discussion of this subject. Notice, I had a bias in favor of the 12 step program as used for various afflictions. This chapter is my response to those requests and from my research. These two chapters on Twelve Steps may seem excessively detailed and lengthy, however, every paragraph has been written with a specific purpose. That purpose is to relate to each of the principles presented to me in favor of the Twelve Step program by its proponents. Twelve Step exercises were not the first *steps* used in the field of mind therapy, Ignatius Loyola in the 1500's established S*teps* of *Spiritual Exercises* in his Jesuit Order, and later the eminent *spiritualist, Swedenborg* (1688 to 1772) included in his writings a spiritual 12 *steps*. However, there is no evidence that the steps of Ignatius were copied by Swedenborg or that the 12 step program of Alcoholic Anonymous was in turn copied from Swedenborg.

Today, "12 steps" are best known for their use in Alcoholics Anonymous sobriety programs. However, the 12 step method is used in a large variety of programs conducted to help people overcome addictions and improper habits. To understand how this came into being we need to tell the story how AA (Alcoholics Anonymous) started and grew into a worldwide organization.

The story is told in detail in *Alcoholics Anonymous* (the blue book) and *Pass It On*, published by Alcoholic Anonymous World Services, Inc., in this chapter it will be presented in a more brief form.

BILL WILSON:

Bill Wilson as a young man had risen in the financial world to a profitable position as a stock analyst of influence in the New York Stock Exchange. With his rise to financial success so to there was a rise of Bill's association with alcohol. Alcohol began to dominate his life to the extent that he was drinking night and day. When the stock market crashed in October 1929, so too did the fortunes of Bill Wilson. For the next five years Bill remained unemployed, supported by his wife.[679] His involvement in alcohol grew deeper with the passing of time.

Promises and attempts to stop alcohol consumption had been in vain, he was not able to stop, and continued the downward spiral toward oblivion. His physician brother-in-law convinced him to seek admission three times to the Towns Hospital for alcohol and drug addictions in New York City, which was known for its "belladonna treatment" (a combination of two hallucinatory drugs) along with hydrotherapy. After the third admission in less than two years he left the hospital sobered for a few months, but reasoned he could take "one" drink on Armistice Day 1934; he quickly found himself back where he started, incessant drinking.

As Bill sat drinking in the kitchen at his home while his wife was away working, he received a telephone call from an old drinking friend requesting permission to come to Bill's home to visit. Bill states that his friend was *sober*; it had been years since Bill had seen him that way.[680] Bill looked forward to drinking again with his friend, Ebby Thatcher. When Ebby came into the house and sat down Bill pushed a drink across the table but Ebby refused the drink. Bill urged him again to take it but a firm refusal was the response. Bill asked "what is all this about?" The reply: "I've got religion." Bill was stunned, but reasoned that it left more drink for himself. Ebby then shared with Bill how two months previously his friend Rowland H., came from the "Oxford Group" as he, Ebby, was in court and the judge was committing him to the insane asylum. The judge was persuaded to suspend the sentence and let Rowland and his friends work with Ebby Thatcher in their religious way. Ebby Thatcher said it worked; for two months he had been dry.[681]

Rowland H. was a recovered alcoholic and had an interesting story as it has to do with the earliest beginnings of Alcoholic Anonymous. Rowland was desperately trying to become sober so he went to Switzerland to be a patient of the psychiatrist C.G. Jung M.D. There he received therapy for a year and returned home. Before long he returned to alcohol. He returned to Switzerland

---

679   Alcoholics Anonymous World Services, Inc, *Alcoholics Anonymous,* Bill's Story, New York City (1939), p. 4.
680   *Ibid.,* p. 9.
681   Alcoholic World Services, Inc., *Pass It On, New York N.Y., (1984), p. 115.*

but Jung told him he had no more help for him and to go home and find a *spiritual* answer through religion. Rowland returned home, joined the *Oxford Group* and became sober. He heard of his friend Ebby and sought him out at the time the judge was going to commit him.

Bill's friend Ebby, had come to Bill to offer him this same path to sobriety, if he was interested. Bill was interested, realizing he was hopeless. In writing about this event Bill reviews his understanding of the forces in the universe. He declares that he was not an atheist:

> ...Despite contrary indications, I had little doubt that a mighty purpose and rhythm underlay all. How could there be so much of precise and immutable law, and no intelligence. I simply had to believe in a Spirit of the Universe, who knew neither time nor limitation. But that was as far as I had gone. With ministers, and the world's religions, I parted right there. When they talked of a God personal to me, who was love, superhuman strength and direction, I became irritated and my mind snapped shut against such a theory.[682]

When Bill looked at and listened to his friend who had been in the process of being committed, to being locked up, because he was totally incapable of personal control. As he heard the testimony of Ebby testifying of his miraculous recovery, Bill then and there had a re-appraisal of his prejudices toward religious people. Here was an impossible change in a human heart. Bill comments in telling his own story that he could accept a power of the universe referred to as Creative Intelligence, Universal Mind, or Spirit of Nature, but could not accept a King of the Heavens no matter if He was said to be the source of love.

At this point Ebby suggested to Bill, why not go ahead and *choose his own concept of God?* What a thought, just to be willing to believe in a *Power greater than himself*, nothing more, Wow! There was no real surrender at this point and Bill continued to drink. Some days later Bill was drunk and in despair, so he sought out Ebby for help. Ebby was not at the mission where he stayed, but Bill attended the meeting that was being conducted at the mission by the Oxford Group. In a drunken condition he kneeled and committed himself to the *God of his understanding*. However, he continued to drink. Bill was at his lowest ebb once again, recognizing he was incapable of climbing out of the pit he had slid into. He admitted himself once again into the alcoholic rehab hospital in New York. Bill tells us he placed himself into the hands of God, *as he understood him*. It was while undergoing treatment with Dr. Silkworth's *Belladonna Cure* Bill experienced a *Hot Flash* spiritual conversion while in the Towns Rehab Center, and he ceased drinking. Immediately prior this sudden conversion Bill Had shouted out:

---

682 Alcoholic Anonymous, *op. cit., p. 10.,* p. 10.

I'll do anything! Anything at all! If there be a God, let Him show himself!" What happened next was electric. Suddenly, my room blazed with an indescribably white light. I was seized with an ecstasy beyond description. Every joy I had known was pale by comparison. The light, the ecstasy — I was conscious of nothing else for a time.[683]

Then, seen in the mind's eye, there was a mountain. I stood upon its summit, where a great wind blew. A wind, not of air, but of spirit. In great, clean strength, it blew right through me. Then came the blazing thought 'you are a free man.' I know not at all how long I remained in this state, but finally the light became more quiet, a great peace stole over me, and this was accompanied by a sensation difficult to describe. I became a living spirit. I lay on the shores of a new world. 'This' I thought, 'must be the great reality. The God of the preachers.'[684]

A question, what is the source of this *Hot Flash* experience? Did the hallucinating drugs he was being prescribed while in the hospital have any effect? Was it from the Creator God of the Universe? Did it come from some other power? The effect was certainly long lasting; and the first time Bill had experienced anything like it.

Wilson had his *hot flash* spiritual awakening, while being treated with these drugs, He claimed to have seen a white light and when he told his attending physician, Dr. Wiliam Silkworth about his experience, he was advised 'not to discount it.' When Wilson left the hospital he never drank again.[685]

He took full responsibility for his ways and turned them over to this new found *Friend*, the new *God-consciousness within*,[686] and the effect was "electric."[687] Bill drank no alcohol from that day forward, December 11, 1934.

Ebby continued to share with Bill the principles that the Oxford Group taught which are identified in *Alcoholics Anonymous Comes of Age* by Bill Wilson. These consist of self-examination for character faults, then admitting and confessing them to some other human, giving restitution to those who you may have harmed, and working as a missionary to help others who are in a similar status.[688]

683   Pittman, Bill, *AA The Way It Began,* Glenn Abby Books, (1988), pp. 163- 65.
684   Pass It On, op. cit., p. 121.
685   Pittman, op. cit., pp. 83-87, pp. 165-167.
686   *Alcoholics Anonymous*, op. cit., p 13.
687   *Ibid.*, p. 14.
688   Wilson, William, *Alcoholic Anonymous Comes of Age,* Alcoholic Anonymous World Services Inc., (1957), p. 39.

OXFORD GROUP:

Let us digress a bit at this time in Bill's story to gain an understanding of the *Oxford Group*. An American Lutheran pastor, Frank Buckman, initiated a spiritual movement starting in the U.S. in 1908, then, moving to England by 1921; it was known as *A First Century Christian Fellowship*. It grew rapidly in numbers and by 1931 was referred to as the *Oxford Group*, and in 1939 was legally incorporated under that name. They were centered in England at Oxford. This movement became *international* with participation of hundreds of thousands in number in many countries of Europe, the Americas, and Asia. There were no membership rolls, no dues, no paid leaders, no theological creed, nor regular meetings. It was a fellowship of people wishing to follow *their God*; chosen by their understanding of a *Higher Power.*

Buchman paid little attention to theology as found in the scriptures, he stressed simplicity of beliefs and emphasized people are sinners, all sinners are capable of changing, *confession* must precede change, with a change God can be *accessed directly*, miracles do happen, and those individuals changed must guide others into change.[689] With the characteristic of minimal theology this movement was accepted by other beliefs with little concern. The goal of this movement was to bring *global peace* through changing people from the heart outward. It concentrated its missionary effort on persons of leadership positions and of wealth. In this endeavor they were very successful.

The minimal theology of the Oxford Group consists of four absolutes: 1) absolute honesty, 2) absolute purity 3) absolute unsefulness 4) and absolute love. Spiritual practices employed were 1) Sharing (confessing) your sins with another person; 2) Surrendering your past, present, and future life unto the control of the Higher Power of one's understanding; 3) Restitution to any one harmed; 4) *Listening* for God's *guidance* and then following it.

It was a custom to *confess one's sins* (sharing) not only to another individual but also in a public forum. The sharing of the sins of members was practiced with the idea that it would help others that as of yet had not changed, to recognize they were sinners and openly confess their sins. The Oxford Group looked at alcoholism as a spiritual "disease— sin" hence the need for a spiritual solution which confession addressed; consequently a *cure* was possible. *Listening for God's guidance* was done daily in early morning by private meditation, prayer, and scripture study. The individual would take pen and paper and write down the directions received from God during the "silence" of meditation.

---

689 Mercandante, Linda, *Victims and Sinners,* Westminster John Knox Press, (1996), pp. 50-51 Reported in Wikipedia.org/wiki//OxfordGroup, p. 20.

BILL WILSON: (continued)

From the time Bill W. reached sobriety and began to proselyte the principles of the Oxford Group until his first success of helping bring another alcoholic to sobriety (Dr. Bob Smith) was fifty drunks and six months later, summer, June 10, 1935.[690] Lois and Bill Wilson attended an Oxford Group meeting in Frederick, Maryland at Francis Scott Key Hotel. James Houck, an Oxford Group member also attended these meetings stated that Bill W. always centered on alcohol and was obsessed with carrying the message of deliverance.

Bill was on a business trip to Akron, Ohio, in May 1935, but the business proposition he came to complete fell through, plunging him into a compulsion to drown it in alcohol. At the Mayflower Hotel in Akron, where he was staying he looked into the cocktail room and was tempted to go in, get drunk and forget this mis-adventurous business trip. He fought off the overwhelming urge, said a prayer, 'received guidance,' and then looked at the ministers' directory board in the hotel. His finger fell on the name of Reverend Tunks who turned out to be acquainted with members of the Oxford Group in Akron. Bill was directed by Tunks to call Henrietta Seiberling; as a new Oxford Group had been meeting at her house for just one month. Bill was invited to join with them in a meeting where he met Bob Smith, M.D. The meeting with Dr. Bob was the beginning of a long association, as well as experiencing his first success in helping another drunk to sobriety.

BOB SMITH, M.D.: (Dr. Bob)

Bob Smith was raised in a small New England town by a religious family. With his family, he attended regularly not only Sunday services but Sunday evening, Monday evenings and often Wednesday for prayer meeting. When he left home he decided not to enter a church again except for special occasions, such as funerals, etc. This pledge he was faithful to.

In his college days he took up drinking for pleasure and he excelled in this new-found pursuit. Following the college years he worked as a salesman selling large hardware products and was able to continue the use of alcohol without interfering in his work. After three years he chose to study medicine. The companionship of alcohol continued with him into the study of medicine. It caused him to have to transfer to another medical school after his second year. He eventually finished school, and then had two further years of hospital internship training. During the internship he was too busy to have time to

---

690   Raphael, Matthew J., *Bill W. and Mr. Wilson,* University of Mass. Press, Amherst, (2000), pp.97-106; *Pass It On,* op. cit., p. 149.

drink. He went into private practice following the internship and once again took up drinking.

Alcohol plagued him throughout his working years. He admitted himself to rehab institutions many times, yet, continued to drink. During these years his wife was faithful to him and continued to search for some method of help. Nothing was of value. In the spring of 1935, Bob had contact with members of the Oxford Group in his town and through Henrietta Seiberling of Akron met a man (Bill W.) who was a recovered alcoholic. This friendship resulted in Dr. Bob's sobriety, starting June 10, 1935, when Dr. Bob took his last drink. This friendship of Dr. Bob and Bill W. resulted in the birth of Alcoholics Anonymous, June 10, 1935.[691]

ALCOHOLICS ANONYMOUS:

Bill Wilson stayed in Akron for some months attempting to resurrect the business project that had brought him to Akron, while also continuing to support Dr. Bob Smith in his ongoing sobriety. Both began to work for other alcoholics in Akron as well as attending Oxford Group meetings. Bill eventually moved into the home of Dr. Bob as he worked on his business project. They began to work on developing a program to be used to help alcoholics gain sobriety. They immediately looked for drunks to share their approach with. A third recovered alcoholic, Bill D., soon joined them in sobriety, then a fourth, Ernie. A partnership was born for working with alcoholics.[692] There was no name for this group; however, they still stayed close to the Oxford Group. After four months in Akron Bill's business adventure failed so he returned to New York.

Bill and Lois attended Oxford Group meetings including various Oxford house parties (large gatherings) from 1934 until 1937. Bill was holding his own meetings for alcoholics at his home during the time he was attending the Oxford meetings. This brought a rift between the two groups in 1935.[693] The Oxford Group in New York advised the alcoholics they were working with not to attend the meetings at the home of Bill and Lois. Bill departed from the Oxford Group in 1937. In 1938 the Oxford Group was asked by Oxford University to change its name to avoid controversy; this it did taking the name *Moral Rearmament* (M.R.A).[694]

In 1937 Bill traveled to Akron, Ohio, to see Dr. Bob. The two men conducted a formal review of their separate work. There were nearly 40 men

---

691   Alcoholic Anonymous World Services, Inc., *Alcoholic Anonymous,* (2001) Fourth Edition, pp. 171-181.
692   *Pass it On,* op. cit., pp. 164-70.
693   *Ibid.,* p. 169.
694   *Ibid.,* p. 171.

in sobriety as a result of their work the past two years. Both Dr. Bob and Bill W. were broke financially but rich in spirit. They came to the realization that it might be possible for their program to eventually circle the globe.

> What a tremendous thing that realization was! At last we were sure. There would be no more flying totally blind. We actually wept for joy, and Bob and Anne and I bowed our heads in silent thanks.[695]

In this meeting, agreement was made for preparing a book to be used in their meetings. A book would make it possible to present a standard program everywhere. As they were working with alcoholics to gain sobriety they had been recommending a book on the beatitudes of the Bible, authored by a *New Thought Movement* minister, Emmett Fox. Several individuals that joined the groups and became ex-alcoholics wrote in their testimonies of having received recommendation from their group leaders to study that book.

In the spring of 1938 Dr. Bob and Bill W. moved forward to produce a text book for their group. The duty for writing fell upon Bill W. The purpose for the book was to have a text that would stimulate interest in sobriety, motivate those desiring to reach this goal and contain the program information followed in the recovery meetings that were presently being conducted. When Bill came to the place in the book writing where he was to form the basic program to follow, he hesitated; he knew it needed to be powerful and thorough:

> There must not be a single loophole through which the rationalizing alcoholic could wiggle out.[696]

So far the recovery programs conducted did not have written material to follow; they simply followed word-of-mouth techniques. There were six basic steps then in use by the Oxford Group as follows:

1. We admitted that we were licked, that we were powerless over alcohol.
2. We made a moral inventory of our defects or sins
3. We confessed or shared our shortcomings with another person in confidence.
4. We made restitution to all those we had harmed by our drinking.
5. We tried to help other alcoholics, with no thought of reward in money or prestige.
6. We prayed to whatever God we thought there was for power to practice these precepts.

---

695   *Ibid.*, p. 178.
696   *Ibid.*, p. 196.

Bill had concern that the six steps as outlined were not definitive enough and needed amplification so as to avoid ambiguity. In December of 1938, while lying in bed with pen and paper he first *relaxed, then asked for guidance,* and then began to write. As he started writing the words flowed out of his mind and within 30 minutes he had formed 12 steps in the place of the original six.[697]

When the book manuscript was finished, 400 copies were printed to be circulated for appraisal. There was strong criticism by the atheists and agnostics in the group of recovered alcoholics reviewing the manuscript prior to printing because of the word "God" being used so frequent. So the word "God" was changed to "Higher Power as you understand it" and or "God as we understand Him" was substituted in most places. Another expression Bill had used was the expression "asking of God on one's knees to having one's shortcomings removed," and this phrase was requested to be removed. Thus the agnostics and atheists were placated. In April of 1939 Alcoholics Anonymous had become a fellowship with its own text and program.

The 12 steps are the backbone of the Alcoholics Anonymous program; the title soon took on the nick-name *Fellowship* and has continued for the past seventy plus years. There was a difference in philosophy from the teachings of the Oxford Group and Alcoholics Anonymous Fellowships; the Oxford Group taught that alcoholism is a spiritual malady and can only be cured by spiritual means; Alcoholics Anonymous takes the stand that alcoholism is a *disease* that needs a spiritual experience to control but does not affect a cure. Hence, once an alcoholic—always an alcoholic so there is need to have continuous fellowship.

The completed book contained the 12 steps. At this time in 1939 the number of recovered people was slightly more than one hundred. They voiced their reason for supporting the publishing of this book.

> We, of Alcoholics Anonymous, are more than one hundred men and women who have recovered from a seemingly hopeless state of mind and body. To show other alcoholics precisely how we have recovered is the main purpose of this book...[698]

PROGRESS

Progress in spreading the 12 step program was slow as were the book sales. There was a gradual increase in locations for the Fellowship meetings and contacts were made in various ways which often led to additional groups starting. On a cold rainy night in the winter of 1940 Bill W. had an unexpected

---

697   *Ibid.,* p. 198.
698   *Ibid.,* pp. 203, 204.

guest. Father Ed Dowling, a Jesuit Priest from St. Louis, also editor of the *Queen's Work*, a Catholic publication. He had come to visit with Bill after obtaining and reading the book, *Alcoholics Anonymous*. The book created a great interest in this priest and he wanted to discuss it with the author. He said he was fascinated by it because of parallels of *12 Steps of AA* to the Spiritual *Exercises* of St. Ignatius, the spiritual discipline of the Jesuit order. Bill stated he knew nothing of the exercises of Loyola. The similarity of spiritual exercises of the Jesuit Order and the AA 12 steps so impressed the local Jesuit organization in St. Louis where Father Dowling was a member, that another priest (an alcoholic) of the order wrote out both the Jesuit spiritual exercises and the 12 steps and posted them together in the *Queen's Work* publication office. A friendship started that night of their meeting which was to grow in depth for the next twenty years. Bill later characterized that evening as the evening he had a "second conversion experience."

On March 1, 1941, *The Saturday Evening Post* published an article on Alcoholics Anonymous 12 step program, and success in sales of the book as well as increased interest of people wishing to participate in the program followed immediately. The country now knew of AA, book orders came in and there was steady progress in expansion in the number of fellowship meeting groups.

A mental state of deep depression afflicted Bill Wilson around 1944 and was to remain with him for ten years. It greatly interfered in his work. He was unable to write more than one half page per day as he worked on his next book *Twelve Steps and Twelve Traditions*. Nell Wing, his secretary, tells that he frequently broke down in tears while dictating to her. He found that many recovered alcoholics a few years following recovery, suffered depression. He wrote letters to many of them in an attempt to help them and himself as well.

In 1953 the Alcoholic Anonymous organization published *Twelve Steps— Twelve Traditions*, a book that had taken Bill W. several years to complete. This book was an extensive treatise and amplification on the 12 steps that had been the backbone of Alcoholics Anonymous' program for gaining sobriety. He added the Twelve Traditions that pertained to the working and governing principles of their organization. These Tradition Steps in 1950 had previously been ratified by the first International Alcoholics Anonymous Convention. This book became a very popular addition to the literature of Alcoholics Anonymous.

Alcoholics Anonymous eventually received acceptance, as a powerful, safe, inexpensive, method for gaining sobriety. This acceptance came from the medical establishment, from religious bodies (especially from Roman Catholicism), and from most secular organizations and general public. It became a worldwide organization, guided by the books *Alcoholics Anonymous* and *Twelve Steps and Twelve traditions.* The program is the same in all countries of the world.

This organization has maintained that it is not a religion but simply a tool which all organizations and religions may safely use without interfering in their religious belief or personal persuasion. Bill Wilson put great effort in writing to choose words and phrases that would keep wide the gate of entrance into AA. He stated that he had to make it work for:

> "...atheists, agnostics, believers, depressives, paranoids, clergymen, psychiatrists, and all and sundry".[699]

The Foreword for the 2nd edition of *Alcoholics Anonymous* in 1955 states there were 6000 groups in 52 countries with 150,000 recovered alcoholics. In March of 1976 the 3rd edition was introduced and 1,000,000 people were meeting in 28,000 groups in 90 countries. By the time of the third edition *Alcoholics Anonymous* had been translated into 43 languages. The 4th edition came off the press November 2001. Comment is again made that the membership had doubled to 2,000,000 since 1976; 100,800 groups were meeting in 150 countries and 15,000,000 books of Alcoholics Anonymous had been printed.

The core principles utilized in the group meetings are the 12 steps. These steps have been used in many other programs for recovery from different addictions and destructive practices; for obesity, narcotic addiction, anger control, sexual perversions, and a variety of programs for anxiety and neurosis. The 12 steps are also in popular use within many churches. Wikipedia in an article on the 12 steps contains the following quote:

> In 1999 Time Magazine declared Bill W. to be in the top twenty of the *Time 100: Heroes and Icons* who exemplified "courage, selflessness, exuberance, super human ability and amazing grace" in the 20th century.[700]

A writer, Dick Burns, a recovered alcoholic now in his eighties, has produced 30 or more books promoting the 12 step program as originating from a Christian organization, *the Oxford Group*, and that the co-founders, Dr. Bob and Bill W. , were near to being Christians. He also has been a staunch defender in print against critics that dispute his characterization of 12 steps being a Christian-based program. Charges of involvement of spiritualism in

---

699 Fitzgerald, Robert, S.J., *The Soul of Sponsorship,* Hazelden, Center City, Minnesota, (1995), p. 58.

700 Time, *Time 100: The Most Important People of the Century,* retrieved Dec. 31. (2007), Bill Wilson reference # 5. Reported in Wikipedia.

the origin of and contained within the 12 steps have been made over the years by a variety of individuals including ministers of the Gospel. Dick Burns in his defense of the principles of the 12 steps has not directly answered critics on this point. To the critics it seems that he side-steps this issue.

The common public concept as well as by many individuals who utilize the 12 steps for use in programs for conditions other than alcoholic addiction is that the program is based upon the Judeo Christian tradition. Since I had spent many years researching spiritualism's rapidly spreading influence in medical therapy several individuals suggested that I had the background knowledge to recognize seeds of spiritualism within the 12 step system if it was present. I received very strong urging to do such a study. I was not anxious to do so as I carried the belief that AA was indeed based in Christian doctrine, was an excellent organization, and was doing a good job in helping recovery for various problems.

I am aware that information that would presumably expose spiritualistic concepts within 12 step therapies would initiate strong reactions. This would bring forth questions in the mind of the reader as to whether I, the author, had become unbalanced and saw ghosts of spiritualism in everything. The subject of the book, *Spiritualistic Deception in Health and Healing,* has been as a whole, well accepted except by those individuals who were involved in a particular therapy exposed. Often I hear that the book is correct in all but a specific therapy which of course was the one this person had belief in. The only defense of a spiritualistic method of therapy ever presented to me in twenty years in sharing my understanding of spiritualism's influence in medicine has been, "well, it works."

I have asked myself the question many times, am I seeing spiritualistic ghosts where they do not exist? In most every seminar I have presented exposing spiritualism's rapidly spreading tentacles, there has been someone who had been involved in New Age or occult practices that came to me and expressed their thanks for my willingness to expose these deceptions and that my material was correct. These comments have helped to calm concern of "over reaction" on my part.

In the remainder of this chapter I will present what I learned in my study on 12 Steps. I will then let the reader decide if the concern expressed of spiritualistic concepts being incorporated within the 12 steps is or is not true.

WAS THE OXFORD GROUP CHRISTIAN?

The proponents of AA have insisted that the Oxford Group was a *Christian movement,* but one could ask upon what basis is this comment made? Pastor H.A. Ironside, in a sermon preached in Moody Memorial Church, testified:

I have gone through book after book, supposedly setting forth the teaching of the Oxford Group Movement, and have not found one reference to the precious blood of Christ in any of them, nor any reference to the fact that the worst sin that anyone can possibly commit is the sin of rejecting the Lord Jesus Christ. 'There is none other name under heaven given among men, where by ye must be saved' (Acts 4:12)[701]

There were practices of the Oxford Group that were not in harmony with Christian theology. These included choosing *a god of your understanding* and not the Lord Jesus Christ the Son of God who came in the flesh, who is the way, the truth, and the life. Also their method of confession, that of personal sins being "shared" in a public forum is not Biblical. The scripture text in James 5 that tells us to "confess our faults one to another" is telling us to confess to our brother when we have faulted him, not to share it with everyone. We are to confess our sins to God and not to mortal man unless we have faulted him.

And the prayer of faith shall save the sick, and the Lord shall raise him up; and if he has committed sins, they shall be forgiven him. Confess (your) faults one to another, and pray one for another, that ye may be healed. The effectual fervent prayer of a righteous man availeth much. James 5: 15, 16

The English word *meditation* often leads to confusion. It has a dual meaning and sometimes it is difficult to differentiate as to which meaning is meant when the word is used. One meaning is referring to a deep thought and study attitude wherein our mind is most active upon a subject; another definition refers to an empting of the mind, a cessation of active thought, placing the thought process in neutral. Often it is necessary to look at the setting in which the word is used to know the intention of the author. Such is the case in its use in writings pertaining to the Oxford Group.

Also it had become a practice of the Oxford Group to hold meditation sessions. Members would sit, pencils in hand, waiting to jot down any "guidance" that might come through during their silences,[702]

An Oxford Group member, C. Irving Benson who was also a minister, gave caution concerning the Quiet Time/guidance in spite of the Bible being read during this period.

701   Ironside, H.A. Pastor, *The Oxford Group Movement Is It Scriptural?,* Loizeaux Brothers, Publishers, New York, (1943), p. 2. http://www.orangeapers.org/orange-Ironside.html

702   Thomsen, Robert, *Bill W.,* Published by Popular Library, a unit of CBS Publication, the Consumer Publishing Division of CBS Inc., by arrangement with Harper and Row, Publishers, Inc. (1975), pp. 215.

The silence becomes a sacrament wherein God comes to us[703].... I wait in self-forgetting silence, contemplating the presence of God.[704]

Pastor H.A. Ironside, a noted fundamental evangelist of the 1930's and 1940's, was very familiar with the Oxford Group and carefully evaluated their teachings. He made the following comment in regards to their meditation practices in a small booklet he wrote entitled, *The Oxford Group Movement: Is It Scriptural?*

> Each (Oxford Group) member is urged...to sit quietly with *the mind emptied* of every thought...waiting for God to say something to them...sometimes they tell me nothing happens, at other times the most amazing things come. Tested by the Word of God, many of these things are unscriptural. They lay themselves open for demons to communicate their blasphemous thoughts to them.[705] (Emphasis in original quote)

Robert Thomsen wrote in his biography *Bill W.* :

> ...that it had become a practice of the Oxford Group members to hold meditation sessions. They would sit, pencils in hand, waiting to jot down any guidance that might come through during the silences and it was extraordinary how many times that winter the message from on high would indicate that Bill Wilson should get himself a job and leave his drunks in peace.[706]

Two women identifying themselves only as "Two Listeners" wrote the book, *God Calling* wherein they received Quiet/Time "guidance" in the manner outlined by the Oxford Group. They tell us they received the words of Christ Jesus on a daily basis.[707] These words they received were not from the Holy Scriptures but out of meditation of "guidance." One of the two "Listeners" wrote the introduction for the book and entitled it *The Voice Divine,* wherein she speaks of the experience of the other "Listener" receiving guidance.

> But with my friend a very wonderful thing happened. From the first, beautiful messages were given to her by our Lord Himself, and every day from then these messages have never failed us. We felt all unworthy and

---

703   Benson, Irving C. , *The Eight Points of the Oxford Group: An Exposition.*
704   *Ibid.,* p. 69.
705   Ironside, op. cit. p. 9.
706   Thomsen, op. cit., p. 215.
707   Two Listeners, *God Calling,* The Voice Divine, Barbour Publishing, Inc. (1949), p.1 http://www.twolisteners.org/Introduction

over whelmed by the wonder of it, and could hardly realize that we were being taught, trained and encouraged day by day by HIM personally, when millions of souls, far worthier, had to be content with guidance from the Bible, sermons, their Churches, books and other sources.[708]

A prior Oxford Group member, then later an AA member, Richmond Walker, wrote a small book, *Twenty-Four Hours a Day*. This book had much in it that was based on the book, *God Calling by the two "Listeners."* He did not refer to Jesus Christ but substituted words that fit a universal spirituality. The book *Twenty-Four Hours a Day,* millions of AA members read.[709] AA history website says of *Twenty-Four Hours a Day*:

> The book explained how to practice meditation by quieting the mind and entering the **Divine Silence** in order to enter the divine peace and calm and restore our souls.[710] (Emphasis added)

Modern Mystics describe "silence" as in *Three Magic Words* by Uell S. Anderson:

> The brain is stilled. The man at last let's go; he glides below it into the quiet feeling, the quiet sense of his own identity with the *self* of other things-of the universe. He glides past the feeling into the very identity itself where a glorious all consciousness leaves no room for separate self-thoughts or emotions. (Emphasis added)

> I turn from the world about me to the world of consciousness that lies within. I shut out all memories of the past, create no images of the future. I concentrate on my being, on my awareness. I slide deep into the very recesses of my soul to a place of utter repose. I know, I know that this is Immortal Self, this is God, this is me, **I AM**, I always was, I always will be. (Emphasis added)

Twenty-four Hours in a Day states:

> There is a **spark** of the **Divine** in every one of us. Each has some of God's spirit that can be developed by spiritual exercise.[711]

---

708   *Ibid.*

709   Lanagan, John, *Alcoholics Anonymous and Contemplative Spirituality,* See John Lanagan Website.

710   AA History, *The 24 Hours a Day* Book . Hazelden Publishing, (1954), http://www.bare-footsworld.net/aa24hoursbook.html

711   Walker, Richard, *Twenty-Four Hours a Day,* Hazelden Foundation, Meditation for the Day, April 30.

The Oxford Group Movement promoted several additional books for study. One was given to Bill W. by Ebby Thatcher shortly after Bill's conversion. This book was *Varieties of Religious Experience* by William James, M.D. James was professor of psychiatry and philosophy at Harvard and a contemporary of Freud and Jung. He, too, (James) was a renowned spiritualist.

> ... Bill learned that even his experience at Towns was not unique. He could never recollect if it had been Ebby or Roland who gave him a copy of William James's *Varieties of Religious Experience*, but he remembered the impact of the book. It was James's theory that spiritual experiences could have a very definite objective reality and might totally transform a man's life.[712]

> ...as Bill Pittman has found, The *varieties of Religious Experience* was "the most often quoted book in Oxford literature,[713]

The Oxford Group considered "sin" as a moral issue and hence confessing a prerequisite to conversion which would be the solution for sin. They also looked at alcohol as a sin and hence with a conversion it could be cured. Their style of conversion did not depend upon a person accepting by faith Jesus Christ and His shed blood as a propitiation for their sins. The entire system of the Oxford Group appears to leave Jesus Christ the Divine Son of God out of equation and so man attempts to save himself.

The doctrine of pantheism—*the Divinity of man* and salvation through progression of the divinity of man is seen in the teachings of the Oxford Group. Will this same teaching be seen in Alcoholics Anonymous teachings? Are these teachings of the Oxford Group *Judeo-Christian doctrine?* That is something the reader must decide!

WERE THE COFOUNDERS, BILL W. AND DR. BOB OF ALCOHOLICS ANONYMOUS CHRISTIANS? DR. BOB SMITH:

Dr. Bob had been raised in a Christian home but had chosen to reject Christianity or any religion when he left home. He only entered a church for a funeral or some similar gathering. His alcohol consumption started in college and grew in intensity through his life.

---

712 Thomsen, Ibid., p. 213.
713 Raphael, Matthew J., *Bill W. and Mr. Wilson,* University of Massachusetts Press, (2000), p. 84.

Chapter 23 - 12 Steps—To Where?
Part 1

383

There is very little written about the doctor and his relationship to Christian fellowship. It is true that he was involved closely with Oxford Group activities for two or more years but I did not find any information that revealed he had accepted Christianity. Dr. Bob had been in the Masonic organization but his membership was suspended in 1934. It was later restored when he gained sobriety. When Alcoholics Anonymous formed he gradually moved away from the Oxford Group. From this association it is known that Bob did have a daily twenty minute period of devotion, reading the scriptures, sitting in quiet meditation with pencil and paper in hand waiting for *guidance*.

We do know from a letter sent by Bill W. to his wife Lois in the summer of 1935 that Dr. Bob, Anne, his wife and Bill W. had been active in séances and other psychic events. *Pass It On* an official book of AA, page 280, tells of a neighbor, friend, and fellow AA member, Tom P., who with his wife frequently joined in *spook sessions* at the Wilson home with Dr. Bob and Bill and their wives; spook sessions were séances and other psychic acts.

Dr. Bob found great interest in and promoted to others while attempting to bring them to sobriety, the book *Sermons of the Mount*. This book is a commentary by Emmet Fox on the Beatitudes of Matthew chapters 5-7. Emmet Fox was a minister of the *New Thought Movement* which was active in New England in 1800's. 'The New Thought Movement's doctrines' were a blend of Christian and Eastern teachings and had wormed its way into many churches of that day feigning as if it would bring a revival and spiritual regeneration. Actually it was a pantheistic *wolf in sheep's clothing* as is revealed by its teachings.

Fox comments that Jesus was the most influential man in the history of the world. For three and one half years of ministry, His influence continued after his absence affecting vast numbers of people, many nations, and entire civilizations. Jesus is not spoken of as the Divine Son of God in his entire book. Promptly from the beginning of the book we are informed that the Bible does not present any plan of salvation, no system of theology, has no doctrines, that all doctrine of churches is man derived, denigrates the seventh day Sabbath, and that the Bible does not teach atonement by the shed blood of Jesus Christ; the Bible is simply a composite of old fragments of writings of authors unknown. The Adam and Eve story is simply an allegory. His book teaches that *man is divine* and is in *progression* toward ("maturity")—godhood, where he will possess everything God possesses.

He tells us that Jesus said the following: "I have said ye are God," and "all of you sons of the Most High." He believed that Jesus actually did miracles but that the power for performing them was obtained by Jesus' understanding of spiritual things, not that he was "God in the flesh." He also teaches that "we are all fundamentally one—all part of the Great Mind." He also teaches that the word *Christ* is not identical with the name Jesus. It only represents "Absolute Spiritual Truth" about any subject.[714]

Does Dr. Bob's activity in séances, the psychic arena, and in promoting these doctrines from Fox's book cause you to question whether or not he was Christian?

BILL W.:

In chapter one of *Alcoholics Anonymous,* Bill W. tells us he was not an atheist and had never been one. He stated he had always believed in some great power above himself and had actually thought on these issues. He did believe that there was some *Spirit of the Universe not bound by time or space*, a *Creative Intelligence, Universal Mind*, or *Spirit of Nature*. His mind was closed to accepting a God that he could have a personal relationship with. He saw Christ as man only, not God in the flesh.[715] He considered himself an agnostic.

Ebby Thatcher, Bill's friend and a member of the Oxford Group, had suggested to Bill W. that he could choose *a God of his own conception* to surrender to. This approach appealed to Bill. What type of God did Bill's conception pick? He spoke of a Power Higher than himself, but was that *Jesus Christ*, the only name (Acts 4:12) under heaven whereby we have salvation? He surrendered himself totally unto the Higher Power he had decided on, the *God-consciousness within.*[716]

> *God-consciousness* was not, however, a term taken from James (William James) , but rather from the *Oxford Group*; it described the nature of personal revelation. Consider, for example, the definition in V.C. Kitchen's *I Was a Pagan* (1934), an Oxford Group testimonial, by a reformed drunkard, that Wilson likely read. 'I am now, in other words,' writes Kitchen, 'receiving super natural aid—not through a nonsensical Ouija Board nor any other spiritualistic 'instrument'— but through God-consciousness— through direct personal contact with the third environment —the spiritual environment I had so long been seeking'.[717]

We will need to explore more of Bill's statements made over time to better determine if he had chosen the God of Christians, *Jesus Christ the Divine Son of God*, or perhaps a pantheistic god. The term *God* is used widely as a synonym for various concepts of a Higher Power. A pagan refers to a universal

---

714 Fox, Emmet, *The Sermon on the Mount,* Buccaneer Books, Cutchogue, New York (1934), pp. 3,4,6,7,11,12,124,125,127,128,149.
715 Alcoholics Anonymous, op. cit., Chapter 1. pp. 11-13.
716 *Ibid.*
717 Raphael, Matthew J., *Bill W. and Mr. Wilson,* University of Massachusetts Press, (2000), p. 79.

energy—a force, the New Ager similarly. A Christian mystic refers to a power he envisions within himself, often referred to as *God Consciousness, Self, Christ Consciousness*, etc. Which God did Bill W. pick? He tells us that it was not needful to consider another person's concept of God, as one's own conception is all that matters no matter what it is. *A Creative Intelligence*, or a *Spirit of the Universe* underlying the totality of things,[718] was all that is needed to begin to get results. Bill makes the following comment:

> *When, therefore, we speak to you of God, we mean your own conception of God. This applies, too, to other spiritual expressions which you find in this book.*[719]
> (Emphasis added)

Where was this God of his conception to be found?

> ...We had to search fearlessly, but He was there, He was as much a fact as we were. We found the *Great Reality deep down within us*. In the last analysis it is only there that He may be found. It was so with us.[720] (Emphasis added)

Here we have a statement, made by the author Bill Wilson in the official book for Alcoholics Anonymous, upholding a pagan—New Age doctrine of the Divine within*, pantheism*. Does that sound like Bill chose the God of the Christian? These are typical terms and expressions I see routinely used in writings from pantheistic Eastern religions and neo-paganism of the West.

Let us look *again*, at Bill's *conversion experience* while he was in Towns Hospital December 11, 1934. This account of the *light experience* is recorded by Robert Thomsen in a biography of Bill and brings out an expression not recorded in the previous rendering of this happening. As Bill cried out in desperation:

> "Oh God," he cried, and it was the sound not of a man but of a trapped and crippled animal. "If there is a God, show me. Show me. Give me some sign."

> As he formed the words, in that very instant he was aware first of a *light, a great white light* that filled the room, then he suddenly seemed caught up in a kind of joy, an ecstasy such as he would never find words to describe. It was as though he were standing high on a mountain top and a strong clear wind blew against him, and round him, through him—but it seemed a wind not of air, but of spirit—and as this happened he had the feeling that he was stepping into another world, a new world of *consciousness*, and everywhere now there was a

---

718   Alcoholic Anonymous, op. cit, p. 46.
719   *Ibid.*, p. 47.
720   *Ibid.*, p. 55.

wondrous feeling of *Presence* which all his life he had been seeking. Nowhere had he ever felt so complete, so satisfied, so embraced.

...Then when it passed, when the light slowly dimmed, and the ecstasy subsided—and whether this was a matter of minutes or much longer he never knew; he was beyond any reckoning of time—the sense of *Presence* was still there about him, within him. And with it there was still another sense, a sense of rightness. No matter how wrong things seemed to be, they were as they were meant to be. There could be no doubt of ultimate order in the universe the cosmos was not dead matter, but a part of the living *Presence*, just as he was part of it.

Now in place of the light, the exaltation, he was filled with a peace such as he had never known. He had heard of men who tried to open the universe to themselves; he had opened himself to the universe. He had heard men say there was a bit of God in everyone, but this feeling that *he was a part of God, himself a living part of the higher power*, was a new and revolutionary feeling.[721] (Emphasis added)

These statements convincingly suggest that the God Bill W. had chosen was a *pantheistic* god, not Jesus Christ the Divine Son of God, the God of a Christian. We will continue reviewing statements made by Bill to his friends and in his writing. The quotation above brought to my mind a comment by E.G. White concerning contemplating the *Presence of God*:

It introduces that which is naught but speculation in regard to the *personality of God* and *where His presence is*. No one on this earth has a right to speculate on this question. The more fanciful theories are discussed, the less men will know of God and of the truth that sanctifies the soul....Those who entertain these sophistries will soon find themselves *in a position where the enemy can talk with them*, and lead them away from God.[722] (Emphasis added)

At this point in looking for an answer to the question of whether or not Bill Wilson was a Christian we need to share with the reader Bill's long time connection with spiritualism. When it began no one can be sure, however, the first written information starts with his association with his wife, Lois. Lois in her autobiography, *Lois Remembers,* recounts fond memories of her church and church family. She came from a family that were members of the Swedenborgian Church (also known as *Church of New Jerusalem* or *New church*) and she had attended this church all her life, and was married to Bill

---

721 Thomsen, op. cit., P. 207.
722 White, E.G., I Selected Messages, Review and Herald Publishing Association, Hagerstown, MD, (1958), p. 202.

in it January of 1918. The mystical aspects of this religion so fascinated Bill and Lois that they vowed to explore it more deeply some time. Her grandfather was a minister in the Swedenborgian church. She mentions the strength and guidance she received from the church's teachings. What is the origin of the Swedenborgian Church and what are its teachings?

Emmanuel Swedenborg (1688-1772) of Sweden was one of Europe's great minds: mining engineer, expert in metallurgy, astronomy, physics, zoology, anatomy, political economics, an author of voluminous writings, Biblical theologian, a spiritualist, seer, and medium. He has been considered the forerunner of modern spiritualism. He was a psychic from childhood and he continued in such all his life. His influence extended to many great names such as Ralph Waldo Emerson, Carl Jung, Helen Keller, etc., and his influence lasted for two centuries. An embodied spirit claiming to be

Christ directed him to re-write every verse of the Bible. He claimed to have direct communications with God, angels, Moses, David, Mary, Martin Luther, Aristotle, the apostles, and many, many other spirits.[723] Notice the quote below:

> ...that night in 1745 his visions began to invade his waking life as well. As he ate, he became aware of frogs and snakes crowding into his private dining room, and an unknown gentleman materialized in a corner to rebuke him for eating too much. Back home in Salisbury Court the stranger appeared again, and introduced himself as Christ, the man-God, creator and redeemer of the world. He then made an important announcement: humanity stood in need of a definitive explication of Holy Scripture, and Swedenborg had been selected to provide it; moreover, to assist him in his labors, he was to be given unrestricted access to the entire spirit world.

> http://www.victorianweb.org/religion/swedenborg2.html (George P. Landow)

Swedenborgians do not believe that salvation is exclusively through Jesus Christ, but that salvation was possible through all religions. He felt that he was destined to bring this doctrine to the world through his writings.

In Swedenborg's book, *Divine Providence,* paragraph 36 he writes:

> ...picture wisdom as a magnificently and finely decorated palace. One climbs to enter this palace by *twelve steps.* One can only arrive at the first step by means of the Lord's power through joining with Him...As a person climbs these steps,

---

723   Catholic Encyclopedia: Swedenborgians; http://www.fst.org/spirit2.htm; http://www.newadvent.org/cathen/14355a.htm

he perceives that no one is wise from himself but from the Lord...the in union with love. (Emphasis added)

This bit of information is interesting because 200 years later Bill W. would be the writer of a 12 step program that would go to the whole world. Is it possible that the origin of both these top scenarios came from the same spiritual source?

What effect of being a member of the Swedenborgian Church had on Lois is not clear, but it is known that she joined Bill on many of his pursuits in the field of spiritualism such as in séances and table tapping, and the Ouija board.[724] The first recorded spiritualism activity of Bill is seen in his letter to Lois in the summer of 1935, the time when Alcoholics Anonymous had its beginning. He had been in Akron, Ohio, for several months staying at the home of Dr. Bob and Anne Smith, the other cofounder of A.A. Bill wrote to Lois stating he had been active in séances and other psychic events with Dr. Bob and Anne.[725]

Pass It On is an official book published by the Alcoholics Anonymous organization telling the life story of Bill Wilson. Chapter 16 shares with us that Bill had a persistent fascination and involvement in psychic phenomena. He had a firm belief in reincarnation and felt everyone had had several lives already and the present life was a "spiritual Kindergarten." It was from this belief that he pursued various forms of occult practices. He believed he could receive energy from another person. He trusted in clairvoyance and other extrasensory phenomena, levitation, Ouija board, séances etc., and played the part of a medium. Spirits would materialize and talk with him.[726]

This 16th chapter also relates that by 1941 he was holding regular Saturday "spook sessions" at his home—Stepping Stones. One room was reserved just for those sessions. It was dubbed the "spook room" and here various psychic experiments were carried out. Different friends and neighbors would join with him in these endeavors. They also practiced "table tapping," performed by several people sitting around a table and placing their hands on the edge of the table and then questions would be asked and answers would return by the table tapping out by alphabet, a letter code, at times the table would levitate. At other times Bill would lie on the couch semi-withdrawn, yet not in trance, and receive messages, sometimes one word at a time slowly and other times rapidly.[727]

He tells of a special time in 1947 that several spirits appeared before him when he was visiting in a home at Nantucket. The visitation of these materialized ghosts occurred when he was alone in the kitchen of the home

724 The Alcoholics Anonymous World Services, Inc., *Pass it On,* New York, N.Y., (1984), p. 277-278.
725 *Ibid.,* p. 275.
726 *Ibid.,* pp. 278,279.
727 *Ibid.,* p. 278.

where he was a guest; the ghosts gave their names and what they had done in life. One of these entities gave the name of "Shaw" and he had been a store keeper on the Island, another gave the name of David Morrow and he had been a sailor, the third called himself Pettingill, a master of a whaler from the Island, then the last another whaling master. Later that day from a monument in the city center and at a museum he found evidence of such people having lived and worked from Nantucket 100 years previously.[728], [729]

On one session of using a Ouija board, Bill wrote the following:

> The Ouija board got moving in earnest. What followed was the fairly usual experience—it was a strange mélange of Aristotle, St. Francis, diverse archangels with odd names, deceased friends — some in purgatory and others doing nicely, thank you! There were malign and mischievous ones of all descriptions, telling of vices quite beyond my ken, even as former alcoholics. Then, the seemingly virtuous entities would elbow them out with messages of comfort, information, advice—and sometimes just sheer nonsense.[730]

A friend and neighbor, Tom P., tells of one particular "spooking session" he attended along with Bill and Lois at the home of his aunt and uncle. An old sunlight faded table was brought into the room. They sat around the table and began "...Knocking the table around and it would ...spell out messages. It would raise and tap."... The table would also levitate. They turned out the lights and took their hands off the table and it "wrapped around inconclusively, and we'd say, 'Oh well, he'll find us another session,' and we all went home."[731] The next day Tom's aunt called to tell them that morning the table was found refinished perfectly. Everyone went to see, to believe.

Tom said he was a problem for these people (Bill and Dr. Bob) because being an atheist and materialist he could not believe in spirits and other worlds. Tom expressed how that Dr. Bob and Bill "believed vigorously and aggressively" in spiritualism. That it was not a fun thing or a hobby; it had a purpose for them. It related to their interest in AA "So the thing was not at all divorced from AA. It was very serious for everybody." Tom also stated that Bill never did anything that was not connected to AA or his own spiritual growth. Tom put it this way, he, Bill, was *one-pointed*.[732] Another author sheds more light on Bill's status as spiritualist:

---

728 *Ibid.*, pp. 276-277.
729 *Ibid.*, p. 278.
730 *Ibid.*, p. 278.
731 *Ibid.*, pp. 279-280.
732 *Ibid.* p. 280.

Wilson himself seems to have been an "adept", that is, "gifted" in the psychic sense; and he served as a medium for a variety of "controls," some of them recurrent. "Controls," in the lingo of spiritualism, are the discarnate (having no physical body) entities who seem to usurp a medium's identity and literally to speak through him or (far more usually) her. Sometimes the control answers questions; sometimes a spirit seems to materialize. In fact, according to the account published in '*Pass it On*,' Bill had one such experience during a trip to Nantucket in 1944.[733] (*Pass It On* gave the date as probably 1947)

A member of the Alcoholics Anonymous and the biographer of *Bill W. and Mr. Wilson*, Matthew J. Raphael speaks plainly in his book page 159:

...it might be said for the cofounder at least, AA was entangled with spiritualism from the very beginning.

After twenty years in AA, Bill and Lois began to break away from the constant duties of AA and in a spirit of controversy about their actions they continued to communicate with spirits. Their séances were not secret and they had many guests that joined with them in their psychic activities. Biographer Susan Cheever in her biography, *My Name is Bill,* relates in chapter 22 *The Spook Room*, something of these *spook* activities.

...Even the sounds from nature seemed to enter the trance. They could hear a silence beyond silence. Then there would be an almost inaudible tap, or Bill's quiet voice would begin to form a letter.

Bill and Lois had a rich past together, and on these evenings they were in the presence of the past, in the company of the Yankee householders clustered around their kitchen tables on cold nights before they had electricity They were in the presence of all their own dead, of Bill's cousin Clarence whose sad violin had been Bill's first fiddle, and the stern Rayette and Ella Griffith, of Lois's beloved mother, and her handsome father who read Swedenborg's teachings to his children in the Clinton Street living room, of all those who had passed on before them.

Bill became acquainted and developed a close relationship with Aldous Huxley, an author (*Brave New World*), philosopher, teacher, and *pioneer of New Age consciousness*. Huxley connected Bill with two Canadian psychiatrists, Humphry Osmond and Abram Hoffer, who were working with alcoholics and schizophrenics in an attempt to break through their resistance to surrender. Bill had been involved in helping the alcoholic surrender himself by a spiritual

---

733 Raphael, op. Cit., p. 159.

means. Their efforts in experimenting with the use of LSD were with the hope of it being useful for the addict. Nell Wing Bill's secretary tells us:

> There were alcoholics in the hospitals, of which AA could touch and help only about five percent. The doctors started giving them a dose of LSD, so that the resistance would be broken down. And they had about fifteen percent recovery.[734]

Bill himself took LSD and gave it to his wife, secretary, friends and alcoholics. (It was not illegal at that time.) Bill was very pleased about the use of LSD and he believed it eliminated barriers erected by "the self" that stood in the way of a person's direct experience of the cosmos and of god (a pantheistic god?).[735]

According to Bill W. *psychic phenomena* of all types as mentioned in the books is found very frequently throughout AA. He shares that besides his early *hot flash* experience, "he had experienced an immense of psychic phenomena of all sorts." Here Bill seems to equate his *hot flash* conversion with other psychic events he experienced throughout his life. Bill believed that:

> ... the cumulative weight of these phenomena validated his belief in *humanity's divine* and therefore *immortal nature*, and he wanted every alcoholic to be able to say, as he could, that their belief in God was 'no longer a question of faith' but 'the certainty of knowledge (gained) through evidence.'[736]

Bill Wilson had an additional character flaw, unfaithfulness to his wife. Author Hartigan tells us that Bill's "interest in younger women grew more intense with age." It became such a problem and embarrassment that:

> ...a "Founder's Watch" committee formed of people who were delegated to keep track of Bill during the socializing that usually accompanies AA functions. They would steer him one way and the woman in another.[737]

Was Bill W. a Christian? That label has been placed on him by multitudes of people. First, what is a definition of Christian? A working definition might be the following: a person who believes in *Jesus Christ as the Divine Son of God* having come in the flesh, born of a virgin, lived a life without sin, died on the cross, His death on the cross paid the penalty for our sins, and by *faith* in the merits of His shed blood we are pardoned by God, empowered to overcome sin into obedience and may have eternal life.

---

734 *Pass It On,* op. cit., p. 370.

735 *Ibid.,* p. 371.

736 Hartigan, Francis, *Bill W.,* St. Martins Press, New York, NY, (2000) p. 177.

737 *Ibid.,* p. 192.

Was this the God of Bill W.? We read in the biography, *Bill W.,* by Francis Hartigan the following:

> His belief in God might have become unshakable, but he could never embrace any theology or even the divinity of Jesus, and went to his grave unable to give his own personal idea of God much definition. In this sense, he was never very far removed from the unbelievers.[738]

> The biggest reason why Bill felt that he lacked faith may have to do with his admission that he was never 'able to receive assurance that He (Christ) was one hundred percent God...'[739]

The Apostle John warned us of those who do not accept the Divinity of Jesus Christ.

> And every spirit that confesseth not that Jesus Christ is come in the flesh is not of God: and this is that (spirit) of antichrist, whereof ye have heard that it should come; and even now already it is in the world. (I John 4:3)

A footnote for chapter 9, #1. Follows:

> At a 1954 AA conference in Fort Worth, Texas, speaking about 'How the Big Book Was Put Together,' Wilson referred ironically to 'the good old book, *Alcoholics Anonymous*: "some People reading the book now, they say, well, this is the AA Bible. When I hear that, it always makes me shudder because the guys who put it together weren't a damn bit biblical.[740]

One more quotation concerning Bill W., and his interest and activities in spiritualism is made in a letter July 31, 1952, by Henrietta Seiberling, the woman who first introduced Bill W. to Dr. Bob in Akron Ohio in 1935.

> He imagines himself all kinds of things. His hand 'writes' dictation from a Catholic priest, whose name I forget, from the 1600 period who was in Barcelona, Spain—again, he told Horace Crystal he was completing the works that Christ didn't finish, and according to Horace he said he was a reincarnation of Christ. Perhaps he got mixed in whose reincarnation he was. It looks more

---

Ibid., p. 123.
739 *Ibid.*, p. 175.
740 Raphael, op. cit., p. 197.

like the works of the devil but I could be wrong. I don't know what is going on in that poor deluded fellow's mind.[741]

Information has been presented to make it possible for the reader to develop his opinion as to whether the claim by people promoting AA, that its cofounders, Bill Wilson and Dr. Bob Smith, were Christians or not. The next question to answer is as to whether AA is founded upon Christian principles and is truly a Christian based.

---

741 http://mywordlikefire.wordpress.com/2008/09/24/seances-spirits-and-12steps/ click on AA listing then Séances, Spirits, and 12 steps, Source of quotation Henrietta Seiberling, 7/31/52 letter, http://www.orangepapers.org/orange-Henrietta_Seiberling.html

CHAPTER 24
12 STEPS TO WHERE? PART IIALCOHOLICS ANONYMOUS AND THE 12 STEPS ARE THEY CHRISTIAN?

From December 11, 1934—the date of the beginning of Bill W. 's sobriety and from June 10, 1935—the date of the start of Dr. Bob's sobriety, the organization Alcoholics Anonymous slowly began to take form, yet without a name for three years. These men from the first days of sobriety were active in assisting other alcoholics to find freedom from alcohol. They immediately embarked upon a relentless missionary campaign of seeking out and to proselytize drunks utilizing the methods for spiritual conversion learned from the Oxford Group. One aspect of the *Oxford Group's* method was to make available a particular book or books to the individual with whom they were working. This was the experience of Bill W. following his "hot flash" conversion in the Towns treatment center.

> Rational light on this mystical event came "the next day", when someone (possibly Ebby) handed Bill a copy of the *Varieties of Religious Experience*, by Willian James M.D., which he found to be "rather difficult reading" but nonetheless devoured "from cover to cover[742]

> It was with them (religious experiences related in the book) that Bill learned that even his experience at Towns was not unique. He could never recollect if it had been Ebby or Nowland who gave him the copy of *Varieties of Religious Experience*, but he remembered the impact of the book. It was James's theory that spiritual experiences could have a very definite objective reality and might totally transform a man's life.[743]

In the previous chapter comments were made concerning this book, i.e., it contains many stories of special spiritual experiences which this author, upon reading the book, is convinced are mostly stories of spiritistic encounters.

---

742   Raphael, Matthew J., *Bill W. and Mr. Wilson*, University of Massachusetts Press, (2000). P. 82.
743   Thomsen, Robert, *Bill W.*, Harper and Row, Publishers, Inc., N.Y., N.Y., (1975) p. 213.

Dr. Bob often chose *The Sermon on the Mount* by Emmet Fox, a *New Thought* minister, for literature support, a book promoted by the Oxford Group that denies the *Divinity of Jesus, but* promotes *Divinity within man.* The New Thought name can be traced to their teaching that the whole outer world—whether it be the physical body, simple things in life, wind and rain, the clouds, and the earth itself are amendable to *man's thought.* The earth had no character of its own, only the character man gives it by his own thinking. This movement was the source of a later concept known as *the power of positive thinking.* Man, it is taught, has dominion over all. Scholars Anderson and Whitehouse comment:

> New Thoughters are fond of such affirmations as...'The Christ in me salutes the Christ in you.' Rather than viewing Jesus as the first and the last member of the Christ family, many New Thoughters believe that Christ is a title that we can all earn by following Jesus' example."[744]

An Internet article May 20, 2008, titled "Alcoholics Anonymous Cofounders Were Not Christians,"[745] and therein are references to individuals who received for reading, Fox's book, *The Sermon on the Mount,* as they were seeking sobriety. Some comments are given below from these individuals.

> In a recorded 1954 interview, early AA member Dorothy S.M. reminisced, "The first thing Bob did was get me Emmet Fox's *"Sermon on the Mount."*[5] Dorothy then recalled how it went with alcoholics who wanted help: 'As soon as the men in the hospital, as soon as their eyes could focus, they go to 'The Sermon on the Mount.'[746]

> Archie T., the founder of Detroit AA, stayed with Dr. Bob and Anne Smith for more than ten months. He became sober in September of 1938. Archie T. recollected, 'In Akron I was turned over to Dr. Bob and his wife. ...I spent Labor Day in the hospital reading Emmet Fox's *Sermon on the Mount,*' and it changed my life.'[747]

This book, *Sermon on the Mount,* teaches that Jesus "taught no theology whatever." On page 3 and 4 it states:

> There is absolutely no system of theology of doctrine to be found in the Bible; it simply is not there.... The *plan of Salvation* which figured so prominently in the

---

744   Anderson, c. Allen, Whitehead, Deborah g., *New Thought and Conventional Christianity* www.gis.net/caa/church.html (archived)

745   http://www.worldviewweekend.com/worldview-times/article. php?articleid=3537 *5 Ibid.,* p.2

746   *Ibid.*

747   www.akronarchives.com/archieT.htm (now off line)

evangelical sermons and divinity books of a past generation is as completely unknown to the Bible as it is to the Koran. There never was any such arrangement in the universe, and Bible does not teach it at all.

Another book promoted by the Oxford Group and that was used in the early work and formation of the organization—Alcoholics Anonymous, was *Modern Man in Search of a Soul* by Carl Jung M.D. In summary, at least part of the literature used to bring spiritual conversion to the alcoholic and patterned after the Oxford Group were two books written by spiritualist mediums, and the other by a minister denying the divinity of Jesus Christ and promoting the pantheistic dogma of the New Thought movement. In the Oxford Group, studies were conducted from the Bible, from the book of James, and I Corinthians 13. However, none of these passages refer to the Divinity of Jesus or that under no other name under heaven could there be salvation. Where do we find Christianity in this scenario?

When Bill W. looked back in the history of AA and its development he gave credit to these books and their authors as being forefathers of AA

> ...both the men Wilson considered forefathers of Alcoholics Anonymous were deeply involved with spiritualism. William James, who was a friend and admirer of Frederic Myers and who himself served as president of the American Society for Psychical Research, spent innumerable hours, in the course of twenty-five years, in séances with Mrs. L.E. Piper, the marvelous trance medium whom the S.P.R. kept practically under house arrest in Boston. It was precisely James's openness to spiritual manifestations in *The Varieties of Religious Experience* that made him simpatico with Wilson. Carl Jung, too, took occultism seriously, beginning with his doctoral dissertation, *On the Psychology and Pathology of So-called Occult Phenomena* (1902: the same year as *Varieties*).[748]

The Varieties of Religious Experience text had considerable influence on forming the 12 steps found in *Alcoholics Anonymous*. The first draft of these 12 steps was lost but they have been reconstructed to similar wording as displayed below:[749]

1.   We admitted that we were powerless over alcohol— and that our lives had become unmanageable;
2.   Came to believe a God could restore us to sanity;
3.   Made a decision to turn our will and our lives over to the care of God;
4.   Made a searching and fearless moral inventory of ourselves;
5.   Admitted to God, to ourselves and to another human being the exact

---

748   Raphael, op. cit., p. 161.
749   Alcoholics Anonymous World Services, *In., Pass It On,* New York, N.Y., (1984), p. 198.

nature of our wrongs;

6. Were entirely ready to have God remove all of these defects of character;

7. Humbly on our knees asked Him to remove these short comings—holding back nothing;

8. Made a complete list of all persons we had harmed and became willing to make amends to them all;

9. Made direct amends to such people where ever possible, except when to do so would injure them or others;

10. Continued to take personal inventory and when we were wrong promptly admitted it;

11. Sought through prayer and meditation to improve our contact with God, praying only for knowledge of His will for us and the power to carry that out;

12. Having had a spiritual experience as the result of this course of action, we tried to carry this message to others, especially alcoholics and to practice these principles in all our affairs.

Bill's first three steps were culled from his reading of James (a spiritualist psychiatrist), the teachings of Sam Shoemaker (Episcopal priest working with Oxford Group), and those of the Oxford Group itself.[750]

That evening Bill had a couple of visitors who looked at his 12 steps. They had objections to the use of the word "God" and his comment on step seven of "humbly on our knees asking Him to remove one's shortcomings." A few days later Bill appeared at the AA office and showed the manuscript again. The same objections arose again. So he changed certain steps as follows.[751]

1. Came to believe that a *Power greater than ourselves* could restore us to sanity;

2. Made a decision to turn our will and our lives over to the care of God *as we understood Him;*

3. Humbly asked Him to remove our shortcomings;

4. Sought through prayer and meditation to improve our contact with God *as we understood Him*, praying only for knowledge of His will for us and the power to carry that out;

5. Having a spiritual *awakening* as the result of these steps, we tried to carry this message to alcoholics and to practice these principles in all our affairs;

---

750 *Ibid.*, p. 199.
751 *Ibid.*

These compromises seemed to placate the atheists and agnostics and made wide the gate leading to acceptance by many people of all races, religions, gender, financial position, social standing,, etc.,,, of the twelve steps. Bill's desire was to make the steps acceptable to agnostics, atheists, Christians, Hindus, Buddhists, Catholics, Masons, or any religious organization and non-believers. The title, Alcoholics *Anonymous,* was chosen after many name considerations.

With the success for alcoholics using 12 step principles many other programs for various addictions, i.e., smoking, obesity, etc., incorporated and adapted the 12 step tactics into their programs. Many churches have utilized this approach in recovery classes they have sponsored.

Let us return to the time that Bill W. was in Towns hospital and had the *hot flash* conversion, the room filled with a great white light and Bill experienced a feeling of a great *Presence.* Was it the same power that inspired him as he *relaxed* and asked for *guidance?* To whom was the request for "guidance" directed to? Was it to the Christian God— Jesus Christ the Divine Son of God? Was it to some unknown god or no god? To a pantheistic god? None of the books containing the story of this event including Bill's own words give us a direct answer. Bill has previously stated that he was not able to accept a *King on High* who he could have a relationship with, yet he could accept a Universal mind, Nature Spirit type god, a pantheistic style god—*The Great Reality deep down within.*

This question, not yet answered, is very important because if the 12 step fellowship method goes to the whole world, the *power source* of Bill's *inspiration* in developing the 12 steps will be the *power* of influence exerted over the world. A result of *sobriety* cannot of itself be the criteria we use to determine the source of *power,* as Satan is given great *power* to heal. He may come as an angel of light in the form of man, even a minister, and deceive even the very elect. The Bible tells us we cannot serve two masters; we must determine if the *power* is of Jesus Christ our Creator God or of His adversary.

Would I expect the power of Jesus Christ the Divine Son of God to be manifest in a person who denies Him, who has been active as a medium contacting spirits of the dead; visited with embodied spirits; who played the Ouija board in a vigorous manner; promoted books written by notorious spiritualist mediums and/or a minister who denies the Divinity of Christ and teaches that we have *divinity within* to bring spirituality to an individual seeking change? If Bill's *inspiration* was not from the Christian God of a 6 day creation, then how could the 12 step method be so beneficial, so effective? As we continue to follow the story of the popularity and growth of AA and the 12 steps in recovery programs this question, "what is the source of power of the spirituality of these steps?" This should be uppermost in our mind.

In 1938, *Alcoholics Anonymous* was published and began to be the written guide used in the fellowship meetings. Progress in increasing numbers of groups and of people continued but slowly. When Father Edward Dowling, the Jesuit priest, from St. Louis, visited Bill W. he said:

> ...we have been looking at this book, "Alcoholic Anonymous."[752]

Father Dowling told Bill he was fascinated with the book because the twelve steps of Alcoholics Anonymous *paralleled the Spiritual Exercises of Ignatius Loyola,* which is the spiritual guide for the Jesuit order. Father Dowling became the spiritual advisor to Bill W.

Who is St. Ignatius Loyola? He was the founder of the Jesuit Order in the early 1500's. His Order had the goal of returning the Protestants as well as the whole world to the fold of the Roman Catholic Church. He is also known as a *Christian mystic.* A comment from author Edmund Paris, in his book, *The Secret History of the Jesuits,* follows:

> Ignatius of Loyola was a first-class example of that "active mysticism" and "distortion of the will." Never the less, the transformation of the gentlemen-warrior into the "general" of the most militant order in the Roman Church was very slow; there were many faltering steps before he found his true vocation....
>
> Blissful visions and illuminations were constant companions of this mystic throughout his life.[753]
>
> He never doubted the reality of these revelations. He chased Satan with a stick as he would have done a mad dog; he talked to the Holy Spirit as one does to another person actually; he asked for the approval of God, the Trinity and the Madonna on all his projects and would burst into tears of joy when they appeared to him. On those occasions, he had a foretaste of celestial bliss; the heavens were open to him, and the Godhead was visible and perceptible to him.
>
> ...From the start, medieval mysticism has prevailed in the Society of Jesus; it is still the great animator, in spite of its readily assumed worldly, intellectual and learned aspects.[754]

What is the origin of his spiritual exercises? A comment is made contrasting the direction that Luther chose in his drive to follow God in comparison to Ignatius' choice is presented.

---

752 *Ibid.,* pp. 241, 242.
753 Paris, Edmund, *The Secret History of the Jesuits* (translated from French 1975), Chick Publications, , Chino, CA p. 17,18.
754 Boehmer, H. professor at the University of Bonn, *"Les Jesuites"* (Armand Colin, Paris (1910), pp. 12-13; Reported in *The Secret History of the Jesuits* by Edmund Paris, p. 18.

Inigo, instead of feeling that his remorse was sent to drive him to the foot of the cross, persuaded himself that these inward reproaches proceeded not from God, but from the devil; and he resolved never more to think of his sins, to erase them from his memory, and bury them in eternal oblivion. Luther turned toward Christ, Loyola only fell upon himself...visions came erelong to confirm Inigo in the convictions in which he had arrived...Inigo did not seek truth in the Holy Scriptures but imagined in their place immediate communication with the world of spirits...Luther, on taking his Doctors degree, had pledged his oath to holy scripture ...Loyola at his time, bound himself to dreams and visions; and chimerical (fantasy plots) apparitions became the principle of his life and his faith.[755]

Ignatius, in choosing to follow the god revealed to him in his visions and apparitions did not choose the same God of Luther but chose a pantheistic god as revealed in the following statement presented by the Catholic *Brentwood Religious Education Service*, April 2005:

Then perhaps we begin to see the examen (prayer and meditation) as so intimately connected to our growing identity and so important to our finding *God in all things* at all times that it becomes our central daily *experience* of prayer. For Ignatius finding God in all things is what life is all about. Near the end of his life, he said that 'Whenever he wished, at whatever hour, he could find God.' (*Autobiography, p.* 99) (Emphasis added)

Being able to find God whenever he wanted, Ignatius was now able to find that God of love in all things through a test for congruence of any interior impulse, mood or feeling with his *true self.* "For now my place is in him, and I am not dependent upon any of the self-achieved righteousness of the Law." (Philippians 3:9)[756] (Emphasis added)

Early in his career Ignatius was arrested three times and imprisoned twice by the Inquisition because of his teachings. He had a special ability to attract young people and this he did on university campuses. What was it that made him so attractive?

...It was his ideal and a little charm he carried on himself: a small book, in fact a very minute book which is, in spite of its smallness amongst those which have

755 D' Auburgine, JH Merle D, *History of the Reformation of the 16th Century, 5 volumes in one.* Grand Rapids, MI, Baker Bookhouse, reproduced from London (1846) edition in (1976), book 10.

756 http://ignatianspirituality.com/ignatian-prayer/the-examen/consciousness-examen/ found in IgantianSpirituality.com , Home>Ignatian Prayer>The Daily examen>Consciousness Examen.

influenced the fate of humanity. This volume has been printed so many times that the number of copies is unknown; it was also the object of more than four hundred commentaries. It is the textbook of their master: the *spiritual exercises*.[757]

Edmund Paris sums up the value and effect of these Spiritual Exercises:

> It is understandable that after four weeks devoted to these intensive Exercises, *with a director* as his only companion, the candidate would be ripe for the subsequent training and breaking. ... Imposing on his disciples actions which, to him, were spontaneous, he needed just thirty days to break, with this method, **the will** and **reasoning**, in the manner in which a rider breaks his horse. He only needed thirty days *triginta dies* to subdue a soul.[758] (Emphasis added)

In the book, *Ignatius of Loyola, The Psychology of a Saint,* by W.W. Meissner, S.J., M.D., p. 87 gives us a glimpse of the influence of Ignatius' Exercises upon the Church for the last four and one half centuries.

> *Spiritual Exercises* is one of the most influential works in Western civilization. It became a guide for spiritual renewal in the Roman church during the entire counter-Reformation and has been a primary influence in the spiritual life of the church ever since, particularly through the efforts of Ignatius' followers in the Society of Jesus. It remains a powerful influence and is the basis for much of the contemporary retreat movement.

> ...It contains a series of practical directives—methods of examining one's conscience, engaging in prayer of various kinds, deliberating or making life choices, and meditating. This program of spiritual development, if you will, is interspersed with outlines and directives for various meditations and contemplations....[759]

Later in the year of 1940, Bill W. traveled to St. Louis to visit Fr. Dowling. Bill noticed in the office of the *Queen's Work,* the outline of the similarities between AA's 12 Steps and Ignatius' Spiritual Exercises. John Markoe a Jesuit priest and an alcoholic had prepared the outline.[760] Bill W. and Ed Dowling continued a close friendship for the following 20 years until the death of Dowling. There were around 150 letters written between these two men during those years as well as many visits with each other. Robert Fitzgerald, S.J. , a member of the order of Jesuits that Ed Dowling belonged to,

757 Boehmer, op. cit., pp. 25, 34-35; Reported in Paris, op. cit., p. 21.
758 Paris. op, cit., p. 22.
759 Meissner, W.W.,S.J., M.D., *The Psychology of a Saint Ignatius of Loyola,* Vail-Ballou Press, Binghamton, New York ,(1992), p. 87.
760 Fitzgerald, op. cit., p. 58.

gathered together the letters spoken of above and published in 1995 the book, *The Soul of Sponsorship,* illustrating their friendship. From this book some following paragraphs share some of their correspondence.

In 1952 Bill W. began to work on a small book which he purposed to be an addition to the literature for Alcoholics Anonymous, *Twelve Steps and Twelve Traditions.* Bill wrote to Ed Dowling in May 1952, requesting a copy of the *Spiritual Exercises* of Loyola, for he wished to study them so as to help him in composing the rest of his essays. Along with the letter requesting a copy of the *Spiritual Exercises* Bill had sent to Dowling copies of his essays, two of the 12 Steps. The book was to consist of an essay of at least 2000 words for each of the 12 Steps and likewise for each of the Twelve Traditions. Bill asked Fr. Ed Dowling who was the Editor of the Catholic journal *Queens' Work* to critique the copies that were sent to him.[761]

Dowling returned a letter to Bill on June 20, 1952, expressing his delight that Bill was going to do an interpretation of each of the 12 steps. He commented that he was sending the *Spiritual Exercises of St. Ignatius* to Bill. July 17, 1952. Bill's return letter speaks of his impression of the Spiritual Exercises received.

> ...Please have my immense thanks for that wonderful volume on the Ignatian Exercises. I'm already well into it, and what an adventure it is! Excepting for a sketchy outline you folks had posted on the Sodality wall years back, I had never seen anything of the Exercises at all. Consequently I am astonished and not a little awed by what comes into sight. Again, thanks a lot.[762]

Bill spoke of the problem he had in writing the essays about the steps. He felt he needed to broaden and deepen the steps for new members as well as those of long term. He had to make them acceptable for atheists, agnostics, believers, depressives, paranoid, psychiatrists, clergymen, and everyone else. How to open wide the entrance into the steps? This was his dilemma. Bill had previously shared that he had good help in writing of the essays by authors Tom Powers, Betty Love, and Jack Alexander. Now he makes the following quote:

> The hoop you have to jump through is a lot wider than you think. But I have good help—of that I am certain. *Both over here and over there.*[763] (Emphasis added)

---

761   *Ibid.,* pp. 55, 56.
762   *Ibid.,* 58.
763   *Ibid.,* p. 59

The author of *The Soul of Sponsorship*, Fitzgerald, on reporting about this letter says "over there" refers to the spirit world. Fitzgerald further comments that the *voice* from the other world, as Bill stated it, came out as if it was an unremarkable comment. Bill was writing about the help he was getting in his writing from Boniface, a spirit entity that was purported to be an Apostle or priest from England that went to Germany, Bavaria, and France as a missionary in the 1600's. Fitzgerald continues his comments about Bill W. and the spirit—Boniface. Bill had chosen not to join the Catholic Church after a year of study because he could not see a Pope having infallibility. Fitzgerald, a Jesuit priest, is puzzled because Bill refuses to join the hierarchical church but was open to receiving help from a dead bishop via his spirit entity. Bill tells his story of Boniface:

> One turned up the other day calling himself Boniface, Said he was Benedictine missionary and English....I'd never heard of this gentleman but he checked out pretty well in the Encyclopedia.[764]

Bill asked Fr. Dowling to check Boniface out for him. Ed Dowling was able to identify Boniface as an apostle of Germany of the 1600's. Dowling cautions Bill with the following words speaking of spirits:

> ...that these folks tell us truth in small matters in order to fool us in larger....[765]

Dowling continued to give caution to Bill concerning the spirits and their messages. He refers to the play *Macbeth* wherein spirit voices—otherworld voices bring temptation to Macbeth to murder the king, Duncan. He tells Bill to read the *Spiritual Exercises* on page 100, the Longridge edition; on this page *Two Standards Meditation* appear in italics. In this text Ignatius views the devil on a throne high above yet surrounded by chaos and smoke, drawing all under his control. To this group will be granted riches, enticements to pride, and other vices. In contrast on a low plain, is seen Christ, inviting any who will come join under His flag and accept humility, poverty and all other blessings. Once each year Father Dowling attended a retreat where he would pray the *Spiritual Exercises* of St. Ignatius, which contain rules for discernment of spirits, as well as rules for discerning God's will. St. Ignatius was visited by, he believed, spirits of the devil as well as members of the Divinity, and he formed these rules to help himself discern which he was being visited by.[766] It is not probable that all of the spirits visiting Ignatius were of the devil?

---

764 *Ibid.*
765 *Ibid.*
766 *Ibid.*, p. 79.

A response to the advice of Dowling to Bill W. came in a letter from Bill dated August 8, 1952. He said he had read the requested passage and accepted the need for caution when communicating with spirits from the otherworld. Yet, he was reluctant to have the church limit his connections with the otherworld. He reasoned that it did not make sense that the devil's spirits could gain access to our world but the saints discarnate spirits did not seem to make it through. Why he reasoned is the opening so wide for the devil's spirits but so restricted for all the good folks. He mentions that he no longer had a compulsion toward the *spook business* but occasionally one gets through without invitation, such as Boniface.[767] In 1955, at a celebration of AA's 20th year anniversary a symbol was displayed which had been chosen to be the logo for Alcoholic Anonymous. The symbol, a circle enclosing a triangle with the words Recovery, Unity, and Service written on each arm of the triangle, was mounted on a banner which floated above the audience. The symbol's meaning is explained:

> ...The circle stands for the whole world of AA, and the triangle stands for AA's Three Legacies of Recovery, Unity, and Service. Within our wonderful new world, we have found freedom from our fatal obsession. That we have chosen this particular symbol is perhaps no accident. *The priests and seers of antiquity regarded the circle enclosing the triangle as a means of warding off spirits of evil*, and AA's circle and triangle of Recovery, Unity, and Service has certainly meant all of that to us and much more.[768]

The 12 Steps constitute the foundation principles of guidance in Alcoholics Anonymous fellowship program—the *spiritual powerhouse of AA*. Father Ed Dowling was the first to recognize the potential for application of the 12 Steps to other *compulsions.*[769] Their use is now found in a large number of recovery-like programs designed to help in overcoming a variety of dysfunctional practices, attitudes, etc., and its use has moved into the church in a big way.

In a previous chapter we reviewed in brief the origin and development of these 12 Steps. Would it not be appropriate to give thought and consideration to the potential that tentacles of spiritualism may have found its way into the 12 Steps? These Steps had their beginning out of the Oxford Group wherein no mention is found of the shed blood of Jesus Christ cleansing us from our sin and they promoted a book in therapy for alcoholism that denies the divinity of

---

767 *Ibid.*, pp. 60, 61.
768 *Alcoholics Anonymous World Services Inc.,* Alcoholics Anonymous Comes of Age, Harper & Brothers, New York, (1957), p. 139..
769 Dowling, Ed S.J., *Grapevine, A.A. Steps for the Under-privileged Non A.A.,* (July 1960); reported in Fitzgerald, Robert, *The Soul of Sponsorship p. 60.*

Jesus Christ. Strong influence came from the books of two spiritualists (Jung and James); the cofounders (Dr. Bob and Bill W.) were from the beginning involved in séances and other forms of psychic phenomena. The initial writing of the steps came following *relaxation* and a request for *guidance* from Bill W. who was an active spiritualist and medium. When the 12 Steps were to be amplified, broadened, and explained in detail in the book, *Twelve Steps and Twelve Traditions,* there was the spirit *Boniface* that Bill said was giving him aid in his writing. Jesuits priests were astonished at the similarity between their *Spiritual Exercises* and the 12 Steps.

While Bill was deeply engrossed in the use of LSD for alcoholics and giving it to many of his acquaintances, Father Ed sent him *Rules for Discernment of Spirits* coming from the second week of Spiritual Exercises. These are recorded in *The Soul of Sponsorship by the Jesuit Priest Robert Fitzgerald,* page 98, and appear below.

> It is the mark of an evil spirit to assume the appearance of the angel of light. He begins by suggesting thoughts suited to a devout soul but ends by suggesting his own. Little by little drawing the soul into his snares and evil designs.

The Bible is very clear and forceful in its warnings against spirit involvement of any kind.

> There shall not be found among you...one who casts a spell, or a medium, or a spiritist, or one who calls up the dead. For whosoever does these things is detestable to the Lord; and because of these detestable things the Lord your God will drive them out before you. Deut. 18: 10-12

Many would say the results speak for itself; there have been millions of people that found sobriety from their association with AA and continue to do so. Is it not a program designed to be neutral to various religions as well as for those of no religion? It is a system that depends on the choice of the member to freely choose the principles of the 12 Steps, there is no hook or coercion. How could a person even suspect spiritualistic influence to be incorporated into the program? Would it not more likely signify that the person holding such thoughts and concerns has a problem and not AA? Up to this time almost all source material used to write these chapters on 12 Steps has come from books that either the AA organization sanctions or from books whose authors are themselves members of AA and/or supporters. Now I will present questions that some have asked who are not members of AA or supporters of, as they evaluated the 12 Steps. First, there is the history of spiritualism association as related in previous paragraphs. The question is asked: will the Creator God, the true God of the universe, use people who are in the service of Satan, as revealed by being a spiritualist medium, etc., to bless His followers with vital information and healing methods? Will the messages and methods passed on by those who are Satan's agents, be free of spiritualistic entanglement? It is needful that we look carefully at certain of the 12 Steps and consider the questions asked by those who have concern that there might be deceptive spiritualistic influence within.

> Do not turn to mediums or spiritists; do not seek them out to be defiled by them. I am the Lord your God. (Leviticus 19:13)

> As for the person who turns to mediums and spiritists, to play the harlot after them, I will also set my face against that person and will cut him off from his people. (Leviticus 20:6)

What is the base for the individual steps? Christian? Pantheistic? Secular? Again the reader must decide, read on. In an attempt to find the answer to the question as to whether or not the originators of, and the AA program itself, is Biblical and Christian based we will look closely at certain specific Steps with that question in mind.

Step # 1:   *We admitted we were powerless over alcohol, that our lives had become unmanageable.*

A. Comments presented by AA in support of the first Step:

When Bill W. was in Towns Hospital December 1934 for his alcoholism, Dr. Silkworth presented his concept that alcoholism was a "disease" (the first professional to do so) and that a person had an allergy to alcohol, which, in turn, caused the uncontrollable urge to drink. Bill W. accepted Dr. Silkworth's opinion that alcoholism as a disease had no moral implications and so Bill was relieved of any guilt that his alcoholism had had anything to do with his personal decision to drink. The medical profession accepted the definition of alcoholism as a "disease" in 1944. However, Bill Wilson felt that a *spiritual power* was what was involved in bringing him to sobriety.

> The tyrant alcohol wielded a double-edged sword over us: first drinking, and then by an allergy of the body that insured we would ultimately destroy ourselves in the process.[770]

---

770 Alcoholics Anonymous World Services Inc. *Twelve Steps Twelve Traditions,* (1952), p. 22.

This first step is stating that the person must come to utter helplessness to be able to move toward freedom of alcohol's hold upon him. Unfortunately these criteria did not work well for those who wished to quit drinking but had not yet reached that state of total helplessness. To remedy this defect in the program, AA simply raised the threshold of what was considered the *bottom* in one's experience. Therefore the belief that one had now reached the bottom long before they actually did reach the worst possible physical condition, made the program acceptable to many heavy drinkers.[771] For therapy of this *physical disease* AA sought after and accepted a *spiritual solution*. We could agree that for most alcoholics there is a need of a physical solution through nutrition, exercise and proper habits of life as well as a spiritual. However, the physical—chemical influence on the body of alcohol is not now understood to be an allergy.

B. Concern over step one.

When man sinned selfishness took the place of love:

> His nature became so weakened through transgression that it was impossible for him, in his own strength, to resist the power of evil. He was made captive by Satan, and would have remained so forever had not God specially interposed.[772]

It is impossible to escape from our habits and behavior by ourselves. Our hearts are ruled by sin and we cannot change such.

> There must be a power working from within, a new life *from above* before men can be changed from sin to holiness. That power is *Christ*. His grace *alone* can quicken the lifeless faculties of the soul and attract it to God, to holiness.[773]

Paul the Apostle experienced the "bottoming out" experience that is referred to in AA's step one. He longed to be free of the enslavement of sin and he cried out:

> O wretched man that I am! Who shall deliver me from this body of death? (Romans 7:24)

---

771 *Ibid.*, p. 23.
772 White, E.G., *Steps to Christ,* Review and Herald Publishing Assoc., Hagerstown, MD, (1892), Ch.2.
773 *Ibid.*

The only way to God is through Jesus Christ.

Step one is a dangerous counterfeit for both Christians and non-Christians. It serves as a substitute for acknowledging one's own depravity, sinful acts, and utter lostness *apart from Jesus Christ*, the only Savior, and the only way to forgiveness (relief of true guilt). Step one is also a substitute for Christians to acknowledge that without the life of the Lord Jesus Christ in them, they are unable to live righteously. Apart from Christ in them, they are unable to please God.[774] (Emphasis added)

Step # 2:   Came to believe that a Power greater than ourselves could restore us to sanity.

A. Comments presented by AA in support of the 2nd Step:

Bill W. the agnostic on Dec. 11, 1934, while in Towns Hospital, readily accepted Ebby Thatcher's invitation to choose a God, a *Higher Power* of his understanding when introduced to the Oxford Group's method of overcoming alcoholism. It did not matter as to what one chose for a God as long as one was selected. It was a way of getting a person to make a step of surrender into the Oxford Group's influence, a foot in the door concept. Once a choice was made then the individual could be exposed to more of their teachings. With this approach a person did not need to accept Jesus Christ the Divine Son of God. One could participate in the Oxford Group's meetings yet could expect to receive the *blessings* of God. In fact, the Oxford Group made no mention of the Divinity of Jesus Christ and recommended a spiritual book for study that taught *divinity within—pantheism*. Alcoholics Anonymous adopted step 2 from the Oxford Group. Bill W. makes it clear in his personal story that is written in the book, *Alcoholics Anonymous*, that he could not accept the God of the Christian, and that Jesus Christ was simply a man. So when it was suggested to him that he could choose his own concept of God, this appealed to him; it was only a matter of being willing to believe in a Power greater than himself, nothing more to start with.

In writing the *big book—Alcoholics Anonymous*, Bill put forth great effort to properly state Step Two to make it acceptable to anyone, so avoiding offense. Jack Alexander, the reporter for *Saturday Evening Post* in 1941, spent a month with the AA fellowship meetings investigating carefully their method

---

774   Bobgan, Martin and Deidre, *12 Steps to Destruction, Codependency/Recovery Dependency, Heresies,* East Gate Publishers, Santa Barbara, CA, (1991), p. 95.

and teachings so that the article he was to write for the *Post* would be accurate and truly reflect their teaching. He wrote the following:

> Describing AA's *higher power*, Alexander noted the alcoholic may choose to think of his Inner Self, the miracle of growth, a tree, and man's wonderment at the physical universe, the structure of the atom, or mere mathematical infinity. Whatever form is visualized, the neophyte is taught that he must rely on it and, in his own way, to pray to that Power for strength.[775]

You may question whether choosing some inanimate object is really suggested or done in AA; the following quotation speaks to this issue:

> ...In fact, initiates who come seeking help, but who have trouble inventing or envisioning a god, are often told they can worship a 'doorknob,' or even the group itself to begin their spiritual journey. The first time we heard we thought it was a joke-some form of esoteric humor. But it is not. We have heard the 'doorknob-deity' *speech* a number of times now. It apparently serves as their *starter-god*. Like the training wheels on a bike-only there until the child is ready for the next big step. Believe in something, newcomers are told; believe in anything; just *believe*.[776]

> We found that as soon as we were able to lay aside prejudice and express even a willingness to believe in a Power greater than ourselves, we commenced to get results, even though it was impossible for any of us to fully define or comprehend that Power, which is God. Much to our relief, we discovered we did not need to consider another's conception of God. Our own conception, however inadequate, was sufficient to make the approach and to effect contact with Him. As soon as we admitted the possible existence of a Creative Intelligence, a Spirit of the Universe underlying the totality of things, we began to be possessed of a new sense of power and direction, provided we took other simple steps.[777]

B. Serious questions and comments that are frequently made concerning the second Step:

Thou shalt have no other gods before me. (Exodus 20: 3)

---

775   Alexander, Jack, Saturday Evening Post, March 1, 1941.

776   Http://mywordlikefire.wordpress.com; Missionaries Into Darkest Alcoholics Anonymous, Feb. 2009.

777   Alcoholics Anonymous World Services Inc., *Alcoholic Anonymous,* (1938), p. 46

I am the Lord, that is my name. I will not give my glory to another, nor my praise to idols. (Isaiah 42:8)

What profit is the idol when its maker has carved it, Or an image, a teacher of falsehood? For its maker trusts in his own handwork when he fashions speechless idols, Woe to him who says to a piece of wood, 'Awake.' To a mute stone, 'Arise!' And that is your teacher? (Habakkuk 2:18-19)

And just as they did not see fit to acknowledge God any longer, God gave them over to a depraved mind, to do those things which are not proper...(Romans 1:28)

If Alcoholics Anonymous is based on Christian principles how is it I can choose a Higher Power that is not the Christian God, and still be Christian? If I choose the pantheistic god known by a hundred different names (universal energy, prana, chi, the Great Reality, god of Nature, Presence, mana, Self, etc.) does that equate to the Christian God and His principles? The same question is asked when choosing an inanimate object, idea, the fellowship group itself, etc., as my god?

These people "Who say to a tree, 'you are my father, and to a stone, "you gave me birth." "For they have turned their backs to Me, and not their face." (Jeremiah 2:27)

The Christian looks at this choice as being critical because some of the following steps directly relate to this choice. The question arises, is this choice simply a trick to get the individual further involved before we spring the Christian God on him or her, or instead to deceptively slip in the god of the pantheist? Many Christians defend AA and may not see it this way, but they are in agreement with a belief system that *lifts up strange gods*, Amos 3:3. In AA all gods are called the *Higher Power* thus relegating Christ our King to commonality, as if He were simply one nameless deity among many— pantheon.

In their Churches on Sunday they call God by that Name above all names: Jesus Christ the Savior. But here, in their all-gods sect, they call Jesus by the term all members use for their various gods. So Jesus becomes a "higher power." Thus has the savior been placed in the pantheon, the temple of the gods.[778]

---

778 (Worldview Times, Missionaries into Darkest Alcoholics Anonymous.) http://www. worldviewweekend.com/worldview-times/article.php? articleid=3574

When I fellowship in AA and we repeat the Lord's Prayer and the Serenity Prayer together, do I in this form of joint worship join with unbelievers in their worship? They worshiping their chosen god and I the Lord Jesus? I am sure many who participate in AA will consider that this verse is not appropriately used in this instance. You decide.

> Do not be yoked together with unbelievers. For what do righteousness and wickedness have in common? Or what fellowship can light have with darkness? What harmony is there between Christ and Belial? What has a believer in common with an unbeliever? What agreement is there between the temple of God and idols? ...Therefore, come out from them and be separate, says the Lord. (2 Corinthians 6: 14-17 NIV)

Step # 3: *"Made a decision to turn our will and our lives over to the care of God as we understood him."*

A. Comments presented by AA in support of the Third Step:

In Twelve Steps and Twelve Traditions, Step Three is likened to opening a door that has been locked; all that is needed is the key. The *key is to give our will,* our power of choice to the Higher Power we have chosen to be our God as we understand. We turn our will and our lives over to the control of that Power. This is a critical step, it is critical because it lets the Power we have chosen be the ruler of our lives.

All the other steps in AA depend upon our effort to conform to the principles of *this step* and to place our trust in our chosen God.[779]

> So how, exactly, can the willing person continue to turn his will and his life over to the Higher Power? He made a beginning, we have seen, when he commenced *to rely upon AA for the solution of his alcohol problem.*[780] (Emphasis added)

The prayer of serenity:

> God grant me the serenity to accept the things I cannot change, courage to change the things I can, and wisdom to know the difference. Thy will, not mine be done.[781]

---

779 Alcoholics Anonymous World Services, Inc., *Twelve Steps and Twelve Traditions,* New York, NY, (1952), pp. 34, 40.
780 *Ibid.,* p. 39.
781 *Ibid.,* p. 41.

B. Serious questions and comments that are frequently presented concerning the third step.

This Third Step in conjunction with step two is the most serious decision one can make in all of the 12 steps. This step is asking me to turn my will, my decision power over to whatever Higher Power I decide upon. The Christian understands two powers in the universe, first,—the power of God the Creator, Jesus Christ the Divine Son of God, and second, the power that Satan has been allowed to exercise. When we choose a God of my understanding, I choose one or the other. No matter what entity I may choose as a Higher Power if it is not Jesus Christ the Divine Son of God I will have chosen the power of Satan for my god. There is no other power to choose from!

Let the reader consider the quotations below:

> The will is the governing power in the nature of man, bringing all the other faculties under its sway. The will is not the taste or the inclination, but it is the deciding power, which works in the children of men unto obedience to God, or unto disobedience. Every child should understand the true force of the will. He should be led to see how great is the responsibility involved in this gift. The will is . . . the power of decision, or choice.

> ...In every experience of life God's word to us is, *"Choose you this day whom ye will serve."* Joshua 24:15. Everyone may place his will on the side of the will of God, may choose to obey Him, and by thus linking himself with divine agencies, he may stand where nothing can force him to do evil.[782]

From the Bible we have this counsel:

> Wherefore, my beloved· as ye have always obeyed, not as in my presence only, but now much more in my absence, work out your own salvation with fear and trembling. For it is God which worketh in you both to *will* and to do of (his) good pleasure. (Philippians 2: 12, 13)

When I surrender my will into the hands of Jesus Christ to be the Lord of my life then His will directs my life in obedience to Him; if I surrender my will into the hands of Satan then he becomes the lord of my life and his will is the power that directs me. Satan has great power and may well do great and wondrous works in my life but eternal life comes only through Jesus Christ the Divine Son of God. Let us reflect once again upon this critical point.

---

782   White, E. G., *Child Guidance*, Southern Publishing Assn., Nashville, TN, (1954), p. 209.

Neither is there salvation in any other: for there is none other name under heaven given among men, whereby we must be saved. (Acts 4:12)

Jesus saith unto him, I am the way, the truth, and the life: no man, cometh unto the Father, but by me. (John 14:6)

We are choosing the Lord of our life in this third step, there is no other choice more important that we will make. We are told that a person makes a beginning toward the goal of sobriety *when one commences to rely upon AA for the solution of his or her alcohol problem.* Does AA become our god? Does not the power to overcome, come from Jesus Christ? Choosing AA does not necessarily involve choosing Jesus as our power and that is the only way to overcome evil.

When we give our will and turn our lives over to the power we chose to believe in, it is important to not have given our permission to spirits—fallen angels, to have sway with us.

Warren Smith, in *Standing Fast in the Last Days*, tells how a psychic woman, who uncannily knew many details about him, told Smith the spirits on the other side needed his permission to work in his life.[783]

Step # 5.   *"Admitted to God, to ourselves, and to another human being the exact nature of our wrongs."*

A. Comments by AA in support of step #5.

After one has made an inventory of all past wrongs, recognized defects of character, and sins then they are to be confessed to some other *human being.* AA declares this is *mandatory* to maintain sobriety. Furthermore, it is said:

...It seems plain that the grace of God will not enter to expel our destructive obsessions until we are willing to try this.[784]

Confess your faults one to another, and pray one for another, that ye may be healed. The effectual fervent prayer of a righteous man availeth much. (James 5: 16)

The suggestion is that only by presenting one's self judged defects to some other person, *not holding back anything* in the confession can one proceed on the road to straight thinking, honesty, and humility. This is a real

---

783 http://www.lighthousetrailsresearch.com/blog/?p=1158
784 *Twelve Steps,* op. cit., p. 57.

test of willingness to confide with some chosen person facts that you may not want anyone else to know.

> Provided you hold back nothing, your sense of relief will mount from minute to minute....Many an AA, once agnostic or atheistic, tells us that it was during this stage of Step Five that he first actually felt the presence of God. And even those who had faith already often become conscious of God as they never were before.[785]

B. Comments questioning confessing all my sins to another human being.

In the study of preparing to write this chapter I discovered that confession not only is taught in the Bible, but has been promoted by the Catholic Church, Ignatius Loyola in the Spiritual Exercises, by the psychiatrists Freud and Jung, Oxford Group, and picked up and practiced by Alcoholics Anonymous. Within these groups confession *is made to man.* The question is asked: Is it Biblical that I confess *all* my sins to my fellow man? Quotations are shared pertaining to this question.

> In the work of overcoming there will be confessions to be made one to another, but the word of God forbids man to put an erring man in God's place, making confessors of frail humanity. We are to confess our faults one to another, and pray one for another that we may be healed. The appointment of men to the confessional of the Roman Church is the fulfillment of the *design of Satan* to confer upon men power which belongs to God only. God is dishonored by the absolution of the priest and by the confession of the soul to man. Confessions of secret sins are made to men whose own hearts may be as sinks of iniquity. *There are sins which are to be confessed to God only*, for he knows the whole heart and will not take advantage of the trust reposed in him; he will not betray our confidence, and if we submit ourselves to him, he will cleanse the heart from all iniquity.[786] (Emphasis added)

> *Many, many confessions should never be spoken in the hearing of mortals*; for the result is that which the limited judgment of finite beings does not anticipate. . . . God will be better glorified *if we confess the secret, inbred corruption of the heart to Jesus alone* than if we open its recesses to finite, erring man, who cannot judge righteously unless his heart is constantly imbued with the Spirit of God. . . . *Do not pour into human ears the story which God alone should hear.*[787] (Emphasis added)

785 *Ibid.*, p. 62.
786 White, E.G., *Signs of the Times,* April 20, (1891), part 5.
787 White, E.G., *Our Father Cares,* chapter 3, (1991), p. 73.

...He who kneels before fallen man, and opens in confession the secret thoughts and imaginations of his heart, is debasing his manhood and degrading every noble instinct of his soul. In unfolding the sins of his life to a priest,—an erring, sinful mortal, and too often corrupted with wine and licentiousness,—his standard of character is lowered, and he is defiled in consequence. *His thought of God is degraded to the likeness of fallen humanity,* for the priest stands as a representative of God. This degrading confession of man to man is the secret spring from which has flowed much of the evil that is defiling the world and fitting it for the final destruction.[788]

If one confesses his faults to the god of his understanding but not Jesus Christ the Son of God, of what value is it? Only Jesus Christ can forgive sin, the devil cannot, and all *Gods of our understanding* outside of Jesus Christ are false gods.

Wilson cautions in *Alcoholics Anonymous,* page 74, that "we cannot disclose anything to our wives or our parents which will hurt them and make them unhappy." He speaks of "perhaps one is mixed up with women in a fashion we wouldn't care to have advertised." In *Bill W. and Mr. Wilson,* author Raphael points out the adulterous behavior of Bill W. which continued during his sober years and with this exception to the rule in confession of all sins, he had made an escape for himself.[789]

The psychiatrist C.G. Jung has written some interesting observations on *confession* as used by the Catholic Church, Ignatius Loyola's Spiritual Exercises, Germany's "Professor Shultz's autogenic training (now called biofeedback), Freud's psychoanalysis, and his own analytical psychology approach to mind—cure. *He compares confession to the Hindu's use of Yoga as the tool to enter into the unconscious,* which he (Hindu) considers a higher level of consciousness. In psychological use its purpose is to open up the *unconscious* to the *conscious* mind. Both approaches suppress our protective inhibitions and open the mind to outside influence and /or control.[790]

He (Jung) elaborates further on the origin of confession use in mind therapy:

> The first beginnings of all analytical treatment are to be found in its prototype, *the confessional.* Since, however, the two practices have no direct causal connection, but rather grow from a common psychic root; it is difficult for an

788   White, E.G., *The Great Controversy,* Pacific Press Publishing Assoc., Nampa, ID, (1888), p. 567.
789   Raphael, *op. cit.,* pp. 128-131.
790   Jung, C.G. , *Psychology and the East from the Collected Works of C.G. Jung, Yoga and the West,* Princeton University Press, Princeton, New Jersey, (1978), pp. 84, 85.

outsider to see at once the relation between the groundwork of psychoanalysis and the religious institution of the confessional.[791]

Jung further tells us that the first stage of psychoanalysis is in essence a *catharsis* (purging) of the mind by confession, with or without hypnotic aid; also this places the mind in the same state as the Eastern yoga systems describe, i.e.,, meditation—open to control by outside powers.

Even if the neurosis is cured there may be a complication that creates a limitation in the use of confession. The patient may be bound to the individual receiving the confession. If this attachment is forcibly severed, there is a bad relapse. This is seen also in hypnosis. Freud first noticed this problem of fixation on the therapists by patients undergoing catharsis. The fixation is similar to that of a child to the father. Notice:

> The patient falls into a sort of childish dependence from which he cannot protect himself even by reason and insight. The fixation is at times astonishingly strong—so much so that one suspects it of being fed by *forces quite out of the common....* we are obviously dealing with a new symptom—a neurotic formation directly induced by the treatment.[792] (Emphasis added)

It appears that the use of confession in therapy is not innocuous.

Step # 11.: "Sought through prayer and meditation to improve our conscious contact with God as we understood Him, praying only for knowledge of His will for us and the power to carry that out.

A. Comments by AA in support of step # 11.

Prayer is an act of supplication and a method of communication addressed to Deity, it may be silent or vocal. There are many forms of prayer and such as is offered to idols, to the pantheistic god or gods of the pagan, to the God of Christians, etc. Praise, gratitude, allegiance, to one's God can be expressed by prayer as well as request for guidance, assistance, deliverance, and blessings. Jesus Christ the Son of God prayed to His Father for guidance and strength and He in turn taught the apostles to pray. Throughout the Bible prayers were recorded of various people and frequent mention was made of specific prayers being offered. Certainly it is fitting for an individual seeking sobriety to be

791 Jung, C.G. , *Modern Man in Search of a Soul,* A Harvest Gook, Harcourt, Inc. San Diego, CA, (1933), p. 31.
792 *Ibid.,* p. 38.

encouraged to pray and pray often asking for the power of God to grant him healing from his malady. There is no other power than Jesus Christ that can truly free us from our afflictions.

There is some awkwardness in the subject of prayer, however, in the 12 Step program. What type of God are we praying to? The God as we understand him can be even an inanimate object, an idea, etc. A quotation from the essay on the Eleventh Step is shared below:

> To certain newcomers and to those one-time agnostics who still cling to the *AA Group* as their higher power, claims for the power of prayer may, despite all the logic and experience in proof of it, still be unconvincing or quite objectionable.[793]

In careful review of Step Eleven's essay, the description of meditation as suggested in the 12 Steps is much closer to the Eastern style meditation than the Christian concept of meditation. To illustrate let us examine several sentences explaining meditation as to be used in the 12 Steps.

> As though lying upon a sunlit beach, let us relax and breathe deeply of the spiritual atmosphere with which the grace of this prayer surrounds us. Let us become willing to partake and be strengthened and lifted up by sheer spiritual power, beauty, and love of which these magnificent words are the carriers. Let us look now upon the sea and ponder what its mystery is; and let us lift our eyes to the far horizon, beyond which we shall seek all those wonders still unseen.[794]

> This much could be a fragment of what is called meditation, perhaps our very first attempt at a mood, a flier into the *realm of spirit*, if you like. ...Meditation is something which can always be further developed. It has no boundaries, either of width or height....But its object is always the same: to improve our conscious contact with God, with His grace, wisdom, and love.[795] (Emphasis added)

Even use of a mantra is slipped in, in an inconspicuous way:

> ...and repeat to ourselves, a particular prayer or phrase that has appealed to us in our reading or meditation. Just saying it *over and over* will often enable us to clear a channel choked up with anger, fear, frustration or misunderstanding, and permit us to return to the surest help of all—our search for God's will, not our own, in the moment of stress.[796] (Emphasis added)

---

793 *Twelve Steps,* op. cit., p. 96.
794 *Ibid.,* p. 100.
795 *Ibid.,* p. 101.
796 *Ibid.,* p. 103.

B. Questions asked concerning and comments made about the Eleventh Step.

In Step *Two* a god of our choice and understanding is chosen; in Step *Three* that god is given a person's *will*, turning one's life over to that power. Confession of sins and faults is made in Step *Five*, to another *human being*. In Step *eleven* prayer and meditation are directed to the power selected in Step Two. No boundaries are placed on meditation and so it can vary from an active thought process, to the Eastern style meditation of silence and emptying the mind wherein the purpose is to make contact with a "god" entity.

In prayer we present what is in our heart in praise, requests, dedication to whatever God of our choice, asking this God to possess us, to put *his will* into *our will* and be the Lord of our life.

How critical it is that we choose the one and only true God, Jesus Christ the Divine Son. In the fellowship meetings I read that the Lord's Prayer and the Serenity Prayer are both prayed out loud in unison by the entire group. The Lord's Prayer begins with "Our father which art in heaven..." A question asked is, if I being a member of the fellowship have not chosen Jesus Christ as my Higher Power yet I pray to *Our Father* of what value is this? The Bible verse John 14:6 tells me:

> Jesus saith unto him: I am the way, the truth, and the life: no man, cometh unto the Father, but by me. If ye had known me, ye should have known my Father also: and from henceforth ye know him, and have seen him.

How can these prayers ascend to the Father when we have denied the Son?

The word *meditation* is of concern to me. Most of us upon hearing the word *meditation* consider an active cognitive process by which we have given study to a word, phrase, or passage and look to God, through the Holy Spirit, to join in blessing us with understanding, to fill our mind with His wisdom. When the meditation practice of the Oxford Group is carefully reviewed it appears to be more of the Eastern pagan practice of *deep breathing, silence, emptying the mind*, as the method of communion with God. Does it open our mind to being possessed by a god not of our choosing? Shall we give control of our mind to the powers of darkness?

> Put on the whole armour of God that ye may be able to stand against the wiles of the devil. For we wrestle not against flesh and blood, but against principalities, against powers, against the rulers of the darkness of this world, against spiritual wickedness in high places. (Ephesians 6:11, 12)

The devil continues to hone his techniques and deceptions to precision. A movement of today referred to as the *Emergent Church* has as its goal to sweep the world into its deceptive dogma; it has also reached out to the 12 step program. The stated goal of the Emergent Church is to be an agency bringing peace to the world through uniting all religions. The power of this movement is through a special style of mystical prayer that is proclaimed to bring God *down* to you; the Christian prayer is to raise man *up* to his God. The prayer method of Rohr and Keating has many names but a more comprehensive name is *contemplative prayer* this prayer movement is actually Eastern meditation in a very smooth disguise. It is sweeping the world.

Two outstanding leaders in this movement, Father Richard Rohr and Father Thomas Keating, both Catholic priests, facilitated a conference in 2008.

> ...to demonstrate to those in 12 Step Fellowship ways to embrace the invitation of the 11th Step to improve our conscious contact with God.... (This) will offer us all a wonderful opportunity *to deepen our contemplative practices.*[797]

The goal of Rohr and Keating is to incorporate their mystical contemplative prayer methods into the 12 Step program. They present the use of a *repetitive phrase*, or word (*mantra*), and a special *breath prayer* at these conferences. Following this Eastern meditation method it is not unusual to hear of people who experience a sense of euphoria, feeling of well-being, and the feeling that they are in the presence of God as a result of these special prayer techniques. They build their foundation of Christianity upon *feelings* and not on *thus saith the Word*. Remember that in the *big book—Alcoholics Anonymous* of AA the central doctrine of the New Age is to be found therein.

> We found the *Great Reality deep down within us*. In the last analysis, it is only there *He* can be found."[798]

CONCLUSION:

AA claims not to be religious, only *spiritual* in nature, is there a difference? The U.S. Supreme Court ruled November 15, 1999, upholding a lower Appeals Court decision, that the AA program *is religious*. Its fellowship meetings are religious in nature; they cite the participants as a body reciting the Lord's Prayer and the Serenity Prayer. They worship a *"Higher Power"*,

---

797   Inner Room Conference" Promotional Material htpp://www.cacradical-grace.org/
798   *Alcoholics Anonymous,* op. cit., p. 55.

confession is a part of the service, testimony is given, and they are instructed to go spread the word. It has been voiced about that it is Christian in orientation and arose from a Christian organization—Oxford Group and its founders Dr. Bob and Bill W. were near Christians. In several months of reading many books which are under the blessing of Alcoholics Anonymous as well as books written by members who are supporters of the organization *I never once found any sentence or reference that acknowledged in any way **Jesus Christ** to be the **Divine Son of God** and that the way to the Father was only through Him.* Forgiveness of sins and removable of character defects happens only through the access of Jesus Christ to God the Father.

The program accepts any and all gods placing itself more closely within pantheism by definition than Christianity. Some critics have called it idol worship, I let you decide. Spiritualistic practices were involved with its cofounders from the beginning and had influence in forming the core program, the 12 Steps. Two fundamental reading texts used by AA were written by spiritualists—Jung's *Modern Man in Search of a Soul* and William James' *The Varieties of Religious Experience*, were:

> ... the sources of many of Wilson's profoundest ideas about religion, philosophy, and psychology.[799]

AA early on used the text by Emmitt Fox, *The Sermon On the Mount*, and which the Oxford Group had used regularly for working with alcoholics. This text denied the Divinity of Jesus Christ, denied that the Bible had doctrine.

A noted writer and editor of a monthly religious journal expressed his conviction that the spiritualistic activities of Bill Wilson and Bob Smith occurred after the establishment of the program of AA. This is not true as Bill's own statement given earlier in this text, dates the summer of 1935 as the start of AA as well as a summer that he and Bob were active in the practice of spiritualism.

> AA was entangled in spiritualism from the very beginning.[800]

The cofounders Dr. Bob and Bill W. were also personally deeply involved in spiritualism in a variety of ways including séances, Ouija board use, table rapping, and automatic writing and as a *control medium*. Bill mentions in a letter to Sam Shoemaker that:

---

799   Raphael, *op. cit.,* pp. 133-4.
800   *Ibid.*, p. 159.

"Throughout A.A., we find a large amount of psychic phenomena; nearly all of it spontaneous....These psychic experiences have run nearly the full gamut of everything we see in the books. In addition to my original mystic experience, I've had a lot of such phenomenalism myself.[801]

Bill had a spirit guide, Boniface, that Bill said helped him in writing *Twelve Steps and Twelve Traditions.* Author Raphael in *Bill W. and Mr. Wilson p. 161, tells us that Bill W. was* committed to *mystical modes* as a way of enduring sobriety. A text extolling the merits of AA makes the following summary:

> The building blocks that Bill W. synthesized into his concept of a fellowship that could help alcoholics were derived from disparate sources: the psychology of Carl Jung, transcendental and existential mysticism, Christian fundamentalism and early notions from American medicine from American medicine about the role of allergy as a cause of alcoholism.[802]

The central core dogma of AA is to be found within the *Twelve Steps and Twelve Traditions,* and is summarized as follows. A person usually comes to an acceptance of his or her inability to control his or her life. A *Higher Power* of one's understanding is chosen to be your God; then a person consecrates and gives their life and *will* to that *Higher Power*. Next an inventory is made of one's faults and these are confessed to another human being; then the chosen *Higher Power* is asked by prayer and meditation to take away those faults; thus allowing that *Higher Power* (no matter what it is) to be ruler of my life.

Marilyn Ferguson, in *The Aquarian Conspiracy* called by the New York Times the New Age Bible, makes a potent point concerning 12 step programs and their influence in transformation of the mind into accepting the neo-pagan belief system. She makes this comment:

> Self-help and mutual-help networks—for example, Alcoholics Anonymous, Overeaters anonymous, and their counterparts, whose twelve rules include paying attention to one's conscious processes and to change, acknowledging that one can choose behavior, and cooperating with "higher forces" by looking inward.[803]

---

801   *Pass It On,* op. cit., p. 374.
802   Mel B., The New Wine, *The Spiritual Roots of the Twelve Step Miracle,* Hazelden Information & Educational Services. (1991) p. 7.
803   Ferguson, Marilyn, *The Aquarian Conspiracy, Personal and Social Transformation in Our Time, J.P. Tarcher, Inc., Distributed by St. Martin's Press, New York, (1980), p. 86.*

In this chapter the history and teachings of the AA program has been presented as their writings have presented it. Contrasting views are also presented. The reader will make up his own mind as to whether or not the 12 Step type programs would be your choice of therapy. I have heard expressed concerns that such programs tend to be looked to as the power for overcoming and take away our confidence in the power of Jesus Christ to cleanse us from our habits and sins. The Creator God is frequently allowed to be replaced, by our enthusiasm, for a *program,* even without our believing such is happening. I share with you statements made by ministers of the gospel relevant to this subject.

> These Christians believe only through attending this all-gods religion can they be free. But it is a strange sort of "free," because they have to attend these meetings *for life.* In fairness, they have been encouraged to participate by their own pastors, family members, and by other Christians who already attend. For seventy years Christians have been part of this movement.[804]

Well, I choose Jesus Christ as my Higher Power, I have given Him my will, I have confessed only those faults that are proper to confess to my fellow man, my prayers are to the God of heaven through the Name of Jesus and I have no part with Eastern style meditation. When I refer to the Higher Power I have in my mind the reference to Jesus Christ the Divine Son of God. So what is the concern?

I have heard the question: do I look to AA for healing rather than the power of Jesus Christ and His healing grace? Do I have more confidence in the 12 Step program than I do for my professed Lord and Savior to keep me in sobriety? Pastor John MacArthur addresses this question in the following comment.

> Others would formally affirm Christ's sovereignty and spiritual headship over the church, but they resist His rule in practice. To cite just one instance of how this is done, many churches have set various forms of human psychology, self-help therapy, and the idea of "recovery" in place of the Bible's teaching about sin and sanctification. Christ's headship over the church is thus subjugated to professional therapists. His design for sanctification, however, is by means of the Word of God (John 15:3; 17: 17). So wherever the *word* is being *replaced with twelve-step programs and other substitutes,* Christ's headship over the church is being denied in practice.[805] (Emphasis added)

---

804   http://www.worldviewweekend.com/worldview-times/article.php? articleid=3574

805   MacArthur, John, *The Truth War,* Nelson Books, division of Thomas Nelson, Inc. (2007), Nashville, TN, p. 159.

We have confidence in the saving power and gift of eternal life through our faith in the merits of the shed blood of Jesus Christ, yet when it comes to freeing ourselves from our sinful habits and addictions it is such a temptation to seek deliverance through the popular methods and programs designed by Satan to deceive us into giving him worship in place of Jesus Christ the Divine Son of God.

> Do not participate in the unfruitful works of darkness, but instead even expose them. (Eph. 5: 11-12)

> Beloved, do not believe every spirit, but test the spirits to see whether they are from God, because many false prophets have gone out into the world. By this you know the Spirit of God: every sprit that confesses Jesus Christ has come in the flesh is from god. And every spirit that does not confess Jesus is not from God; this is the spirit of the antichrist, of which you have heard that it is coming, and now it is already in the world. (1 John 4: 1-3)

The book *Steps to Christ* has twelve chapters which reveal the way to salvation through Jesus Christ our Creator and the thirteenth is a chapter of celebration of the freedom in Christ Jesus. Steps of themselves are not the concern; it is the teaching in the step that could deceive one into choosing unawares a power other than the Divine Son of God. Having great fellowship and continued sobriety is not proof positive that the power of overcoming is of heavenly origin.

These chapters on 12 steps, similar to the chapters on psychology, were submitted to a variety of individuals including professionals in mind—therapy, for their response to the content. The feedback was positive as well as negative. The negative responses tended to dismiss or discredit concerns about the strong spiritualistic history of the founders. It was expressed that no spiritualistic practices had been observed in those attending recovery programs. In fact a stronger fellowship seemed to come from attendance with a recovery group or program than occurs at their church. This may very well be, however, the concern is whether that is a fellowship that leads to eternal life by faith in the shed blood of Jesus Christ the Son of God. If one does choose to participate in AA or a 12 step program then beware of those steps that harbor risks exposed in this chapter. The next chapter contains a personal story of three recovered addicts who developed a recovery program that features Jesus Christ as the power by which we may overcome through the use of His Word. Enjoy.

CHAPTER 25

RECOVERY IN THE UNDERGROUND OASISTHE UNDERGROUND OASIS STORY:
AS TOLD BY DALE JOHNSTON

The Underground Oasis is a safe place in the desert of this world. It is a place all of us who are involved in this ministry longed to find when we were lost in our addictions. We all tried numerous programs to get and stay clean but each one failed. Yes, we could maintain for a few months, but no matter how diligent we were at changing our behavior, we found it never changed who we were. We were told that once an addict...always an addict.

I used to hate going to AA and NA meetings where I had to introduce myself by saying, "Hi, my name is Dale and I'm an addict." I knew that was not who I was! I also knew that it was not who God had created me to be. I was created to be much more than an addict. I am a child of God, a God who loves me. I hated the failure identity I was claiming but didn't know what to do about it.

Late one night in November of 2004, my brother, Steve "Mad Max" Fund, called me and asked if I could meet with one of his employees who was just coming down from a 2 week meth binge and was suicidal. Johnny was 42 years old and had been "slamming" (using meth by needle) for 20 years. He was at the end of his resources and saw no other way out than to end his life. I had recently met Leo Bristol, who had spent 15 years in prison due to his addiction to meth and who recently had been baptized. I knew him as a powerful *God Man* who could relate well to Johnny's current condition. We spent 2 hours with Johnny and I watched as Leo connected with him on a very personal level.

Leo had been the biggest and most feared meth dealer in our community for years. He would be sentenced to prison for 3-5 year stints but would return to the old life as soon as he was released. But during his last 5 year sentence, Leo had a very personal encounter with Jesus. When the cell door slammed behind him the last time, he fell to his knees and said:

> God, I'm tired of this life. I'm tired of doing drugs and going to prison. If you are real, you have to do something right now to save me.

Instantly there was a knock on his cell and a blue arm, one covered with prison tattoos, was reaching though the bars to shake his hand. This person said:

> Brother Leo, the Lord has directed me to ask you to come and join our Bible study.

From that day on, his life would never be the same. Upon his release, he and I had been praying in the same way, that God would direct us to a specific ministry that would make a difference in the lives of these hopeless people.

When we finished praying and intervening with Johnny that night and were walking towards the door, Johnny said something that would forever change our lives. He said simply:

> I have a lot of friends who need to hear what you all just shared with me.

It was like God just hit us with a clap of thunder. We all felt the same thing. This was our ministry. We were joined by a young man by the name of Kirk Shea, who desired to be part of this outreach and who also had been deeply involved in the drug life.

We wanted to develop a recovery program that boldly proclaimed God as our Higher Power; the God who is able to heal us from any and all destructive dependencies and habits. We are not talking about just being clean and sober. We are talking about being free. There is a big difference. We believe that God has the power to heal us, not just make us clean and sober. He is in the business of bringing victory to those who are hopeless and helpless.

"Biggin" is one of our members who runs our UO program in a neighboring town and is fond of saying:

> I was once a hopeless dope addict…now I am a dopeless hope addict!

How to develop a program that was relevant to the needs of this drug culture was a daunting task. None of us knew where to start, so we did the most logical thing. We prayed. We asked God to open the door to a program that would glorify Him. One week later while walking through a book store the title of a book caught my attention. It was a book by Neil Anderson and Mike Quarles entitled *Freedom From Addiction...Breaking the Bondage of Addiction and Finding Freedom in Christ.* It was exactly what we needed to help us see that God's way to freedom did not depend on me *working a program* but on understanding who I was in Christ and that He accepts me as I am, not as I should be. That through His power I am dead to sin and alive through Jesus. The Underground Oasis prayer says:

> Lord I give you permission to work in my life today. I know I am dead to sin and alive in you. And today I choose to believe what you say is true regardless of how I feel.

So many of our decisions as addicts have been based on emotions and feelings that are not reliable. So we teach that God's promises are true. Believe what He says about you...do not rely on how you *feel*.

We all understood that our program had to be a format that would be familiar to those who had been used to the traditional 12 step program. But we were determined to put God into the process—not just a nameless *Higher Power*. So we rewrote the 12 steps inserting God into the Program and attempting to take out the secular humanistic approach that stressed mothering more than behavior modification. Our goal was to clarify the perception of God's character; to teach about relationship with Jesus, not just using white knuckle effort to help overcome addictions. We also wanted to abolish the belief that you could choose anything from the light bulb to the doorknob as your Higher Power and expect that power to keep you clean and sober.

Our meetings are three nights per week, Monday, Wednesday and Friday evenings. After four plus years of this schedule we found ourselves extremely busy. The courts recognized us as a viable program and we receive court mandated people who are required to attend a recovery meeting. We do not care why they come or who sends them. They often hear the truth of the Gospel for the first time at the Underground Oasis. I began feeling that God wanted us to do more than just have three meetings a week. But I was unsure of exactly what could be done to be more involved in helping these people who were struggling with their addictions.

In February 2009 I buried a young man who had died of the effects of years of substance abuse. He was 41 years old. His name was Parley. He was so deeply entrenched in the drug world that it finally killed him. He would come to Oasis and pray for deliverance, but he could never follow through. I worked with him for 6 years, long before we started the Underground Oasis. He would show up at church on the Sabbath and would be a faithful member of the Oasis program for a while and then disappear back out into the drug world.

On his death bed I was blessed to be able to assure him of God's grace and love. He was able to accept God's forgiveness and died in assurance of the resurrection. His last words to me were:

My life has not amounted to anything Dale, please tell my friends to live life God's way and not to end up like me.

When I did Parley's memorial service, 55 people showed up from our town that I did not recognize. They turned out to be the *night people*. They were meth addicts who had no place to go except the bars and other crack houses. Even if they wanted to get clean, they had nowhere to go. I met some of the most beautiful young people whose hair was falling out, their teeth were rotting and they had open sores on their bodies. My heart went out to them and it was then that God began to speak to me about doing something to address this tragedy.

Mad Max owns the building in which we had been holding our meeting, and I approached him about my idea. Although the story is long and involved the outcome is that in the spring of 2010, a place opened up on Main Street here in LaGrange, Oregon. It is a 24 hour, 7 days a week *safe place* for those who are trying to maintain their sobriety. It is staffed by our Underground Oasis members and each night we have facilitators who are there to reach out to the young people who come.

If you want to get pulled out of your comfort zone, come and spend a few hours with us. Some of the most precious young people you will ever meet will be there. Their stories are heart rending. Their lives have been strewn with wreckage. Most do not have parents who care. Many have parents in prison. Many are homeless. There are many very young single mothers. In our town of 13,000 there are over 70 homeless teens.

Underground Oasis is working on a grant to build a teen safe house for these children. There is a plaque over the door of our meeting place now that reads "The Parley Room." Parley's life is going to make a difference now.

The story goes on. When God opens the door for ministry you can never stand still. God leads you into a deeper relationship and a deeper ministry than you ever expected.

AT THE UNDERGROUND OASIS, WE DO NOT CARE ABOUT WHERE YOU'VE BEEN; WE CARE ABOUT WHERE YOU'RE GOING.

By Dale Johnston Co-originator of Underground Oasis

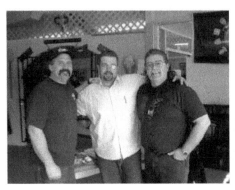
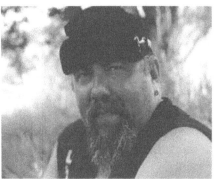

Kirk, Leo, Dale   *Mad Max*

Figures 42, 43.

A BIBLE BASED GUIDE TO FREEDOM

The process of learning occurs by increments. Mathematics is learned by starting with the most basic rules and then adding to those with additional principles. We often use the term *steps* to refer to this process. Alcoholic Anonymous proceeded in its recovery program by a step by step program. In II Peter I:4-8 Peter takes us step by step through an ascending set of character building characteristics known as Peter's ladder, which bears fruit for Christ. A little book by E.G. White entitled *Steps to Christ* illuminates the way to be in Christ through a step by step spiritual growth process. So, too, has Underground Oasis formed a series of steps based solely on scripture and Biblical principles to bring recovery and freedom to the addict.

Underground Oasis program is very similar to the steps outlined in *Steps to Christ;* the steps may not be in the exact same sequence but overall cover the same principles. Both are designed to lead a person to the recognition of Jesus Christ as the Son of God and that by *faith* in the merits of His shed blood at the cross we may be transformed into His likeness and receive salvation. At the very first lesson in Underground Oasis program a bold proclamation is made that the Creator God of the Universe, the King of Kings and Lord of Lords is the Power by which lives are changed and it will be the only Power recognized in the program. And that the word *God* when used in the recovery sessions always refers to Jesus Christ the Divine Son of God, the only name under heaven whereby we may be saved. Prayer to this God is always made at the beginning of every meeting. If the phrase *Higher Power* is ever used, unless stated differently, it also only refers to Jesus Christ.

Each participant is considered to be a child of the King, and upon introduction is to be recognized as such and not as an alcoholic or an addict of some habit—a failure in humanity. Yes, there is the all true fact of the problem burdening the person seeking recovery; one must face up to it and be honest about it. However, rehearsing each time one is introduced or introduces one's self, by stating that he or she is a failure only strengthens that conviction and interferes with accepting that a person is a loved and valued child of God. It keeps one in bondage where God promises that in Christ there is freedom from the sinful nature.

This course teaches that addictive problems are an *identity* problem; who are we? It presents four basic truths as to who we are:

1. I am accepted in Christ: I am bought with a price, I Corinth 6:20; Redeemed, Col. 1:14; Justified, Rom. 5:1; complete in Christ Col. 2:10
2. I am secure in Christ: Free from condemnation Rom. 8:1; I cannot be separated from Christ.
3. I am significant in Christ.
4. I am free in Christ.

The introduction the first night is:

> This is a Christ centered ministry. This program may not be for you, but then, again, it may be just the thing you need to help overcome your destructive dependencies and habits. If you have tried everything else and it has not worked, why not give God a chance.

It is made clear that the leader conducting the class is not attempting to bring a *religion* to those in attendance, or to suggest that *religion* can save them from their addictions, but that a *friendship with God can*. The leader, holding a Bible, shares that those who have been attending, love what is in that book as it has brought them freedom from their addictions. It is boldly proclaimed that the program is *Bible* based.

Does this boldness of a Bible based approach cause those seeking help to reject and flee from the meetings? That has not been the experience of Underground Oasis. They have programs in six states and have been operating for several years and I am told that people bolting from a meeting because it is Bible-based has been rare.

Underground Oasis takes the first step by helping the attendees understand that God loves us just as we are, Christ died for me even while I rejected Him. A person under addiction is brought to recognize and admit that *he is powerless* to pull him or herself up out of this human failure. There is no power within self that can do it. One is led to understand that my problem is the end result of sin and *living apart* from the Creator God of the Universe. It is a result of not knowing one's true identity, that you are a child of the King of Kings and Lord of Lords. This King loves us even in our state of bondage and slavery and He is willing and anxious to break that bondage and give us freedom.

The Biblical book of Romans chapter 7 describes the condition of man, often though he is a proclaimed believer in God, he is also in the slavery and bondage of sin, addiction, dependency, frustration, failure, condemnation, etc., it is referred to as *carnal*, and being *in the flesh*. Man in his mind wants to do what is right but his *self*, *carnal*, being *in the flesh* keeps him from doing it and he does what he does not want to do. Then we have the story of victory over this condition through the *Spirit*, of being *in Christ Jesus* in Romans chapter 8. For a person to be *in* Christ Jesus means that he or she has accepted Christ as his or her Savior. The person trusts Him implicitly and has decided to make Christ's way of life his or her own way. The result is a close personal union with Christ.

The name *Underground Oasis* was chosen for this recovery program because of its special meaning. The following definition is given by the Underground Oasis organization.

The Oxford Universal dictionary defines the word "oasis" as a "fertile spot in the desert."

> Throughout history, weary travelers would find refuge at an *oasis*; a refuge from the extreme heat as their caravans crossed the vast wasteland. There they could regain their strength and rest their animals before continuing on through lonely seas of sand. ...The *Underground Oasis* is a safe refuge for today's weary travelers, who are struggling through our own wasteland of addiction. A place where we can find rest, a rest that can only be found through Jesus Christ. He is our fertile spot in the desert of this world. From His Word we can drink freely giving us the strength and regeneration that is needed to break the chains that bind us; a place where we can again become clean, productive members of society. Fertile ground for the fruits of the Lord and sharing with others what Jesus Christ can do for us.

> Here at the *Underground Oasis*, we don't care about where you've been. We care about where you're going. OASIS by Kirk Shea.

Anonymity in Underground Oasis is maintained just as it is in Alcoholics Anonymous, however, when being introduced or introducing oneself it is counterproductive to refer to being a failure, an alcoholic, a doper, a rage-aholic etc., as repeating such creates a deeper impression on the mind that one is what one calls himself. The introduction to be used is *I am a child of the King*, struggling with the uncontrollable use of alcohol" or whatever the addiction is. Behavior is consistent with belief. Truth as it is in Christ is the key to receiving power that breaks from slavery and bondage.

The following quotation is the nightly welcome presented to the attendees of a meeting of Underground Oasis.

> Hello, my name is_____. I'd like to welcome everyone to the Underground Oasis. We dedicate this time and program to God and our loving savior Jesus Christ. Our prayer is that everyone here will receive a blessing as well as the hope and tools needed to overcome any and all destructive habits and dependencies. Thank you for coming.

Belief in and accepting a power *above self* is mandatory to overcoming. The apostle Paul shares with us the way out of being *in the flesh.*

> Therefore, there is no condemnation to those who are hid in Christ by faith. For the Holy Spirit has given me a new life in Christ and has freed me from the controlling power of my sinful nature which always stands ready to put me back on the road to death. No matter how holy and good the law of God is, it is powerless to save me from my sinful self. But what God's law could not do, His Son did. God sent Him to earth to take on human nature, to condemn sin and to overthrow its power. He did this so that by His obedience the righteous requirements of the law could be transferred to us who no longer follow our sinful human natures, but shape our lives according to the Spirit. Romans 8:1-4 (Clear Word)

As a result of accepting the power of Jesus Christ to bring us from death to life we then undergo a *transformation.* We still have those sinful impulses but we now have a *Power from above* that is able to give us a new heart so as to overcome the sinful drives and replace them with healthful patterns in life. This is *a process* for most people and involves a daily walk in Christ, a daily surrender of self, as we meet again and again our impulses. As we resist through the power of God we replace the old impulses and drives with new ones that are in harmony with the righteousness of God. By regular attendance to the meetings that continue to present Bible truths, support is gained by allowing the Holy Spirit to bring about a transformation of our hearts and life.

There are only *two powers* in the Universe, the Power of God, and that power which God has allowed Satan to possess and manipulate. When we give our *will, volition,* or *power to choose* to a power, it is either to Jesus Christ the Divine Son of God or to Satan; there are no other powers. If we have chosen some power outside of Jesus Christ as our *Higher Power*, or *God of my understanding*, we have chosen by default Satan.

Through a process of repentance and confession a person brings to light his hidden faults. These faults that have involved others are made right; there are other wrongs that only God is to receive confession about. It is offensive to God to have man divulge every aspect of his life to another human. We are to be our own conscience, not to allow others to decide for us what is right or wrong. Wrong use of confession has given Satan great influence over mankind for millennia.

To summarize the experience of participating in the program conducted by Underground Oasis I will place below, words presented to the participants concerning prayer as a part of delivery and overcoming.

> The commitment has been made. The line has been crossed. We have chosen to get right and not be left behind. We've realized through our past that we are unable to care for our self with the knowledge and will power we have, let alone be guided by it. We've decided to turn our will and life over to the care of God as He reveals Himself to us.
>
> Now our daily task is to ask God for guidance and power to achieve the peace, serenity and love we have always searched for but were never able to attain. We receive this through personally inviting our Lord and Savior to take control of our life. We ask to be molded, forgiven and accepted, by studying God's Word. Believing it, achieving to it and relying on it, reveals God's will for our new life with Christ. We start to realize we are special and have a purpose. We can be sure that God desires a blessing for us. We start to act on this knowledge and pray for the power to carry it out. As our new life with Christ begins, we realize that many of our old thoughts and habits, including our compulsions and addictive behaviors, do not automatically vanish all at once. What has happened is that from God's viewpoint, we have been forgiven and now have a right to enter into His presence. We now have the right to ask Him for the power needed to begin the complete regeneration and transformation of every part of our lives... The power needed to change every area of life that falls short of Christ's glorious idea of how we can live for Him.

If the God we serve was capable of Creating the universe, earth, and man, if he is capable of re-creating man and raising him from the dead and giving him eternal life, is He not also able to give us deliverance—freedom from sin and bondage? We trust Him to redeem us, to translate us to heaven, but when it comes to seeking deliverance from the results of a sinful nature with its bondage and slavery we tend to look to man's programs, and not to the power of the Creator of the Universe.

> Then said Jesus to those Jews which believed on him, if ye continue in my word, (then) are ye my disciples indeed; and ye shall know the truth, and the truth shall make you free. (John 8: 31, 32)

CHAPTER 26

BABYLONIAN SPIRITUALISTIC MYSTERIES–
COMPATIBLE WITH THE ATONEMENT?

Atonement means "at-one-ment" with God. Salvation is the act of God in restoring man to be in harmony with his Creator. The 17th chapter of John records the great prayer of Jesus just before He started His night in the Garden of Gethsemane. He prayed:

> That they all (His disciples) may be one; as thou Father, art in me, and I in thee, that they Also may be one in us: that the world may believe that thou hast sent me. John 17:21

In heaven, a great battle for the loyalty of the angels occurred between God and Lucifer who desired to be in the place of the Son of God. That battle spread to this earth when man sinned.[806] Sin separated God from man, so that there could be no direct communication, no salvation while in the separated state. Only by the *atonement* of the Son of God could there be a restoration of communication, blessings, or salvation from God for man. Satan became the:

> *Prince* of this world. This great controversy of the ages continues today. God uses only truth, righteousness and love in defending Himself.[807]

He expects the same defense by His believers. From the very start, all of Lucifer's accusations against God were based in *falsehood*, *deceit*, and *self-glorification*. These same principles he has taught his followers to utilize. The name *tree of knowledge of good and evil* contains much of the secret of Satan's methods. He has been able to convince man that within himself (man) exists all the knowledge of the universe and all man has to do is to learn how to bring it out.

The first *supplement* to attaining a higher level of consciousness, health, and becoming wise like God was the fruit offered to Eve. Some supplements are still being sold with nearly the same degree of promise. Eve already

---

806   Rev. 12.
807   White, E.G.; *Patriarchs and Prophets,* Pacific Press Pub. Assn., Nampa, ID, (1958), chapter 1.

had all that the serpent was offering except godhood and she knew that was impossible, but on the *testimony of one, the serpent,* and without any evidence that it was so, she believed the lie, she bought into it.

The devil wishes to take the place of God in the minds of men. To do so, he must take their minds off knowing who their Creator is. He devised a story for the origin of man which portrayed man as being formed by the balancing of a great (imaginary) two-part opposing energy (chi, yin–yang) or force that was proclaimed to be throughout the universe. When the balance of the two parts was perfect, then the universe, earth, and man were formed. God the Creator, who has power and life within Himself, is left out of this story. And so Lucifer, in truth, takes the credit for creation. These are *Babylonian Mysteries,* that is, secrets of astrological concepts. If we choose to utilize any of the modalities for health and healing that are based on this false premise, after we have been exposed to the truth about these astrological teachings, we are actually accepting this theory as the truth.

Immortality was promised to Adam and Eve on the condition of obedience. If they sinned they would lose eternal life. Satan's lie that *you will not die* had to be explained to man because man did die. To cover this obvious untruth the doctrine of reincarnation was formed.

In the early history of the Adventist church, spiritualism entered the medical work through the dogma of pantheism. This was called by Ellen White the *alpha of apostasy.*

> Be not deceived; many will depart from the faith, giving heed to seducing spirits and doctrines of devils. We have now before us the alpha of this danger. The *omega* will be of a most startling nature.[808]

Should we consider the movement of present-day Eastern mysticism and sympathetic remedies as a part of the omega apostasy? God has allowed man to choose whom he will serve. This book has been written to help us see clearly that at times when we feel we are following God and using His methods, we may actually be deceived and be partaking of a counterfeit. The consequences are eternal. E.G. White, in the book, *Early Writings,* page 88, speaks of the delusion that Satan will bring to the world through the influence of *spiritualism.*

> I saw the rapidity with which this delusion was spreading. A train of cars was shown me, going with the speed of lightning. The angel bade me look carefully. I fixed my eyes upon the train. It seemed that the whole world was on board, that

---

808   White, E.G.; I *Selected Messages,* Review and Herald Publishing Assn., Hagerstown, MD, (1958), p. 197.4.

there could not be one left. Said the angel, "They are binding in bundles ready to burn." Then he showed me the conductor, who appeared like a stately, fair person, whom all the passengers looked up to and reverenced. I was perplexed and asked my attending angel who it was. He said, "It is Satan." He is the conductor in the form of an angel of light. He has taken the world captive. They are given over to strong delusions, to believe a lie, that they may be damned. This agent, the next highest in order to him, is the engineer, and other of his agents are employed in different offices as he may need them, and they are all going with lightning speed to perdition.

How can I determine that the method of *natural healing* that I am being offered is not of Satan's origin? After all, I seem to have improved with the method and others swear by it. The most frequent comment I hear is: "It helped me," or "My friend was helped by it," or "It works."

The criteria as to whether a method is of Satan or not, does not include whether or not an individual was benefited. People do get better and apparently receive healing at times. The issue is whose power brought healing? Another comment often heard is: Well, I just take the good out of it.

Any technique distinctly connected to the occult cannot be considered neutral.

Participating in these methods may be the first step to altering our concept of our origin, and the beginning of the changing of our world view. When a technique has its origin in pantheistic concepts and astrological beliefs, just accepting that it may do something desirable is actually unconsciously accepting this belief.

At times, a mixture of scientific medicine is combined with *holistic* methodology so as to stimulate the question, is it good or not? I would ask you to search out the answers to the following questions and make a determination. The report, *The New Age Movement and Seventh-day Adventists* by the Biblical Research Committee of the General Conference, July 1987, lists the following criteria which we may use to determine whether a treatment method is valid. These questions were first printed in *Mystical Medicine* by Warren Peters M.D.

1. What and where are its roots?
2. What (other healing modalities) does it keep company with in clinical use and in the books and literature describing it?
3. Does the method claim to activate the *innate powers within myself,* or does it direct me to recognize the *power of the Creator God* in healing?
4. Is its method of action in harmony with the known laws of physics and science?
5. Does it claim to balance, polarize, manipulate, unblock, and correct energies, electromagnetic frequencies, or vibrations?

6. Is it a technique that involves altering my consciousness or rational thought process, so as to impede control of my mind and whose power controls me?

The most powerful deterrent to becoming bewitched by Satan's deceptions in health and healing is to know God's methods so well that it becomes easy to detect the counterfeit. We are told that:

> ...disease is an effort of nature to free the system from the effects of violating the laws of health.[809]

God's remedies involve the use of pure air, sunlight, temperate use of good substances, avoiding the injurious, rest, exercise, proper diet, the use of water inside and outside the body, and trust in Divine power.[810] Trust involves being obedient to the Creator's physical and spiritual laws.

The rapid spread of Neo-paganism across the world, and especially here in America, has been, to a great extent, related to the dogma and modalities involved in health and healing practices of the so-called *alternative methods*. The devil has used these methods as the *right arm of his message*. Satan presents his health and healing program so that it appears *natural* and that it is the same method God has given us. The difference can be ascertained by looking for the explanation of the source of the power for healing. If it is from some *energy* within us, and if we are doing some act to balance that power from within, then it is of the counterfeit.

We, too, believe that the health message is the right arm of the gospel. There is a difference however. The difference is that we trust in a living God as our Creator, and that His power sustains and restores us to health when we choose to place ourselves in harmony with His physical and spiritual laws, and ask Him to bless our efforts.

The history of medicine should help give us the answers we need in making a correct choice in methods of health and healing. Wherever the system of medicine has been built upon the *energy* concept, the health of that country remained primitive. Over millennia those nations using such methods saw no improvement in health and healing. As soon as the scientific method, based upon the laws of physics and chemistry—God's physical laws, are instituted in the approach to health and healing, quick and great improvements occur. Keep in mind the change China experienced when they made changes directed by scientific understanding of disease and its cause. The traditional Chinese

809 White, E.G.; *The Ministry of Healing,* Pacib c Press Pub. Assn., Nampa, ID, (1905), p. 127.
810 *Ibid.,* p. 127

medicine had been available and used in medical treatment for the people for more than 3500 years. With just a little use of scientific methods (cleanliness of water, body, and environment) the life span doubled in 50 years' time.

We have a written history of medical systems of several past and present civilizations and the story is the same in all of them. When an approach to health and healing based on God's physical laws and methods is utilized we see profound improvements. We have evidence of the advantage of following the messages God gave to the SDA church through Ellen White. Review chapter 3 *The Story of Our Health Message.*

If we remember that systems like that of Ayurveda were designed by men on the basis of intuition, contact with spirit guides, and astrological concepts of origins, it should be easier to make the right choice in the selection of our health and healing methods.

> Already there are coming in among our people spiritualistic teachings that will undermine the faith of those who give heed to them. The theory that God is an *essence* pervading all nature is one of Satan's most subtle devices. It misrepresents God, and is a dishonor to His greatness and majesty.[811]

Christ's death on the cross met the conditions of the *atonement.* His work on earth was accomplished, and He won the kingdom. Following Christ's resurrection, He ascended to the heavenly courts to hear from God the Father that His atonement for men's sins was sufficient.

> ...The Father ratified the covenant made with Christ, that He would receive repentant and obedient men, and would love them even as He loves His son....[812]

Christ returned to earth for 40 days, after which he returned to heaven and there entered the heavenly sanctuary to be our High Priest, and

> ...finishing of the atonement, and preparing of the people to abide the day of His coming.[813]

The application of the atonement made on the cross for each of us is now taking place in heaven. If we believe on the Son of God and have *no other gods before us,* He will, at the time of our judgment, present His life to the Father in

---

811   White, E.G.; *Evangelism,* Pacific Press Pub. Assn., Napa, ID, (1946), p. 601.

812   White, E.G.; *The Desire of Ages,* Pacific Press Pub. Assn., Nampa, ID, (1898), p. 790.

813   White, EG.; *Christian Experience and Teaching,* CD of E.G. White Writings, (1922), p. 56.

place of our sinful lives. Let us guard carefully so that we not allow *other gods before us* by becoming entangled in Satan's deceptions in health and healing.

> The spiritualistic theories concerning God make His grace of no effect. If God is an essence pervading all nature, then He dwells in all men; and in order to attain holiness, man has only to develop the power within him.[814]

The answer to the original question, *are the Babylonian Mysteries of health and healing compatible with the atonement?* The answer is stated below:

> *These theories, followed to their logical conclusion, sweep away the whole Christian economy. They do away with the necessity for the atonement and make man his own savior. These theories regarding God make his word of no effect.*[815]

That should answer the question of compatibility.

---

814 White, *The Ministry of Healing* op. cit., p. 428.3.

815 *Ibid.*, p. 428.

APPENDIX A
ELLEN G. WHITE

Throughout this book the reader will frequently see in the footnotes at the bottom of the page the name *E.G. White*. Ellen Gould White (1827-1915) was an author of many books on spiritual as well as medical subjects. She began writing on health subjects from the mid 1800's and continued until her death in 1915. Her writings on health were not in harmony with medical science during her lifetime; in fact they were at odds with the established concepts of scientific medical care, diet, and nutrition. However, they have stood the test of time and in the past 40 plus years have been shown scientifically to be the best health guides ever given. Almost everything she wrote in the field of health and healing has been scientifically verified. No statement she made in regards to health and healing has been shown to be untrue—all this from a lady with only three years of schooling.

Those people who have even partially followed her advice and guidelines for health have been blessed. Science has shown that those who accept and follow those guidelines from midlife onward will experience less disease of all types as well as enjoy an extended life of 11-12 years longer than their contemporaries.

Not only did this woman have wisdom in proper lifestyle, health, and healing, but she also wrote on the subject of this book—spiritualism in health care. During her life time the names we now see in reference to therapeutic practices that are called alternative and or complementary methods for healing were not known. However, the principles by which these practices (energy balancing methods) are explained by their adherents, she understood with a depth that is surprising. If a person were to search out all of her writings on spiritualistic modalities of healing, all a person needs to know on this subject would be found. For this reason I have included many quotations she made in reference to spurious healing methods and the explanations she gave revealing their spiritistic nature.

Ellen White's writings on health are in harmony with the science of physics, chemistry and physiology. She gave strong directions to those teaching health principles to be sound in the science of the physical laws of the universe, which, in turn, are in harmony with the physical laws of God, as He is their Author. She warned of counterfeit healing methods that have explanation of their action rising from a false story of creation. Truly, God put wisdom into this individual's understanding of which we would be wise to take notice.

APPENDIX B
BIBLE TEXTS RELATING TO SPIRITUALISM

Astrologers: Daniel 2:10, Isaiah 47:13, Daniel 1:20, Daniel 2:2, Daniel 2:27, Daniel 4:7, Daniel 5:11, Daniel 5:15

Baalzebub: II Kings 1:2, 3, 6, 16

Bewitched: Acts 8:9, 11, Galatians 3:1

Charmer: Deuteronomy 18:11, Psalms 58:5, Isaiah 19:3

Divine: Genesis 44:15, I Samuel 28:8, Proverbs 16:10, Ezekiel 13:9, 23, Micah 3:6, 11

Divination: Numbers 22:7, Numbers 23:23, Deuteronomy 18:10, II Kings 17:17, Jeremiah 14:14, Ezekiel 8, 9, Ezekiel 12:24, Ezekiel 13:6, 7, Ezekiel 21: 21-23, Acts 16:16

Diviners: Deuteronomy 18:14, 1 Samuel 6:2, Isaiah 44:25, Jeremiah 27:9, Jeremiah 29:8, Micah 3:7, Zechariah 10:2

Familiar spirits: Leviticus 19:31, Leviticus 20:6, Deuteronomy 18:11, I Samuel 28:3, I Samuel 28:9, II Kings 23:24, Isaiah 8:19, Isaiah 19:3, II Chronicles 33:6

Magicians: Genesis 41:8, 24, Exodus 7:11, 22, Exodus 8:7, 18, 19, Exodus 9:11, Daniel 1:20, Daniel 2:2, 27, Daniel 4:7, 9, Daniel 5:11

Miracles: Revelation 13:14, Revelation 16:14, Revelation 19:20

Necromancer: Deuteronomy 18:11

Prognosticators: Isaiah 47:13

Serpent medium: Genesis 3:1-5

Soothsayers: Joshua 13:22, Isaiah 2:6, Daniel 4:7, Daniel 5:7, 11 Micah 5:12

Sorcerers: Acts 13:6, 8 Exodus 7:11 Jeremiah 27:9 Daniel 2:2 Malachi 3:5, Revelation 21:8, Revelation 22:15

Sorceries: Isaiah 47:9, Isaiah 47:12, Acts 8:9, Acts 8:11, Revelation 9:2,

Stargazers: Isaiah 47:13

Times: Leviticus 19:26, Deuteronomy 18:10, Deuteronomy 18:14, II Kings 21:6, II Chronicles 33:6

Witch: Exodus 22:18, Deuteronomy 18:10

Witchcraft: II Kings 9:22, Micah 5:12, Nahum 3:4, I Samuel 15:23, II Chronicles 33:6, Galatians 5:20

Wizards: Deuteronomy 18:11, Leviticus 19:31, Leviticus 20:6, I Samuel 28:3, 9, II Kings 21:6, II Kings 23:24, II Chronicles 33:6, Isaiah 8:19, Isaiah 19:3

Other texts: Acts 19:19, I Timothy 4:1, Ephesians 6:12, Colossians 2:8, II Thessalonians. 2:9, 10 I John 4:1, I Revelation 18:23, I Corinthians 10: 20-21; Deuteronomy 32: 16-17; Revelation 16: 1314

APPENDIX C

A CRITIQUE OF: "VIBRATIONAL MEDICINE, THE HAND BOOK OF SUBTLE-ENERGY THERAPIES, THIRD EDITION" BY RICHARD GERBER M.D.

The motto of Loma Linda School of Medicine, *To Make Man Whole*, refers to man as a physical/mental/spiritual being. In the past thirty or more years the term, h*olistic medicine,* has become a common expression. It too refers to a body/mind/spirit relationship. However, there is a difference between the two expressions. We need to look at the teachings, as to the origin of man, to understand this difference.

The Biblical story of man's creation tells us of a living Being, God, the Source of life, who formed man from dust of the earth and breathed into him the breath of life.

> By the word of the Lord the heavens were made and all the host of them by the breath of His mouth. (Psalm 33:6 NKJV).

To make man *whole* is to direct man to live in harmony with God's physical laws, as well as His spiritual laws.

The word h*olistic* refers to being in harmony with the world of nature, including the god of pantheism. In chapter 4 of *Exposing Spiritualistic Practices in Healing,* the pagan's view of creation is presented in brief. That theory tells us in very simplistic terms, that the creation of man and the universe came about through evolution of a *god-force*. This allowed every entity of the universe to be a part of each other, as each is a part of this *god-force*, (also known as vital force, chi, prana, universal energy, and a hundred other terms). The theory contends that all matter is made up of *primordial* energy and/or light and that *material substance* is *frozen light*.[816] This *vital energy* is said to be of contrasting divisions, positive/negative, masculine/feminine, yang/ yin, and is also considered to possess *vibrational* (*frequency*) *energy*

---

816   Gerber, Richard, M.D., *Vibrational Medicine, The #1 Handbook of Subtle-Energy Therapies,* Bear & Company, Rochester, Vermont, 2001, p. 59.

characteristics. Each substance, animate and inanimate, is supposed to emit an electromagnetic vibrational frequency peculiar to it alone.[817]

Holistic medicine refers to the teaching of and/or use of various treatment methods for illnesses that form healing methods based on this theory. This concept has its origin and propagation from Eastern religions and Western occultism's theosophy, and has not been verified by present day science.

The basis of vibrational energetics as a method of diagnosing and treating disease along with use of acupuncture, qi gong exercises, pulse diagnosis, etc., is a result of an attempt to connect and blend pantheistic healing methods with modern science.

Richard Gerber, M.D. , is recognized as a prominent advocate of this movement. In 2001 he published his third edition of *Vibrational Medicine, The #1 Handbook of Subtle-Energy Therapies.* The prior editions had sold more than 125,000 copies. The purpose of his book is to foster the belief that the ancient paganistic systems of healing are nothing more than, *when understood,* extensions of present day scientific methods. Dr. Gerber and other authors of similar texts readily acknowledge that their hypotheses and theories are not in harmony with the present understanding of the sciences of medicine, physics, and chemistry. The goal of Dr. Gerber is to close this gap in understanding.

Dr. Gerber is to be lauded for aspiring to more natural methods in health and healing that will depend less on pharmaceuticals and more on our own systems to correct disorders. He is highly trained in internal medicine, and states that he still finds it necessary to use the knowledge and methods for treatment from his specialty training. However, his book leads in a direction that a Christian must ponder and question. As I read the preface to this 600 page book I am impressed that Dr. Gerber has a deep belief in Eastern mysticism, and his writings purpose to convince the reader that it is truth.

During his medical school days Dr. Gerber enrolled in a class called *A Course in Miracles,* which changed his spiritual viewpoint. He tells us that as he went further in the course he began to awaken psychic abilities within himself. The comment is made that he understood that:

> "A Course in Miracles" had been *dictated* via a psychic or by telepathic means to a psychologist from a "high spiritual source."[818]

As a result of his study of *The Course in Miracles,* and from other reading, two concepts developed in his mind. First, humans are more than just physical beings--they are also spiritual beings with consciousness on higher planes than

---

817   *Ibid.,* p. 171.
818   *Ibid.,* p. 29.

recognized in this life and that this higher mental state continues after death. Secondly:

> There are those 'in Spirit' who seek to communicate with individuals still in physical incarnation.[819]

These communications are said to be twofold in nature: 1) To make us aware of *life after death;* and 2) to relay information that pertains to:

> ...healing, soul growth, and personal spiritual evolution.[820]

Curiosity had been awakened in him by this new knowledge and he sought a deeper understanding of "technical channeled information" from spirit channeled sources. Dr. Gerber shares with us the fact that he and his wife are clairvoyant. He states:

> I would like to point out to the readers of *Vibrational Medicine* that I believe this book is the result of cooperation between healers and researchers on the physical plane and beings who exist on the higher spiritual planes. This cooperation has made possible the transmission of a wealth of information that is needed on the planet at this time. Many of the sections of this book are actually 'messages from spirit' channeled through various sources.[821]

Vibrational medicine does not arise from research in science that reveals the human system to have focalized areas of electromagnetic energy (chakras, see chapter 7) that in turn produces an aura outside of the body. Nor does research find specialized channels (acupuncture meridian system) throughout the body that carries a non-measurable, non-demonstrable energy (chi, qi) that can be manipulated by pressure or needling particular points on the body. There has been no reporting of energy faster than light. Yet these beliefs, which are a result of messages from *spirits* by channeled sources and from ancient pagan religious dogma, form the basic principles of vibrational medicine. Much of this theory has already been presented in this book. My purpose for this appendix is to show that *by accepting even fragments* of this teaching as true, it can initiate change in our world view (concepts of our origin and destiny), and to which power we place our allegiance. Dr. Gerber in chapter 3 of his book uses the title, *The Birth of Vibrational Medicine.* Herein is presented the prediction that conventional medical/surgical medicine will experience a

---

819 *Ibid.*, p. 31.
820 *Ibid.*
821 *Ibid.*, p. 37.

revolution and electromagnetic healing will take its place. This will occur as physicians understand,

> ...that the human organism is a series of interacting multidimensional energy fields.[822]

A presentation and illustration of the proclaimed seven different frequency levels of universal energy is given in chapter 5 of this book. Level 1, refers to all matter (substance) in the universe; 2nd level, etheric and astral bodies; 3rd level, mental and causal bodies; and progresses upward to level seven. This level has several names such as Supreme Self, Jewel, etc. (the level of *godhood*). These different frequency levels are said to make connection with the different levels of chakras, the higher frequency level of energy which are said to connect with the respective higher chakra.

Dr. Gerber explains this relationship as follows: The chakras act as *transformers* converting energy (hypothesized to be) traveling at a far greater speed than light to a slower speed; the top chakra receives, then converts the highest energy frequency, level seven, to the next lower chakra and again the frequency is reduced by that chakra.[823] This reduction of frequency may continue downward strengthening each chakra until the energy frequency is converted to the speed of light, which is level 1 (the materialized physical body). These chakras (*transformers*) are said to also act in the opposite direction, transforming energy frequency upward via the chakras, this is accomplished through meditation. By many life times of meditation the seventh frequency level may be perfected, resulting in "god-hood."

Remember, the lowest level of energy is that of which all material substance is said to consist of. The next level, ethereal, is believed to be an electromagnetic template of the physical body and guides growth and restoration. Changes or influences on the etheric body or energy supposedly precedes and effects changes either positively or negatively in the physical body.[824] At these etheric and higher levels of frequencies, the belief is that outside electromagnetic fields influence a person's *electromagnetic bodies*. Such influences are said to restore balance to the etheric and other bodies, and in turn, health to the physical body. Dr. Gerber quotes a psychic source:

---

822   *Ibid.,* p. 91.
823   *Ibid.,* p. 171
824   Karagulla, S., Energy Fields and Medical Diagnosis, in *The Human Aura,* ed. N. Regush (New York:Berkeley Publishing, 1974); Reported in Richard Gerber M.D., *Vibrational Medicine 3rd Ed,* Bear and Company, Rochester, Vermont, (2001), p. 126.

There is a direct link between the nervous, circulatory, and meridian systems (acupuncture pathways) partly because ages ago, the meridians were originally used to create these two parts of the physical body. Consequently, anything that influences one of these systems has a direct impact on the other two areas. The meridians use the passageway between the nervous and circulatory systems to feed the life force into the body, almost extending directly to the molecular level. *The meridians are the interface or doorway between the physical and ethereal properties of the body.*[825] (Italics added by Dr. Gerber)

From the book *Vibrational Medicine*, I read:

All matter, both physical and subtle [etheric, astral bodies, etc.] has frequency. Matter of different frequencies can coexist in the same space, just as energies of different frequencies (i.e., radio and TV) can exist nondestructively in the same space.[826]

From this concept various alternative healing methods claim to affect health by their vibrational properties, such as flower essences, aromatherapy, gem elixirs, color therapy, sound therapy, homeopathy, and subtle energies from plant food. The concept is that subtle vibrational frequencies (faster than light energy) of plants, gems, colors etc., can be transferred to the chakras. Through homeopathy, vibrations are claimed to be transferred via the water used in dilution in preparing the homeopathic remedy, even if there are no molecules of the original substance left in the solution due to dilution.[827] Dr. Gerber illustrates in a diagram: the relationship of flower essences, which are supposed to have a high frequency of energy and influence the higher chakras and, in turn, consciousness; gem elixirs (solutions of ground up gemstones) tend to influence the middle and lower level chakras; while homeopathy is said to affect primarily the acupuncture meridian system which is said to connect the higher energy levels to the physical body.[828]

Vibrational Medicine, Chapter VIII, "The Phenomenon of Psychic Healing," presents the history of the origin of Therapeutic Touch. It is believed to exist on the hypothesis that subtle energy is sensed by and/or passed through hands to another person even without actual physical contact. The explanation for psychic healing is that the mind of the therapist can pass

825 Gurudas, *Flower Essences and Vibrational Healing,* channeled by Kevin Ryerson (Albuquerque, NM: Brotherhood of Life, Inc., 1983), p. 29; Reported in, Richard Gerber M.D., *Vibrational Medicine 3rd Ed.,* (2001), p. 126.
826 Gerber, op. cit., p. 171.
827 *Ibid.*, pp. 88–89.
828 *Ibid.*, p. 272.

healing vibrational frequencies of subtle energy from him/herself to another person over distance.[829]

Another common practice in alternative medicine is the use of machines or instruments that are purported to measure and/or correct subtle energy frequencies within the body. There are two different instruments that are used to measure the energy of acupuncture meridians and their points: one is called, *AMI machine*, which is supposed to reveal an imbalance (yin/yang) in the acupuncture meridian system; and another machine that is referred to as the VOL machine (Electroacupuncture According to Voll), and measures subtle energy of individual meridian channels and/or acupuncture points. The operators of this machine claim it is able to reveal the energy status of specific organs, even to the ability of an organ, such as the pancreas, to form its specific digestive enzymes, lipase, protease, etc.[830] The VOL machine goes beyond diagnosing energy imbalance, it is said to be capable of finding the cause of imbalance as well as possible cures.[831]

An additional style of instrument frequently used in alternative medicine since the early 1900's is referred to as a "radionic black box." Such a machine is said to accurately diagnosis various subtle energy level dysfunctions. The successful use of these instruments depends upon the "psychic ability," known as "Radiaesthesia," of the radionic practitioner. A substance referred to as "a witness" from the patient, such as hair, a spot of blood on paper, a picture of the patient, some object handled by the person, etc., will be placed in the instrument for analysis of the body's energy-balance. Also, a substance, *a witness*, can be sent long distances for analysis without loss of accuracy. If a spot of blood were to be sent for examination, that blood spot could continue to reflect the current energy status of that person without need for fresh samples. The substance sent for inspection provides a two-way link with the practitioner and patient so that not only the subtle (faster than light) energy status of the patient is revealed over distance, but the practitioner is able to return healing energies with the proper frequency to bring healing.[832]

There are other instruments that may be encountered that operate on the vibrational hypothesis such as the Homo Vibra Ray and Rife Beam Ray machines. Both of these are promoted as capable of making a diagnosis by analysis of frequencies and provide treatment by correcting the same. It is interesting that Dr. Gerber considers these various instruments as *"electronic pendulums."*

---

829   *Ibid.*, p. 287.
830   *Ibid.*, p. 207.
831   *Ibid.*, pp. 206–208.
832   *Ibid.*, p. 235.

Dr. Gerber looks to a Dr. William Tiller, a retired former professor at Stanford University and former chairman of the Department of Materials Science at Stanford:

> ...as perhaps the leading theorist in the subtle energetic field.[833]

He credits him for the hypothesis of energy frequency faster than light, (10^{10-20} times the speed of light for astral travel). Dr. Tiller has coined a new word to describe subtle energy, *magnetoelectric energy*, which is just another synonym for universal energy.

Astral travel, out of body experiences, near death experience, life after death, reincarnation, higher consciousness, Supreme Self, "god-hood", are all explained on the hypothesis of *universal energy* and its supposed various frequency levels. The ultimate deception of what this mode of thought leads to is best illustrated by the following quote from Dr. Gerber.

> People through the centuries have accepted Jesus as the one true son of God. This is, in fact, a *misinterpretation*. What Jesus came to teach us is that we are all the children of God. ...we who are the evolving souls or fragments of God's consciousness are *divine* brainchildren.[834]

That's it, the end of the journey, from partaking of the fruit from the tree to *god-hood*.

> For God doth know that in the day ye eat thereof, then your eyes shall be opened, and ye shall be as gods, knowing good and evil. (Genesis 3:5).

> For we wrestle not against flesh and blood, but against principalities, against powers, against the rulers of the darkness of this world, against spiritual wickedness in high places. (Ephesians 6:12).

Is it possible that we could be accepting these spiritualistic teachings by participating in the healing modalities built upon this premise? They were not included in the healing methods presented to this body of Seventh-day Adventist believers in 1863. The system of universal energy was already millennia old at that time but the only mention of this system was to *beware of it*. We cannot serve two masters, we must make a choice. We have been blessed with heaven sent directions for health and healing. Time and science have verified that it is the correct way, so why look to "Baalzebub, god of

---

833   *bid.*, pp. 151, 155–171
834   *Ibid.*, pp. 493–494.

Ekron" to seek guidance? When Joshua took the children of Israel into Canaan he challenged them with the following words:

> And if it seems evil unto you to serve the LORD, choose you this day whom ye will serve; whether the gods which your fathers served that were on the other side of the flood, or the gods of the Amorites, in whose land ye dwell: but as for me and my house, we will serve the LORD. (Joshua 29:15)

APPENDIX D
DIVINING FOR WATER

Christopher Bird, in his book, *The Divining Hand*, tells of a miner and diviner of metals who would dowse with his arm outstretched and fist clenched. His arm would shake when near a vein of metal, and his whole body shook when he was directly over it. The miner was asked why he does not shake and vibrate when he is working in the mine and next to the vein all the time. He answered:

> If I do not 'orient' my thoughts specifically to finding a vein of ore, I get no reaction when I cross over a vein or work near one.[835]

A very common practice is to *witch* for water before a well is drilled or dug. Witching is most often done by using a forked tree branch. Many well drillers will not drill until someone has witched for water. There is a very strong belief in this practice, even within the Christian church. To suggest to people that the power in this act is of the occult, and not of science, is to ignite an argument. Those who have accepted dowsing as being scientific do not easily change their minds. It is believed that there is some physical force connecting the tree branch, the person doing the witching, and the water in the ground. The explanation as to why some people can do it and others cannot, is proclaimed to be due to differences in the electrical activity in our bodies.

These explanations are wishful thinking. The science of physics has not been able to demonstrate any of these claims. The more one studies the variety of ways of witching for water, and divining for other objects or information, the easier it is to be persuaded that there is no physical explanation for divining. For instance, some utility crews will use two copper wires bent at a right angle and held in each hand. One part of the wire held in the hand will be at 90 degrees to the ground, the other part bent at a 90 degree angle so as to be horizontal to the ground. When a water or gas pipe is located underground, the horizontal wires will swing and cross, not dip down as is done with the tree branch.

Witching may be done with a forked stick, a strait rod, wires bent at a 90 degree angle, a plain stick held in the palms of outstretched arms, a coin

---

835   Bird, Christopher, *The Divining Hand,* New Age Press, Black Mountain, NC, (1079), p. 110.

resting in the palm of the hand, outstretched hands alone, or just the mind with no tools of the trade. The stick may point up or down, or it may vibrate or oscillate. The wires may turn inward or they may turn outward; they may also turn opposite each other as they are held in the hand. A wire may oscillate up and down, sideways, or in other modes of gyrations. The hand may shake; a coin in the palm may turn over. The stick may turn round and round in the palm of an outstretched hand, or be thrown clear out of the diviner's hands. When divining with no instrument, the taste of water may be the sign that water, or whatever is being dowsed, is beneath the dowser. The diviner chooses what method he wants to use, and before he divines he decides the reaction that is to occur with his instrument.

Witching may be done from a map thousands of miles from the area of interest. It may be done for any substance, fluid, solid, mineral, or water. It can be done for any object on earth. It may even be done for an underground tunnel. Bird, in his book, *The Divining Hand,* tells of the use of the divining rod by Marines in Vietnam to find tunnels. Divining by map was used to locate prisoners of war, and the location of Viet Cong prisons. Any question under the sun could be asked, and would receive an answer as long as it involved a *yes* or *no* response. A gentleman once came to my office for treatment of a very swollen and painful shoulder. After injection with medication it promptly healed. He later returned and told me I had ruined his "bobbing arm." I asked what a bobbing arm was. He stated that when the arm was very tender he was able to more accurately sense the pull on the wire he would use in witching for water. Later he came to my home to demonstrate to me his technique for witching.

He took a bucket and turned it upside down using it for a stool. Sitting on the bucket he took a strong, stiff wire about a meter long, and bent a coil on the end to hold a light bulb. A bulb was placed in the coiled wire, and the wire was held on his knee, pointing out in front of his knee about 25 inches, with the light bulb on the end. He held a pencil in the other hand and placed a tablet on the free knee. The wire began to bend up and down causing the light bulb to rise and fall 8–10 inches. He would count the number of times it would flex until it stopped. When it stopped the wire began to bend back and forth in horizontal moves. After 10-12 moves this way, the wire would stop and begin to bend up and down again. He counted the up and down moves, and he also counted the horizontal moves, recording them. The up and down moves represented one foot for each bend, and the horizontal moves represented the volume of water at that depth. The distance was thus calculated to each level where water would be found, and an estimate given for the volume at the different levels. I asked him why it was that in America each *bob* of the wire is counted as a foot and in Europe each *bob* of the wire is calculated as one meter? He had no answer.

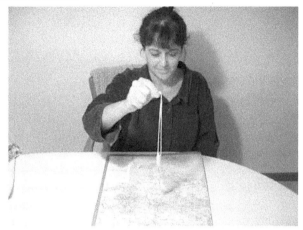

Figure 44. Map dowsing

Later I found the answer to the question. A relative came to visit whom I learned belonged to a dowsing club of "water witches." I asked him the same question, and this is his answer:

That is no problem, a person doing the *bobbing* just determines in his mind what measurements he is going to use before he starts.

Many who are involved in divination for metal or water continue their attempts to find some scientific association or answer so that dowsing will be accepted by the scientific world. However, there seems to be no common ground with science.

APPENDIX E

THE NEW AGE MOVEMENT AND SEVENTH-DAY ADVENTISTS

Prepared by the Biblical Research Institute General Conference of Seventh-day Adventists 12501 Old Columbia Pike, Silver Spring, MD 20904, July 1987

I. INTRODUCTION:

In recent years some Seventh-day Adventists have participated in a variety of strange experiences. Are these phenomena harbingers of the coming outpouring of the Holy Spirit (as sometimes claimed), or do they disclose a subtle attempt by Satan to ensnare unwary members of the remnant church? A few instances will highlight the nature of the problem:

- A nurse places her hands in certain positions on her own abdomen for twenty-minute periods several times a day. Although formerly a sufferer from chronic constipation, she now has relief by correcting the disordered electrical currents of her body.
- A concerned mother swings a pendulum over her cancer-afflicted son to discover what herbs are needed to cure his diseased condition.
- A lady suspends a lead crystal pendant over a handful of vitamin C Pills to determine her daily dosage. The number varies from day to day.

- Books on iridology, a psychic method for diagnosing disease through the iris of the eye, on sale in a college-operated supermarket. Another popular volume on the same shelf: *Magnetic Therapy: Healing in Your Own Hands*, by Abbot George Burke. The author refers with approval to the studies of Dr. Franz Mesmer (from whom the term "mesmerism" derives) and traces his research through pagan thought to Isis, a famous goddess of ancient Egypt.
- A young man in ill health is tied to a tree with his back to its "window" or "door." The aperture has been located by means of a pendulum. It is believed that electrical energy will flow into the patient to bring renewed vigor.
- A gentleman, attending a Pathfinder dinner, dangles a nail tied to a string over a small amount of food in his hand to discover what he may safely eat. In a similar manner a child checks her lunch at the school cafeteria.
- After a Five-Day Plan to Stop Smoking clinic meeting, a participant places a cigarette behind his ear and extends his arm out from his side. The director grasps the arm and easily moves it back to the participants' side. The gentleman removes the cigarette from his person and extends his arm again. Now his arm becomes rigid and the director is unable to move it. The phenomenon is cited as striking evidence against the use of tobacco.
- The practitioner places one hand on the patient's pain-wracked leg and with the other directs a pendulum over several pictures depicting a variety of diseases. The positive spinning of the pendulum over a picture of tuberculosis of the bone indicates this disease as the cause of the patient's affliction.
- House wives, shopping for groceries, hold their pendulums over lettuce and other products to determine freshness or wholesomeness.
- A lady on medication for epilepsy is told by an herbal practitioner that toxoplasmosis is probably the cause for her epilepsy (toxoplasmosis is a disease caused by the presence of parasitic microorganisms known as toxoplasmas). The patient is assured that the disease can be killed by using "vital therapy."

"Vital therapy" is based on the belief that the right side of the body, including the hand and foot, is electrically positive; the left side is negative. "To draw out" from the sick person the practitioner places his left hand with the palm open toward the body of the patient; the right hand is held palm open and downward, parallel to the ground. This allows the "bad electricity" to flow away from the patient. "To put in" natural life-force the practitioner places the right hand over the patient and holds the left hand up over his head with the palm facing directly upward and the fingers curved as though holding a ball. This allows energy to flow into the patient. It is this flow of energy that does the healing; it can be balanced or increased by these motions of the hands.

Participants in a 14-hour video-tape course entitled, "Achieve Your Potential," are taught to exercise the "God Power" that "everyone" has "within."

These experiences could be multiplied. They all involve Seventh-day Adventist church members; in certain instances, personnel in denominational churches and schools. Professional and college-educated persons are engaged in these practices as well as individuals with lesser educational backgrounds. Actually, the above experiences have a common denominator: We believe they reflect an intrusion here and there of some aspects of the so-called New Age movement into the ranks of Seventh-day Adventists.

II. THE NEW AGE MOVEMENT: SOME BELIEFS

The roots of the New Age movement may be traced to the 1960's when many American young people became enamored not only with the occult but also with the oriental religions and their explanations of reality. Thus a movement began. In the last two decades Western occultism has linked with Eastern mysticism to present a new face to modern society under the general name of the "New Age movement."

The New Age movement, however, is not a denomination with a structured organization and a central headquarters. Actually, the "movement" is a broad coalition of religions and organizations which hold in common similar views of reality. Theories and practices based on the so-called "ancient wisdom" have penetrated virtually every area of contemporary life: science, business, health/medicine, education, psychology, religion, politics, the arts, and especially entertainment. In fact mass entertainment and the media in general have made many concepts of the New Age philosophy familiar household terms.

The foundational belief which ties together the diversified groups of New Agers is the unbiblical world view of pantheism. Pantheism once knocked on the Adventist door through the teaching and influence of Dr. J.H. Kellogg, superintendent of the Battle Creek Sanitarium in Michigan, as well as others. We believe it is knocking again today in more insidious ways. Whereas Kellogg emphasized that *God* was in everything (flower, tree) and in people (cf. the title of his book, *The Living Temple*), the modern emphasis is on a universal *consciousness* (cf. Hindu, *world soul*; Christian Science, *divine mind*) or *energy* as the true reality that undergirds all nature and which may be manipulated. There is a subjective emphasis on activating a person's *higher powers* as the source for insight and healing rather than looking to an external, transcendent God and to objective guidelines that exist outside oneself. The word "pantheism" itself is not used in New Age literature. However, the terms employed by writers presenting the New Age world view simply mask this unbiblical teaching.

Why would modern humanity, after achieving such great feats through the scientific methods, be attracted to pantheism? For one thing, there are not many options, as Robert Burrows, editor of publications for Spiritual Counterfeits Project, points out:

> The religious options open to humanity are limited: We can believe in no God and be atheists. We can believe in one God and be theists. Or we can believe that all is God and be pantheists.

> Of these three, pantheism has been humanity's major preoccupation throughout history....In the absence of revealed religion; humanity gravitates to natural religion, assumes nature is all that is, and deifies it and humanity accordingly. ("Americans Get Religion in the New Age," *Christianity Today*, May 16, 1986, 17)

According to Norman L. Geisler, professor of Systematic Theology at Dallas Theological Seminary, "Western society is experiencing an ideological shift from an atheistic to a pantheistic orientation." Strange as it may seem the two perspectives have much in common since both take a naturalistic approach to the world.

> (1) Both deny an absolute distinction between Creator and creation. Both deny there is any God beyond the universe. (2) Both deny that a God supernaturally intervenes in the universe (by miracles). (3) And in the final analysis both believe that man is God (or Ultimate), though not all atheists admit this. ("The New Age Movement," Bibliotheca Sacra, January-March, 1987, 79-80)

It is clear that any religion or movement that puts man at the center and underscores his self-centeredness will appeal to the sinful heart equally well whether the orientation of the religion is atheistic or pantheistic. Consequently both schools of thought are directly opposed to the God-centered faith of Christianity.

According to Dr. Geisler at least fourteen doctrines are typical of the New Age groups (though some do not embrace all of them.) A pantheistic coloring is given to most (Ibid., p. 85):

1. An impersonal god (force). Some designate this as "mind"
2. An eternal universe

3. The illusory nature of matter
4. The cyclical nature of life
5. The necessity of reincarnations
6. The evolution of man into Godhead
7. Continuing revelation from spirit beings beyond this world
8. The identity of man with God
9. The need for meditation (or other consciousness-changing techniques)
10. Occult practices (astrology, mediums, etc.)
11. Vegetarianism and holistic health
12. Pacifism (or anti-war activities)
13. One world (global) order
14. Syncretism (unity of all religions)

If confronted with a clear statement of faith (such as listed above), most Seventh-day Adventists would perceive immediately that these New Age teachings are foreign to the Christian religion. Indeed, they clash with the plainest teachings and claims of the Christian Scriptures. But the approach of New Age ideas and practices has caught the attention of some Adventists by more subtle means. Before examining the ways by which specific inroads have been made in the church, we turn to two important biblical teachings that impact on this topic.

III. BIBLE BACKGROUNDS The Existence of Evil Angels

The Bible teaches the existence of an evil personage known as Satan and his hosts of devils. These supernatural beings are in constant warfare against God, the human race, God's people, and all that is holy and good.

Christ, as God the Son, created all things. "For in him all things were created, in heaven and on earth, visible and invisible, whether thrones or dominions or principalities or authorities—all things were created through him and for him" (Col. 1:16). Thus, it is evident that Christ created the angels (cf. also Ps 148:2, 5). The angels presently in heaven form an innumerable multitude of intelligent beings (Rev 5:11) who joyfully serve the Creator as He directs (Ps 103: 19-21; Heb 1:14).

Devils (also referred to as demons and unclean spirits) were once part of these angelic armies whom Christ created at some point in eternity past. However, under the leadership of Lucifer (Satan) these angels rebelled against the authority of God and were expelled from heaven (Isa. 14:12-15; Rev 12:7-9; 2 Peter 2:4). As fallen angels they form the dark forces of evil which war against God and the human race.

The connection of the visible with the invisible world, the ministration of angels of God, and the agency of evil spirits are plainly revealed in the Scriptures, and inseparably interwoven with human history. There is a growing tendency to disbelief in the existence of evil spirits, while the holy angels that "minister for them who shall be heirs of salvation"...are regarded by many as spirits of the dead. But the Scriptures not only teach the existence of angels, both good and evil, but present unquestionable proof that these are not disembodied spirits of dead men....

Evil spirits, in the beginning created sinless, were equal in nature, power, and glory with the holy beings that are now God's messengers. But fallen through sin, they are leagued together for the dishonor of God and the destruction of men. United with Satan in his rebellion, and with him cast out from heaven, they have, through all succeeding ages, co-operated with him in his warfare against the divine authority. We are told in Scripture of their confederacy and government, of their various orders, of their intelligence and subtlety, and of their malicious designs against the peace and happiness of men. (*The Great Controversy,* 511, 513)

From the beginning of their operation in the earth demonic forces under Satan have been connected intimately with all forms of pagan idolatry and the occult practices involved. Israel was warned strictly not to unite with the pagan idolaters in their religious rites. The reason was underscored: If they participated in the rites of paganism and in the practices of the occult, they would thereby commit themselves to the service and control of the demons (cf. Rom 6:16). Note the implication of the following passages:

They stirred him (God) to jealousy with strange gods: with abominable practices they provoked him to anger. *They sacrificed to demons which were no gods....* (Deut. 32:16-17)

They served their idols, which became a snare to them. *They sacrificed their sons and their daughters to the demons;* they poured out innocent blood, the blood of their sons and daughters, whom they sacrificed to the idols of Canaan; and the land was polluted with blood. (Ps 106:36-38)

I imply that *what pagans sacrifice they offer to demons* and not to God. *I do not want you to be partners with demons.* You cannot drink the cup of the Lord and the cup of demons. You cannot partake of the table of the Lord and the table of demons. (1 Cor. 10:20-21)

The occult-mystical philosophy of ancient forms of paganism lives on today in the modern activities of the New Age movement. Some practices like Spiritualism continue on, unchanged, more or less; however, New Agers emphasize the presence of good spirits who can guide and empower the human mind. Then, there are new practices, adapted to the interests and concerns of modern society. We will consider some of these.

We believe the Christian needs to be warned that the same unbiblical philosophical base and the same demonic power lie behind many of the practices now being offered contemporary society by the occult-mystical oriented New Age programs. The same possibility of coming under occult oppression—under Satanic deception, domination, and control—is as real now as in ancient times. On this point God has given end-time Christians specific cautions:

> Now the Spirit expressly says that in later times some will depart from the faith by giving heed to deceitful spirits and doctrines of demons. (1 Tim 4:1)

The biblical world view

Today's secularized society is ripe for Satanic delusions. Since in any era the church must cope with intrusion of worldly culture and philosophy, we are safe in saying that some/many in the church stand in a similar danger.

To a large extent the modern scientific mind has abandoned the Bible and its claims and the authority of the God revealed there. Secular humanity likewise rejects belief in a personal being known as Satan or in the existence of evil spirits. Quantum physics now views fundamental reality "as a seamless web of vibrant, pulsating energy" (Burrows). This has led certain physicists who have accepted New Age occultism to identify this fundamental energy with Eastern mysticism's pantheistic "god"—consciousness, life-force, or mind that it alleges permeates the universe. Thus the New Age movement has developed as an endeavor to join modern science, the occult and Eastern mysticism into one world system of pantheistic belief.

This current thrust toward a pantheistic view of reality clashes with the clear, unambiguous testimony of the Bible. We summarize a few of its basic teachings:

1. *The Bible affirms the existence of a personal God who, as Creator, stands outside and separate from His creation.* Jesus taught us to address God as "our Father." By contrast pantheism perceives "god" as an impersonal force, energy, or "mind" permeating all nature, including ourselves.

2. *The Bible affirms that men and women are creatures—created by God in His own image but distinct from Him and dependent upon Him for existence.* Humanity is in no sense divine, although it is called to reflect

God's character. By contrast pantheism sees the human as an extension of "god." The divine essence within is the person's true self; he is "god" and through a series of lives humanity will evolve into a more mature understanding of its godhead.

3. *The Bible affirms the reality of the external world of nature and the universe and acknowledges all things as the handiwork of the* Creator. "I look at the heavens, the work of thy fingers, the moon and the stars which thou hast established" (Ps 8:3). "And God saw everything that he had made, and behold, it was very good" (Gen 1:31).

4. *The Bible affirms that the human family has sinned against God by transgressing His will as revealed in His Law. It further affirms that the sinner can be redeemed only through his personal acceptance of the merits of the sinless life and atoning death of the Savior, Jesus Christ.* Pantheism rejects the Christian gospel and its premises. Humanity is essentially good, not fallen nor a transgressor of God's laws. Pantheists argue that the problem lies in our forgetting that humanity is divine. The goal is for each to discover his or her essential deity.

5. In pantheistic thought ultimate salvation is unification with "god" after a series of lives and reincarnations. Jesus is regarded as a great religious teacher influenced by the "Christ Spirit" which has dwelt in others as well. It is denied that Jesus died for man's sin. In fact, a consistent pantheist would argue that Jesus never died at all, but while in the tomb solved the problem of the ages by transmuting his human flesh into divine flesh.

The Bible affirms the value of prayer-communion between the believer and God.

Have no anxiety about anything, but in everything by prayer and supplication with thanksgiving let your requests be made known to God. And the peace of God, which passes all understanding, will keep your hearts and your minds in Christ Jesus. (Phil 4:6-7)

In any time of need the believer is encouraged to approach God in prayer through the intercession of Christ, our understanding high priest (Heb. 4: 14-16).

Pantheism denies this kind of prayer relationship between two distinct beings— between God and the believer. Since the human is held to be essentially divine, *prayer* takes the form of a kind of *meditation.* Various techniques for *consciousness-altering* are employed to enable the meditator to move through levels of consciousness until he is able to invoke, or to come into union with, or to tap the god-energy within. By contrast Christian meditation directs the mind of believers to the Creator God who is external to them.

6. *The Bible affirms the presence of evil angels, confederated under Satan, who war against God and humanity.* Pantheism denies the presence of evil in the universe. It claims, however, that the cosmos is a multidimensional reality and that it is inhabited by spirits who are viewed as sources of power and guidance. Hence the New Ager is open—but blind—to the deceptions of evil angels.

7. *The Bible affirms the reality of death and a final judgment of mankind.* It is appointed for men to *die once*, after that comes *judgment* (Heb. 9:27). Pantheism denies both events. Life is upward and mobile through a series of reincarnations. The Bible knows nothing about a series of lives and reincarnations by which one gradually *improves* as he moves toward full reunion with *god.*

> The Bible teaches that one may be fully saved in this present life through the acceptance of Jesus Christ and in union with Him. Should the believer die before the actual return of Christ in His kingdom of glory, he will be resurrected then with an immortal body. The living saints will be translated; both groups will be gathered to Christ at that great event and will remain with Him eternally (1 Thess. 4:16-18; 1 Cor. 15:51- 55). This earth, renewed by the Creator's hand, will become the eternal home of the redeemed (Rev 21: 1-5; Matt 5:5).

8. *The Bible affirms the reality of miracles by the power of God. It also recognizes that Satan and the evil angels work apparent miracles through their agencies* (Exodus 7:10-12, 20-22; 8:6- 7; Matt 24:24; Rev 16:13- 14). Pantheism attributes physical phenomena such as the curing of disease to the activating of latent "higher powers" within the human mind or to the manipulating of the aura of energy which is alleged to envelop each person and object. The above Bible affirmation does not negate the fact that the mind and the body are intimately related (cf. psychosomatic medicine). Some diseases are related to mental attitudes. Thus their cures are effected by changes in thinking rather than through direct miracles by a supernatural agency. Ellen White has written:

> Disease is sometimes produced, and is often greatly aggravated, by the imagination. Many are lifelong invalids who might be well if they only thought so....Many die from disease the cause of which is wholly imaginary.
>
> Courage, hope, faith, sympathy, love, promote health and prolong life. A contented mind, a cheerful spirit, is health to the body and strength to the soul....

In the treatment of the sick the effect of mental influence should not be overlooked. Rightly used, this influence affords one of the most effective agencies for combating disease. (*The Ministry of Healing,* 241)

It is evident from this brief summary that the Christian faith revealed in the Holy Scriptures is in open conflict with the pantheistic-oriented beliefs that undergird the New Age movement. Christians must reject New Age practices and procedures which derive from or support a pantheistic world view contrary to the teachings of the Bible.

IV. HOLISTIC HEALTH Health and Wholeness

One aspect of the New Age movement that can prove alluringly deceptive to Seventh-day Adventists is its emphasis on holistic health. Adventists long have believed in the "wholeness" of the human being. We know that mind and body interact, thus the individual should be treated as a whole person. However, New Age holistic health means "wholeness" on pantheistic grounds ("All is One"; "We are all God") and not the Bible's view of the nature of man. There is a sharp difference.

In recent years a strong movement has developed in the United States to establish medical centers that unite physicians practicing scientific medicine with the practitioner of occult and eastern healing arts. In 1979 the *Journal of the American Medical Association* reported the existence of more than 500 such centers/clinics in the country headed and staffed by physicians and 10,000 holistic health care practitioners (November 16, 1979). Thus, *ancient* (that is, occult-Eastern) methods of healing and modern medicine are joined.

In 1977 the prestigious Johns Hopkins University opened its doors to lectures in *psychic healing* and other *unconventional treatments*. According to news reports Dr. Lawrence Green, head of the school's division of Health Education, "helped organize a series of seven lectures at the Baltimore, Maryland, school that included demonstrations and talks by practitioner in psychic healing, laying on of hands, yoga, meditation and nutritional therapy" (cited in spiritual counterfeits Project Journal, August 1978, 6). Later in the same year (1977), the New York Times reported:

An unorthodox therapy in which nurses attempt to make sick patients feel better by "laying hands" on them is being introduced in hospitals and nursing schools throughout the country.

In many ways similar to the laying –on of hands that is practiced by faith healers and mystics and that is scoffed at by medical science, the therapy is being taught at the graduate level by Dr. Dolores Krieger, a nurse and a professor at the New

York University School of Education, Health, Nursing and Arts Professions (Ron Sullivan, "Hospitals Introducing a Therapy Resembling 'Laying on of Hands,'" New York Times, November 6, 1977, cited in *Spiritual Counterfeits Project Journal*, August 1978,7)

It should be observed that Dr. Dolores Krieger (R.N., Ph.D.), an advocate of Eastern mystical energy concepts, was tutored under a psychic by the name of Dora Kunz. She openly admits the source of her therapy: "I had been taught the technique of laying on of hands by Kunz" ("Therapeutic Touch and healing Energies From Laying On of Hands," 28-29, cited in John Weldon and Zola Levitt, *Psychic Healing* [Chicago: Moody Press, 1982], 22).

Unlocking potential

Success has become the goal for contemporary professionals. Natural desire provides access to the modern mind for New Age thought under the guise of Human Potential seminars. A variety of courses are offered to enable the professional to activate his latent "higher powers." Varying approaches have been devised, but they commonly include some form of meditation accompanied by physical, breathing, and relaxation exercises. The Eastern mystical context from which these techniques are drawn to bring about states of consciousness usually is omitted. The participant is led to think he is tapping a "reservoir of magnificence" within himself. (See Burrows, *Christianity Today*, May 16, 1987, 17, 19-20

The Bible acknowledges that the Creator has endowed human beings with many talents and abilities. It challenges every person to improve these. There is, therefore, a true realization of the human potential from a Christian perspective. However, there is a difference between developing ability by study and practice and attempting to tap an alleged inner power by mystical forms of meditation. From a Christian perspective a developed ability brings honor to the Creator; from the New Age perspective any development is self-centered and brings honor to the person.

But a greater danger may lie in the meditative process. The unstated goal behind such techniques (whether the participant senses it) is to alter consciousness to achieve union with the *god* or *god-power* within. But in such a state of passive neutrality the mind could be subject to Satanic invasion and delusion.

Registered nurse, Sharon Fish summarizes David Haddon's remarks on Transcendental Meditation on this point:

In his analysis of TM, David Haddon notes that the alteration of consciousness which results from practicing the various forms of Eastern meditation can have adverse spiritual effects. Sensory perception gradually shuts down with the repetition of a word or mantra, for example, and the conceptual activity of the mind ceases as the brain shifts gears to neutral. This passive state, Haddon notes, resembles that sought by mediums in order to make contact with spirits. . . "(David Haddon, "Transcendental Meditation Wants You, Eternity [November 1974], 24-25, cited in Sharon Fish, "Holistic Health and the Nursing Profession," *Spiritual Counterfeits Project Journal*, August 1978, 41)

Meeting stress

Emotional and physical stress are characteristic of contemporary society. The need to cope with these also has opened doors to the New Age holistic health approach. Americans, who once flocked to psychiatrists, encounter groups, or chiropractors, now go to teachers of Transcendental Meditation, yoga classes, and biomedical feedback labs where they learn to control muscle tension by meditation into an altered state of consciousness (see *Spiritual Counterfeits Project Journal*, August 1978, 29-40). Transcendental Meditation, yoga, and biomedical feedback (some forms of the latter may be neutral) are three of the most common stress reducers popularized in holistic health.

Another is "Guided Imagery." For example, a nurse first leads her patient into a relaxed mood by means of deep breathing exercises. The patient then is invited to close her eyes and accompany the nurse on a beautiful walk in her imagination as it is described to her. In the course of the imagined stroll the two arrive at a fence enclosing a pleasant meadow. They enter, and the patient is told that this is to be her own private meadow. Walking across the grass, they come to a large tree and sit down under its shade. Then touch it. The nurse tells the patient to let the strength of the tree flow through her, to express her fears, and to cry if she needs to. Then, in imagination, they return home. Now the patient is informed that this imaginary walk has provided her with a personal experience, and whenever she cannot take the pain, she should return to the meadow in her mind and talk to the tree. (See *Spiritual Counterfeits Project Journal*, August 1978, 39).

We recognize kindness in this technique and a rational attempt to divert the mind of a suffering person from pain to something more pleasant, but from a Christian point of view it bypasses the privilege of prayer and the Christian's personal relationship with God. Instead of sharing her pain and her need with God through prayer, the patient is told to consult with an imaginary tree and not to be afraid to cry before it. This particular example reveals the shallow dimensions of pantheism: there is no personal God to whom one can turn. The participant ends up talking to an illusion—her imagined tree: in reality talking to herself.

It may be asked whether there is really any danger to spiritual experience for a Christian to adopt a holistic technique for bringing about relaxation or reducing stress. Dr. Kenneth R. Pelletier, Assistant Professor of Psychiatry at the University of California, School of Medicine in San Francisco and a prominent advocate for holistic health, candidly addresses this question. Let Christians take note:

> A person entering into meditation has already in some sense committed himself to an accompanying philosophical system. This factor of the individual's attitude as he approaches meditation practice cannot be underestimated in understanding the positive effects of such practice. (*Mind as Healer, Mind as Slayer: A Holistic Approach to Preventing Stress Disorders* [New York: Dell Publishing Co., 1977], 195, cited in Brooks Alexander, "Holistic Health From the Inside," *Spiritual Counterfeits Project Journal*, August 1978, 16)

Sharon Fish summarizes Dr. Pelletier's further remarks thus:

> Pelletier notes that though the information received from the body by the mind in biofeedback is neutral and various forms of meditation may be engaged in without adhering to a particular belief system, *this is the exception rather than the rule.* In the apparent simplicity of each technique, he says, lies a common search for a deeper meaning as a person moves from early meditative states to deeper and deeper states of meditation, it should be clear, states Pelletier, that meditation is more than a simple means of stress reduction and that each system of healing is based on certain philosophical assumptions....

> While the practice of meditation will probably not lead most people to the extreme of demonic contact or possession, there are other spiritual effects. As Pelletier and other advocates of holistic health have noted with enthusiasm, there is often a change in one's belief system that accompanies meditation—a change that reflects the assumptions of pantheistic theology underlying most of the proposed healing techniques. ("Holistic Health and the Nursing Profession," *Spiritual Counterfeits Project Journal*, August 1978, 40, 41, emphasis added)

Diagnosing and healing disease

Psychic healing has always been an important aspect of the occult. The current holistic health emphasis is no exception. It presents a bewildering array of techniques for diagnosing and healing disease. We list only a few of the better known ones such as: Radionics or Radiaesthesia (use of objects, pendulum, black box, etc.), acupuncture, acupressure, reflexology, applied kinesiology, iridology, herbal therapy, color therapy, gem therapy, etc.

We recognize that a scientific basis is argued for some of the above, yet these and scores of other practices in holistic health are closely related to either an occult, humanist, or Eastern world view that is anti-biblical. Therein lays the danger to the Christian who is tempted to adapt these techniques to his biblical world view. We believe that in most cases this is not possible.

We wish to underscore this warning. Conservative Christians who have studied holistic health over the last two decades (see appended bibliography for a few examples) are convinced that its diagnosing and healing procedures are based squarely on occult and mystical concepts. *While some elements in holistic health may be matters of indifference, no distinctive occult technique can be viewed as "neutral" even when separated ostensibly from its roots.* (Emphasis added) Note the following assertions by the editor of the *Spiritual Counterfeits Project Journal*:

> The original purpose of this article was to answer the question: To what extent does the holistic movement commonly recognize occult metaphysics and Eastern mystical spiritual experience as an operation basis for its activities and its self-understanding? Most of the evidence available for inspection indicates that the answer can be given without qualification: Overwhelmingly. It appears that the movement as a whole is dominated, if not controlled, by a consistent and systematic form of spirituality that is radically antithetical to biblical Christianity....
>
> It is probable that none of the Eastern or occult healing techniques are "neutral" in themselves, even when ostensibly divorced from overt philosophical statements; the metaphysical framework from which they emerge is so pervasive and encompassing that every detail of practice is intricately related to elements of the underlying belief system. As a result, the technique taken as a whole will carry overtones and implications of the metaphysical system from which it is derived, even if that system is not *explicitly* attached. (Brooks Alexander, "Holistic Health From the Inside," *Spiritual Counterfeits Project Journal*, August 1978, 15-16)

We believe the above conviction will be confirmed as we proceed.

The Magnetic Energy Field. An assumption that is fundamental to many of the diagnosing and healing techniques of holistic health is the belief that every individual (all objects as well) is enveloped in an energy field. This energy, sometimes designated as the "aura," is viewed as *external* to the human body, although it is alleged to be composed of seven rays issuing from seven centers within the body. The energy field is presumed to act as a medium for the interplay of other energies with which it may interact. It is obvious that such a view follows logically from the movement's pantheistic orientation which teaches that force or energy is the fundamental reality that permeates and binds the universe together.

When illness occurs in the body, it is alleged that the magnetic energy field around the sick person is disturbed and an imbalance is developed. The holistic health practitioner can manipulate this magnetic field of energy both to determine the nature of the disease and to treat it. The healer may be present with the sick person or actually at a distance from his subject. In this case he may diagnose and heal by working with a picture or writing of the patient or some object he has handled.

It is claimed that some practitioners, as *sensitives*, can perceive subjectively the aura and its balance or imbalance. Others may view the aura objectively through the Kilner screen (a special type of glass). Here the occult *slip* is showing. In actual fact, *the magnetic energy field or aura cannot be scientifically demonstrated.* It can be perceived only by persons who are sensitives or mediumistic.

Ellen G. White Statements on Body Electricity. Some Seventh-day Adventists have been led to believe that the writings of Ellen White endorse the various holistic health techniques and their philosophical premises. This is based upon several of her statements where she alludes to the electrical currents of the body. We will examine this point briefly, noting meanwhile that although both sources may use some common terminology, the differences in the meaning are profound. Ellen White speaks of electrical currents in harmony with the biblical world view; holistic health writers speak from a pantheistic orientation. We cite Mrs. White's principal statements without attempting to be exhaustive:

> The sensitive nerves of the brain have lost their healthy tone by morbid excitation to gratify an unnatural desire for sensual indulgence. The brain nerves which communicate with the entire system are the only medium through which Heaven can communicate to man and affect his inmost life. *Whatever disturbs the circulation of the electric currents in the nervous system lessens the strength of the vital powers, and the result is a deadening of the sensibilities of the mind.* In consideration of these facts, how important that ministers and people who profess godliness should stand forth clear and untainted from this soul debasing vice! (*Child Guidance*, 447; see also *Testimonies*, vol. 2, 347)

> God endowed man with so great vital force that he has withstood the accumulation of disease brought upon the race in consequence of perverted habits, and has continued for six thousand years. *This fact of itself is enough to*

evidence to us the strength and electrical energy that God gave to man at his creation. It took more than two thousand years of crime and indulgence of base passions to bring bodily disease upon the race to any great extent. If Adam, at his creation, had not been endowed with twenty times as much vital force as men now have, the race, with their present habits of living in violation of natural law, would have become extinct. (*Testimonies,* vol. 3, 138-39)

This class fall more readily if attacked by disease; the system is vitalized by the electrical force of the brain to resist disease. (*Testimonies*, vol. 3, 157)

The influence of the mind on the body, as well as of the body on the mind, should be emphasized. *The electrical power of the brain, promoted by mental activity, vitalizes the whole system, and is thus an invaluable aid in resisting disease.* (*Education*, 197, emphasis added)

Physical inaction lessens not only mental but moral power. The brain nerves that connect with the whole system are the medium through which heaven communicates with man and affects the inmost life. *Whatever hinders the circulation of the electric current in the nervous system, thus weakening the vital powers and lessening mental susceptibility, makes it more difficult to arouse the moral nature. (Education*, 209, emphasis added)

Although the tracks of truth and error lie nearby at times, it is clear from these statements that Ellen White gives no support to the pantheistic view that the individual is surrounded by an aura of energy comparable to a halo or magnetic energy field. Her statements pertain to "the circulation of the electrical current in the nervous system" *within the physical body of the individual.*

Although Mrs. White wrote the statements before the advent of modern medicine, the presence of these electrical impulses can be scientifically demonstrated now. Electrocardiographs and electroencephalographs are well-known in conventional medicine. The tracings of these natural electrical impulses generated within the body can assist the modern physician with his treatment of disease.

But Ellen White never suggests or implies that an *external* aura of electrical energy surrounds every person and object. Nor does she teach that such can be manipulated to determine or heal human sickness. To superimpose views of holistic healers upon her clear-cut statements is to distort what Ellen White actually is saying.

Ellen G. White's View on Occult Healing. But Ellen White did recognize that occult healers claimed to heal through the manipulation of electrical currents. In fact, she claimed that the healers were "channels for

Satan's electric currents." In an article entitled "Shall We Consult Spiritualist Physicians" (part of Testimony 31, published in 1882) she spoke to this issue, basing her remarks on King Ahaziah's appeal to Baalzebub the god of Ekron for healing (see 2 Kings 1):

> *The heathen oracles have their counterpart in the spiritualistic mediums, the clairvoyants, and fortunetellers of today.* The mystic voices that spoke at Endor are still by their lying words misleading the children of men. *The prince of darkness has but appeared under a new guise....* While they (modern people) speak with scorn of the magicians of old, the great deceiver laughs in triumph as they yield to his arts under a different form.

> *His agents still claim to cure disease. They attribute their power to electricity, magnetism, or the so-called "sympathetic remedies." In truth, they are but channels for Satan's electric currents.* By this means he casts his spell over the bodies and souls of men.

> I have from time to time received letters both from ministers and lay members of the church, *inquiring if I think it wrong to consult spiritualist and clairvoyant physicians*. I have not answered these letters for want of time. But just now the subject is again urged upon my attention. *So numerous are these agents of Satan becoming, and so general is the practice of seeking counsel from them, that it seems needful to utter words of warning....*

> *Not a few in this Christian age and Christian nation resort to evil spirits rather than trust to the power of the living God. The mother, watching by the sickbed of her child, exclaims: "I can do no more. Is there no physician who has power to restore my child?" She is told of the wonderful cures performed by some clairvoyant or magnetic healer, and she trusts her dear one to his charge, placing it as verily in the hands of Satan as if he were standing by her side. In many instances the future life of the child is controlled by a satanic power which it seems impossible to break....*

In the name of Christ I would address His professed followers: Abide in the faith which you have received from the beginning. Shun profane and vain babblings. *Instead of putting your trust in witchcraft, have faith in the living God.* Cursed is the path that leads to Endor or to Ekron. The feet will stumble and fall that venture upon the forbidden ground. There is a God in Israel, with whom is deliverance for all that are oppressed. Righteousness is the habitation of His throne....

Angels of God will preserve His people while they walk in the path of duty, but there is no assurance of such protection for those who deliberately venture upon Satan's ground. An agent of the great deceiver will say and do anything to gain his object. It matters little whether he calls himself a spiritualist, an 'electric physician,' or a 'magnetic healer.' By specious pretenses he wins the confidence of the unwary....

Those who give themselves up to the sorcery of Satan may boast of great benefit received thereby, but does this prove their course to be wise or sage? What if life should be prolonged? Will it pay in the end to disregard the will of God? All such apparent gain will prove at last an irrecoverable loss. *We cannot with impunity break down a single barrier which God has erected to guard His people from Satan's power.* (*Testimonies*, vol. 5, 193-4, 197-99, emphasis added)

The counsel is clear. In harmony with the Bible Ellen White recognizes the presence of Satan and evil angels behind the occult systems of healing. To pursue recovery from sickness at such sources simply opens the door to satanic deceptions and control. The Ellen G. White writings give no support to the holistic health's pantheistic view or reality and emphatically reject this approach to healing.

V. PSYCHOMETRY AND RADIONICS/RADIAESTHESIA

We return now to some techniques associated with assuming that a magnetic energy field or aura surrounds every object and every person, and how this assumption is employed for diagnosing and treating disease in holistic circles.

Psychometry, a holistic method of diagnosing a patient's illness, rests on the assumption that the energy radiating from the patient (his aura) attaches itself to objects he may handle. It is alleged that the practitioner— even at a distance— can gather "impressions" by touching the object and thereby determine the person's illness and prescribe for its cure.

Radionics or Radiaesthesia are names given to that branch of holistic health that uses some device to diagnose disease. The device may be in the form of a pendulum, a black box (Abrams' Box), or some complicated machine. The common pendulum may be constructed by tying a weight to the end of a piece of string. The weight may be most anything: a lead crystal ball, a metal object such as a nail, machinist's nut, or metal button—or even a plastic button. It is explained that the pendulum ascertains the condition of the aura surrounding the body. Disturbances or imbalances in the aura which the pendulum detects indicate the presence of disease in the body. When held over a given organ of the body, a clockwise movement (positive) of the pendulum indicates the organ is healthy. A counter-clockwise movement (negative) indicates an imbalance in the magnetic energy field and a diseased condition of the body. If no movement occurs in the pendulum, it may indicate to the practitioner that the ill person does not have sufficient vital force or energy to affect the pendulum.

The pendulum is used in a variety of ways to diagnose disease. It is also used in determining what medication or herbs the patient should take, or what foods he should or should not eat.

The *black box* (or Abrams' box, named after its developer, Dr. Albert Abrams, d. 1924), contains devices for measuring electrical current. A drop of blood or a hair from the patient is placed within the box. The box is viewed as a complex form of pendulum since it functions on the same theory that it can detect disturbances in the patient's aura. Strange as it may seem, practitioners using the *black box* have made supposedly accurate diagnoses even when they had forgotten to place blood samples in the box! (See John Weldon and Zola Levitt, *Psychic Health* (Chicago: Moody Press, 1982), 56-57.

It is admitted openly by knowledgeable persons within the holistic health movement that success in diagnosing disease is not dependent on the pendulum, black box, or one of the more sophisticated diagnostic machines. It *depends, rather, on the human operator, the practitioner*. If diagnosing by these devices were a matter of working with genuine electrical currents in the body—such as are picked up in an electrocardiograph reading—then anyone could determine disease by these methods. However, this is not so. The pendulum and box will not work for some. The fact is—and this is emphasized by those within the movement—that *we are dealing with psychic healing and not conventional scientific medicine. It takes "sensitives" or psychics to obtain results from psychic or occult methods of treating disease.*

> Note these plain statements by the Theosophical Research Centre, an influential organization within the occult movement:
>
> But no good will be done either to medical or psychic research by denying or ignoring the psychic and psychological factors involved in their (pendulum, box, etc.) use....
>
> These criticisms do not imply that cures do not appear to take place in association with the use of these machines. What we wish to emphasize is that the diagnoses and treatments involved should be considered as psychic or extra-sensory phenomena, and that the claims made as to their being based upon purely physical science and its known laws cannot be substantiated. (*The Mystery of Healing* (Theosophical Publishing House 1958_, 63-65, cited in John Weldon and Zola Levitt, *Psychic Healing* (Chicago: Moody Press, 1982), 61-62)

VI. BIBLE COUNSELS

It may be helpful at this juncture to summarize two specific points that emerge in this brief survey on diagnosing and healing disease in the holistic health manner.

1. From a strictly scientific viewpoint the holistic health approach to the diagnosing and treating of human sickness is highly irrational.

In fact no magnetic energy field can be shown to exist externally to the body, enveloping it like an atmosphere or halo. Consequently, no pendulum or other device can determine the internal condition of the physical body by detecting an imbalance in a non-existent energy field. At times the pendulum is not even made of material that will conduct electricity. In addition, the belief that an object handled by a sick person absorbs rays of energy from him which (at a touch) can replay to the practitioner information concerning the patient's physical condition is not viable.

2. Proponents of holistic healing admit that their approach is psychic healing, that is, occult healing. This is the only basis upon which it can be fully understood.

The techniques used function within the framework of a pantheistic world view which holds that there is only one fundamental reality at the base of the universe: energy or force (some call it *mind, consciousness, god*). Thus the same essence of energy runs through practitioner, pendulum, patient, or any other object. If healing takes place—and it often does—it is not due to the restorative powers of the Creator God of the Bible, but to the dark powers that stand behind the occult.

The Canaanites were deeply involved in the occult—in all its forms. It was an integral part of their idolatry. As we saw earlier from the Bible, the devil and his forces of evil angels—are intimately associated with these systems. Consequently, God warned His people strictly not to adopt the occult practices of the surrounding nations:

> You shall not practice augury (*nahas*, "divination") or witchcraft. (Lev. 19:26)

> When you come into the land which the Lord your God gives you, *you shall not learn to follow the abominable practices of these nations.* There shall not be found among you any one who burns his son or his daughter as an offering, anyone who practices divination [*qasam*], a soothsayer, or an augur (*nahas*), or a sorcerer, or a charmer, or a medium, or a wizard, or a necromancer. *For*

whoever does these things is an abomination to the Lord; and because of these abominable practices the Lord your God is driving them out before you. You shall be blameless before the Lord your God. For these nations, which you are about to dispossess, give heed to soothsayers and to diviners (*qasam*); but as for you, the Lord your God has not allowed you so to do. (Deut. 18:19-14)

The exact meaning of every Hebrew term listed in Deuteronomy is not presently known, but it is clear that the Levitical code prohibited all forms of divination, magic, and spiritism—the whole range of occult practices.

The Hebrew word *"nahas"* rendered *"enchantment/enchanter"* in the KJV and *"augury/augur"* is one of the Hebrew words that carry the meaning *to divine*—to determine the future or to discover hidden knowledge by occult means. Joseph's servant claimed that his master could *"divine"* (*nahas*) with his silver cup (Gen 44:5). Another term, qasam, also means *"to divine."* Nebuchadnezzar *"divined"* (*qasam*) which nation he should attack first (Judah or the Ammonites) by consulting a quiver of arrows, figurines, and an animal liver (Ezek. 21:21).

While these procedures appear irrational to us—and they are—we must not forget that Satanic agencies stand behind these actions. In occult practice divining may take a variety of forms. It links itself naturally with two large areas of human concern: (1) the desire to know the future, and (2) the desire to diagnose and cure disease. Psychic healing has always been an important aspect of the occult.

It can be seen readily that the diagnosing of disease by means of a pendulum, a black box, or by one of the several holistic health techniques is simply a form of occult divining. The practitioner swinging a pendulum over the body of the sick person is not practicing scientific medicine; in reality he is using an occult instrument to "divine" the cause of the illness. It is admitted within the holistic health movements itself that it takes a psychic or a person who is open to develop the sensitivity of a psychic to be successful with these methods. It is clear from the Bible counsels that psychic healing—diagnosing disease by *"divining"*—is simply another form of the forbidden occult.

We believe it is dangerous reasoning for Christians to think they can adopt and adapt them from their original context—as though healing rested in the technique only, a procedure which at times may be irrational in itself. We question whether an occult practice can be superimposed upon a Christian base without bringing to the patient (in time) a false world view or making such persons liable to oppression from the demonic powers who originated the occult-mystical practice in the first place.

God has not changed. He strictly forbad ancient Israel to adopt occult practices. We believe He would say the same things to Seventh-day Adventists Christians today:

> For whoever does these things is an abomination to the Lord;... You shall be blameless before the Lord your God....God has not allowed you so to do (Deut. 18: 12-14).

VII. SEVENTH-DAY ADVENTIST MEDICAL EMPHASIS

In her comments on King Ahaziah's sin in seeking healing from Baalzebub the god of Ekron (2 Kings 1) *Ellen White warns that spiritism may take many different forms*:

> There are many who shrink with horror from the thought of consulting spirit mediums, but *who are attracted by more pleasing forms of spiritism.* Others are attracted by the teachings of *Christian Science, and by the mysticism of Theosophy and other Oriental religions.* (*Prophets and Kings*, 210, emphasis added; see *Evangelism*, 606 for a slightly different phrasing.)

The setting and phrasing imply that Christian Science, Theosophy, and Oriental religions are some of the "more pleasing forms of spiritism." It is indeed significant that this grouping encircles religions that entertain the world view of pantheism. In other words, pantheistical oriented religions compose some of the "more pleasing forms of spiritism." This warning, therefore, is especially applicable to Seventh-day Adventists living in the close of the twentieth century who face the challenge of the New Age movement—a union of Western occultism and Eastern mysticism—and its emphasis on holistic health.

The séance is only one avenue by which the dark powers seek to promote spiritism. The holistic health emphasis of the New Age movement appears also to foster one of the "more pleasing forms of spiritism." Its inroads into the church raise just cause for concern.

Ellen White continues in the next paragraph (after the above citation) with an observation about the link between "all forms of spiritism" and their "power to heal."

> The apostles of nearly all forms of spiritism claim to have power to heal. They attribute this power to electricity, magnetism, the so-called *sympathetic remedies*, or to latent forces within the mind of man. And there are not a few even in this Christian age, who go to these healers, instead of trusting in the

power of the living God and the skill of well-qualified physicians.... (*Prophets and Kings*, 211, emphasis added)

It is significant that Ellen White contrasts *occult-mystic healers* and their claims to heal by electrical energy with *well-qualified physicians* who have been trained in scientific medicine.

From our beginning health and healing have been important to Seventh-day Adventists. Ellen White's major, comprehensive vision on health was given in 1863, the same year that the General Conference organized. Her first written presentation appeared in a 30 page article entitled "Health," published in *Spiritual Gifts*, vol. 4, in 1864. There she amplified this material in six articles entitled "*Disease and Its Causes*" for a series of pamphlets which were printed in 1865 under the general caption, "How to Live" (see *Selected Messages*, bk. 2, p. 410 for a reprint). While these messages recognized the wholeness of the human being (body, mind, and spirit), they presented this position from a biblical world view and the approach to health and healing was along rational lines.

The writings of Ellen White on health are voluminous. Her summary work, *The Ministry of Healing*, was published in 1905. Well-known compilations include *Counsels on Health, Counsels on Diet and Foods, Medical Ministry*, and *Temperance*. None of these works give the slightest credence to occult-mystical techniques of diagnosing and healing. Instead they emphasize the Bible's world view of God, man, the nature of sin, and the divine plan to save sinners. A sound, rational approach is taken to understand the cause for disease and to ameliorate its condition.

Early in their history the Lord guided Seventh-day Adventists to establish a health institution. "I was shown," said Ellen White, "that we should provide a home for the afflicted and those who wish to learn how to take care of their bodies that they may prevent sickness" (*Testimonies,* vol. 1, 489). In 1866 the Western Health Reform Institute opened in Battle Creek, Michigan (later known as the Battle Creek Sanitarium), the first of many medical units (clinics, sanitariums, hospitals, dispensaries) that would eventually encircle the globe.

In 1895 the doors of the American Medical Missionary College opened in Battle Creek, Michigan, offering a four-year course leading to the M.D. degree. In 1909 a charter was secured under the laws of the state of California authorizing the College of Medical Evangelists (now Loma Linda University) to grant degrees in the liberal arts and sciences, dentistry, and medicine. Since there still remained questions in the minds of some just what God intended by "a medical school," the administrators addressed a letter to Mrs. White in January 26, 1910, which asked in part the following:

We are very anxious to preserve unity and harmony of action. In order to do this, we must have a clear understanding of what is to be done. Are we to understand, from what you have written concerning the establishment of a medical school at Loma Linda, that, according to the light you have received from the Lord, we are to establish a thoroughly equipped medical school, the graduates from which will be able to take State Board examination and become registered, qualified physicians?

Mrs. White's reply was received the following day. It read in part:

The light given me is, we must provide that which is essential to qualify our youth who desire to be physicians, so that they may intelligently fit themselves to be able to stand the examinations required to prove their efficiency as physicians....

The medical school at Loma Linda is to be of the highest order,... and for the special preparation of those of our youth who have clear convictions of their duty to obtain a medical education that will enable them to pass the examinations required by law of all those who practice as regularly qualified physicians, we are to supply whatever may be required, so that these youth need not be compelled to go to medical schools conducted by men not of our faith.... (See *Review and Herald*, May 19, 1910, for both letters, cited in part in Dores E. Robinson, *The Story of Our Health Message* [Nashville: Southern Publishing Association, 1943], 326-27)

The medical work of the church includes not only the profession of medicine but other phases of the healing arts such as nursing, dentistry, dietetics, and various paramedical fields, and health education. Adventists emphasize five specific areas of the health care field:
a. Medical education
b. Health education (health evangelism)
c. Clinical medicine (operating through sanitariums, hospitals, clinics, dispensaries, private practice, nursing homes, senior citizens homes)
d. Preventive medicine
e. Medical relief (food and medicine distribution)

In response to the light given Seventh-day Adventists through the prophetic gift we have proceeded to train medical personnel and qualify them with the best scientific training possible so that they may pass all necessary government regulations. This training has been scientific and rational and in harmony with the world view of the Christian Scriptures. We have not trained our youth in methods of psychic healing. Throughout our history as a denomination we have rejected both the philosophy and the techniques of occult-mystical healing. It is the only position consistent with the Christian faith.

Vegetarianism and herbal therapy. While an emphasis on these is found in holistic health, they are not really distinctive to it. The Creator provided a vegetarian diet for mankind at the beginning (Gen 1:29). The use of herbs to assist in healing has developed naturally. Ellen White notes: "The simplest remedies may assist nature, and leave no baleful effects after their use." (*Selected Messages*, bk. 2, 249). Again she says:

> There are many simple herbs which, if our nurses would learn the value of, they could use in the place of drugs, and find very effective. Many times I have been applied to for advice as to what should be done in cases of sickness or accident, and I have mentioned some of these simple remedies, and they have proved helpful. (Ibid., p. 295)

While there is a proper and intelligent use of some simple herbs in certain situations, our people should be warned of the dangers that may arise from the free use of herbal remedies and concoctions advised by scientifically untrained person. Herbal treatments by laymen untaught in the science of pharmacology can be just as radical today and as poisonous as the use of the most dangerous drugs employed in Ellen White's time.

The modern preparation of medications to meet human illnesses is a scientific study. It involves an intimate knowledge of physiology and the biological process, pathology, and chemistry, as well as considerable experimentation and testing in the laboratory. Employing the scientific method here is a necessity if a safe and useful product is to be produced.

On the other hand popular herbal medicine—such as may be seen in the literature advocating herbal remedies in health food stores and shopping mall bookstores—often is based on outdated information, folklore, superstition, wishful thinking, or even fantasy. More important than that; the uninformed use of herbal medication can lead to serious sickness. Some herbs are carcinogenic; some are toxic to the human system, producing serious side effects.

Again, we are led by the counsels of Ellen White to "preventive medicine"—to a daily way of living that involves a nutritious diet, an abundance of exercise, water, sunshine, air, and rest, a temperate lifestyle and an abiding trust in God. For simple sicknesses, let simple remedies be used; for serious disease, "the skill of well-qualified physicians" (*Prophets and Kings*, 211) may be needed. Skilled medical personnel have their place. "There were *physicians* in Christ's day and in the days of the apostles. Luke is called the beloved physician. He trusted in the Lord to make him skillful in the application of remedies." (*Selected Messages*, bk. 2, p. 286).

VIII. CONCLUSION

Although the New Age movement is of recent origin in the United States, it is a revival in new forms of the "ancient wisdom" of paganism. It is a modern union of Western occultism and Eastern mysticism fully committed to a pantheistic world view. The movement is a complex of religions and organizations, and to some degree its views and practices have penetrated nearly every area of our culture.

The New Age movement presents a serious challenge to Christians because its world view is unbiblical. Yet its emphasis on holistic health has led many Christians, including some Seventh-day Adventists, to adopt certain of its techniques and therapies. The bewildering array of techniques and therapies, and seminars and workshops—some of which appear quite neutral in tone—has produced confusion in Christian circles about whether the holistic health aspect of the movement would be dangerous to Christian faith and experience. As in most deceptions, truth and error are mixed in varying proportions.

Clearly the Bible condemns ancient occultism and identifies the power behind it as demonic (Satan/evil angels). Its teachings likewise deny pantheism and the false views developed from that source. Since neither of these false philosophies has changed from ancient times, the Bible's condemnation of both remains valid for Seventh-day Adventists regardless of what new guises they may assume. In a similar manner the writings of Ellen G. White reject both occultism and pantheism and foretell the appearance of similar teachings in modern times in "more pleasing forms of spiritism."

For Seventh-day Adventists the Bible and the Spirit of Prophecy writings should be sufficient to safeguard members from New Age deceptions. We are a health-conscious people, realizing that physical health has an effect on our spiritual well-being. From its beginning our church has upheld a rational approach to health care and has qualified its medical and paramedical personnel with the best scientific training possible. Occult or psychic healing has never been accepted as consistent with our biblical world view. However, in recent years, some members have become enamored and involved in holistic health to the point that they are reluctant to believe that they are in any spiritual danger. In concluding this review we would like to address briefly three claims commonly raised in the connection.

1. *It works*. "I had such and such a problem. The practitioner diagnosed and treated me by using the pendulum, and I enjoy good health now."

There is no question that healings take place with the use of occult methods. That is what makes them deceptive. We have observed already that according to the Bible the dark powers are well able to work miracles and to do wonders. It is not in the healing or the miracle that the evidence is to be sought. Both God and Satan can heal. Consequently, the Christian must look beyond the miracle or healing to the teachings being endorsed. Healing by occult-mystical world view places both the practitioner and the patient on Satan's ground to be oppressed by him at will.

Dr. Kurt Koch (now deceased), a German Lutheran pastor of some forty years' experience, discovered the following solemn fact in counseling people involved in the occult:

These four examples from Christian counseling show the fact which has been observed a hundred-fold, that the pendulum therapy can accomplish certain relief and healings in the organic field. This organic relief must be paid for with disturbances in the psychic field. (Kurt Koch, *Between Christ and Satan* [Grand Rapids: Kregel Publication, ND], 52)

Ellen White makes similar observations. Again we cite a portion of the testimony entitled, "Shall We Consult Spiritualist Physicians?"

His (Satan's) agents still claim to cure disease....In truth; they are but channels for Satan's electric currents. By this means he casts his spell over the bodies and souls of men....

...she (the mother) is told of the wonderful cures performed by some clairvoyant or magnetic healer, and she trusts her dear one to his charge, *placing it as verily in the hands of Satan as if her were standing by her side. In many instances the future life of the child is controlled by a satanic power which seems impossible to break....*

Those who give themselves up to the sorcery of Satan may boast of great benefit received thereby, but does this prove their course to be wise or safe? What if life should be prolonged? What if temporal gain should be secured? Will it pay in the end to disregard the will of God? All such apparent gain will prove at last an irrecoverable loss. We cannot with impunity break down a single barrier which God has erected to guard His people from Satan's power: (*Testimonies*, vol. 5, 193, 194, 199, emphasis added)

2. The technique is neutral. It is argued that a holistic health practitioner may interpret its use in one manner; the Christian healer may interpret its use in another manner.

Our study of this subject concludes that a technique *distinctively* linked to an occult-mystical background cannot be treated as neutral. For example, no Christian can regard the Ouija board as neutral. This is a distinctive occult instrument that will always be linked with demonic powers of spiritism.

Psychometry and the use of the pendulum are other examples of distinctive occult procedures. Apart from an occult-mystical explanation they are irrational. They make sense only in the occult context. As admitted by their advocates, these methods are examples of psychic healing that can never be explained on a scientific basis. It takes a psychic or someone sensitive to developing psychic powers actually to achieve healing by these means.

Forms of meditation that alter consciousness are linked inseparably to Eastern mysticism. Can the Christian safely adopt these procedures by cutting away their roots? Those in the holistic health movement have observed: "There is often a change in one's belief system that accompanies meditation—a change that reflects the assumptions of pantheistic theology underlying most of the proposed healing techniques" (*Spiritual Counterfeits Project Journal*, august 1978, 41, emphasis added).

We repeat an earlier observation: God explicitly forbad Israel to adopt the occult techniques of the pagan Canaanites (Deut. 18:9-14; Lev 19:26). Consequently we Adventist Christians function like a holistic healer by using techniques and therapies that are the distinctive property of the occult-mystic program. Nothing can prevent the demonic powers from intruding into the processes to affect either the practitioner, the patient, or both.

3. **Gray areas.** The complexity of the New Age movement and the numerous practices of its holistic health emphasis inevitably present a mix of the true and the false. While its philosophical base is anti-biblical, it has incorporated certain practices of proven value. For example, vegetarianism, deep breathing exercises, and possibly some relaxation techniques may not be distinctively occult or mystic. Such a blend presents a deceptive face to the inquiring Christian. Dr. Warren Peters suggests some criteria to assist the Christian in analyzing a given holistic health practice or therapy. We adapt the following statements from his publication, *Mystical Medicine*, 41-42. The Christian should ask:

1. Where did it come from: In other words, what is its source? Does it have psychic roots?
2. What company does the technique keep? Who uses it and what other therapies are included?
3. What is the ultimate direction to which this therapy leads? Am I led toward Jesus Christ or away from Him? Do I still need Him as a Savior, or have I become my own savior? Does the therapy or technique follow the known laws of physiology? It is important to study the physiology or methods of action that have been delineated by those not involved in the therapy itself. The explanation given by the one pushing his technique, who profits from the product or the method, is rarely reliable.
4. We would add this further question: Does a given meditation technique

alter my conscious-ness and close down my rational thought processes to such a neutral, passive state that I would be open to Satanic intrusion? The mind, under the influence of the Holy Spirit, is my only means for detecting truth and error. I am never wise to let it slip out of my personal control.

Robert Burrows adds these further suggestions:

> Because of the variety of New Age programs, it is impossible to list criteria that would serve as a basis for recognizing the unbiblical world view that undergirds them all. *World view is, however, the key ingredient. Knowing your own is essential for detecting another's....*
>
> Be particularly world-view attentive if a therapy, seminar, or workshop is (1) explained in terms of harmonizing, manipulation, integrating, or balancing energies or polarities, (2) denigrates the value of the mind or belief; and (3) makes extravagant claims—if it seems too good to be true, it probably is.
>
> Americans Get Religion in the New Age," *Christianity Today*, May 16, 1986, 23, emphasis added)

Seventh-day Adventists have long taught that baffling delusions would precede the Second Coming of Christ (2 Thessalonians 2:9-12). Jesus Himself warned: "False Christs and false prophets will arise and show great signs and wonders, so as to lead astray, if possible even the elect" (Matt 24:24).

Our review of the New Age movement has led to the conclusion that it embodies one of the "more pleasing forms of spiritism preparing our society for the final deception. Members and health –care personnel presently advocating or participating in holistic health or in other programs of the New Age movement should give serious thought and prayer regarding their involvement. All such persons—patients and practitioners alike—should separate themselves from the movement and its distinctive practices.

APPENDIX F
(2009) GENERAL CONFERENCE INSTITUTION MANUAL GUIDE LINES

A copy of a very small section from a 900+ page General Conference manual for church institutions reveals the recommendation for medical institutions to refrain from using questionable healing practices as exposed in this book. The Medical Ministry Department recognizes the spiritualistic influence that such therapeutic methods bring into the SDA medical institutions.

General Conference of Seventh-day Adventists Health Institutions Working Policy-2009

FH 20 Statement of Operating Principles for Health Care Institutions

1. Christ ministered to the whole person. Following His example, the mission of the Seventh-day Adventist Church includes a ministry of healing to the whole person—body, mind, and spirit. The ministry of healing includes care and compassion for the sick and suffering and the maintenance of health. Adventist health care institutions (hospitals, medical/dental clinics, nursing and retirement homes, rehabilitation centers, etc.) should teach the benefits of following the principles of health.

   The relationship of spiritual and natural laws, man's accountability to these laws, and the grace of Christ which assures victorious living are to be integrated into ministry. (See also A 15 35, What Total Commitment to God Involves for the Hospitals and Healthcare Institutions.)

2. Health care institutions should function as an integral part of the total ministry of the Church. These follow church standards, maintaining the sacredness of the Sabbath by promoting a Sabbath atmosphere for staff and patients. Routine business, elective diagnostic services, and elective therapies should be avoided on Sabbath. Church standards also include the promotion of a balanced vegetarian diet free of stimulants and alcohol, in an environment free of tobacco smoke. Control of appetite shall be encouraged, use of drugs with a potential for abuse shall be controlled,

and techniques involving the control of one mind by another shall not be permitted. The institutions are part of the ministry of the Church with activities and practices pervasively identified as the unique Christian witness of Seventh-day Adventists.

3. The activities of the devil are rampant, both within and without the Church. The Church is warned (Col 2:8) "Beware lest any man spoil you through philosophy and vain deceit, after the tradition of men." Because of the great controversy between good and evil, Health Ministries encourages church members to avoid practices rooted in non-Christian philosophy and belief. The Church and its institutions should promote and provide competent and caring service that respects the dignity and rights of patients.

Adventist health care and ministries are to promote only those practices based upon the Bible or the Spirit of Prophecy, or evidence based methods of disease prevention, treatment, and health maintenance.

"Evidence-based" means there is an accepted body of peer reviewed, statistically significant evidence that raises probability of effectiveness to a scientifically convincing level. ***Practices without a firm evidence-base and not based on the Bible or the Spirit of Prophecy, including though not limited to aromatherapy, cranial sacral therapy, homeopathy, hypnotherapy, iridology, magnets, methods aligning forces of energy, pendulum diagnostics, untested herbal remedies, reflexology, repetitive colonic irrigation, "therapeutic touch," and urine therapy, should be discouraged.***

4. In harmony with Christ's loving reaffirmation of freedom of choice, and the dignity of humankind, Seventh-day Adventist health care institutions should give high priority to personal dignity and human relationships. They should seek to provide an efficient, safe, and caring environment conducive to the healing of mind, body, and spirit.

Education in healthful habits of living, as well as supportive care of the patient and family through the dying process is integral to Adventist health care.

5. Health care policies and medical procedures must always reflect a high regard and concern for the value of human life as well as individual dignity.

6. Seventh-day Adventist health care institutions operate as part of the community and nation in which they function. In representing the love of Christ to these communities, the health of the community and the nation is a concern of each institution. Laws of the land are respected and the regulations for the operation of institutions and licensure of personnel are followed.

7. The institutions welcome clergy of all creeds to visit their parishioners.

8. The mission of institutions in representing Christ to the community, and especially to those who utilize their services, is fulfilled through a compassionate, competent staff which, in the performance of their duties, upholds the mission, practices, and standards of the Seventh-day Adventist Church.

9. A regular program to assist the staff in keeping up-to-date professionally, growing in understanding, and in sharing the love of God shall be instituted. Staff development and support of formal education is a priority.

10. Institutions must operate in a financially responsible manner and in harmony with the Working Policy of the Seventh-day Adventist Church.

11. Primary prevention and health education shall be an integral part of the health emphasis of Seventh-day Adventist health care institutions.

12. The administration and operation of Seventh-day Adventist health care institutions shall include consultation with the Health Ministries Department on a regular and continuing basis. Consultation shall include the mission/conference, union, division, and General Conference Health Ministries Departments as circumstances and occasion may indicate.

APPENDIX G
A Physician Explains Drugs, Herbs, and Natural Remedies

At almost every seminar I have conducted on the subject of spiritualism in medical care, also at book signing endeavors someone will come to me, usually with a sarcastic tone and ask the question: *Well, what about drugs?* I may answer: "what about them", so as to better draw out the understanding of this subject by the individual asking the question. The insinuation toward me is that I should have included the use of pharmaceuticals as spiritualism in the information I had shared with those in attendance. (See chapter 17 "Those Who Do Magical Arts" for a discussion of the Greek word from which our word "sorcery" has derivation.)

This subject has been the source of much contention for many years. Dr. Mervyn Hardinge was concerned over this subject and the controversy surrounding it during his years as a physician and an instructor in pharmacology in the school of medicine at Loma Linda. After retirement he had the time to do the research needed on this topic and to present it in the book *A Physician Explains Ellen White's Counsel on Drugs, Herbs, and Natural Remedies.* I highly recommend to any person having interest in this subject to secure his book at an Adventist Book Center and read it from cover to cover. It is a fascinating discourse and most enlightening. It answered the questions I had on this subject.

Ellen White from the mid 1860's onward spoke strongly against the use of "drugs" for therapy in illness. The following are snippets of quotes concerning use of drugs: "Parents sin against their selves as well as against their future children"; "Drug medication as it is usually practiced is a curse"; "Drugs never cure"; "The Lord is strongly opposed to the use of drugs in our medical work." etc., etc..

These statements seem strange when we realize anesthetics which would be poisonous gasses—drugs, are used to put people to sleep for surgery and bone setting. She never spoke against surgery and did say that angels and Christ attended Dr. Kellogg in surgery. These questions have caused great controversy since they were stated. However, she said to not let such be a controversy. Dr. Mervyn Hardinge researched this subject to find answers to this paradox, after he retired from directing the Loma Linda School of Health. He then wrote a book sharing with us what he learned from his research.

LETTER FROM EDGAR CARO TO E.G. WHITE: 1893(third year medical student)

> Several of the students are in doubt as to the meaning of the word *drug* as mentioned in the article by E.G. White, **How To Live,** he said "Does it refer only to the stronger medicines as mercury, strychnine, arsenic, and such poisons, the things we medical students call *drug*, or does it also include the simpler remedies, as potassium, iodine, squills, etc.? We know that our success will be proportionate to our adherence to God's methods. For this reason I have asked the above question. (Edgar Caro letter, 1893, quoted in 2SM p. 278).

E.G. White's answer: "Your questions, I will say, are answered largely, if not definitely, in *How to Live.* Drug poisons mean the articles which you have mentioned. The simpler remedies are less harmful in proportion to their simplicity; but in very many cases these are used when not at all necessary. There are simple herbs and roots that every family may use for themselves and need not call a physician any sooner than they would call a lawyer. I do not think that I can give you any definite line of medicines compounded and dealt out by doctors that are perfectly harmless. *And yet it would not be wisdom to engage in controversy over this subject"* (letter 17a, 1893, quoted in 2SM 279). (Emphasis added)

Points made:

1. Mrs. White named as drugs, opium (which contains codeine and morphine), calomel (which is a form of mercury), and nux vomica (strychnine).
2. "Drug poisons mean the articles which you have mentioned." Terms used in the letters: "stronger medicines" used by Edgar, "drug poisons" used by White.
3. Caro: "Does it refer only to the stronger medicines... or does it also include the simpler remedies?" White: "Drug poisons mean the articles which you have mentioned." (This answer excludes the simpler medicines.)
4. Simpler remedies: "The simpler remedies are less harmful in proportion to their simplicity." She points out that they are not harmless and must be used with caution.

White considered the common herbs (catnip tea) used by laity and also the same substance used by a physician under a Latin name as a "simple". (19 MR 48)

White speaks of using "catnip tea, hop tea, strong coffee, and dark tea," as medicine only. (Letter 12, 1888, quoted in CD 490; manuscript 3, 1888, quoted in 2SM 301,302; letter 20, 1882, quoted in 2SM 302,303.)

5. **"And yet it would not be wisdom to engage in controversy over this subject"** (2SM 279)

However, this controversy has existed through the years, not only in US, but in all countries where Mrs. White's writings are translated. It (the controversy) is often emphasized, aggravated and transported from US, Australia and other countries to other countries. It has at times caused severe conflict between believers, even to the degree to bringing about divisions. These divisions tend to be of two groups, 1) physicians and people who chose to conservatively use medication yet still believe and follow lifestyles that are preventive in nature. 2) Physicians (very few) and people (many) who believe that everything prescribed by a physician is considered a drug and harmful, and restrict their use to medicinal herbs, hydrotherapy, and other "natural" remedies.

E.G. White strongly condemned the harsh, poisonous preparations dispensed for treatment of the sick. This included minerals and poisonous herbs. She did not include in this advice the more simple remedies, yet cautioned that with proper living habits and diet there would seldom be a need to use the simplest remedies.

APPENDIX H
SATAN'S GROUND

Often, after I have presented information that exposes a particular technique of healing as having a spiritualistic connotation, I receive the comment that because a technique may have been used over time in an occult or pagan setting; does not of itself incriminate the therapy. This comment usually comes because the individual speaking is persuaded of the benefits of a particular discipline of treatment and believes there is some physiologic explanation for its working power. It seems that little or no caution in accepting a therapy that has a long history of being a part of a religious belief seems to be prudent with these individuals. Their insinuation to me is that to be concerned of the spiritual connection is equivalent to being on a *witch hunt*."

The Biblical Research Committee of the General Conference of Seventh-day Adventists in 1987 presented a paper on their study of the New Age Movement and Seventh-day Adventists (See Appendix E). The issue: can we consider any technique that has long been a part of occultism, Hinduism, or some other pagan religion as neutral or safe, even if we disavow any aspect of the religion or belief system in our use of the technique? A technique which originated out of a belief system and used as an integral part of it? Would this be what E.G. white refers to as *Satan's ground*.

The Committee's conclusion on this matter was that in their judgment there is no neutral or safe use of such a method. There is too strong a connection to the mind-set of its prior origin and usage to be entirely free of the spiritual influence of its past. It constitutes "Satan's ground."

Ellen G. White's View on Occult Healing. Ellen White did recognize that occult healers claimed to heal through the manipulation of electrical currents. In fact, she claimed that the healers were "channels for Satan's electric currents." In an article entitled "Shall We Consult Spiritualist Physicians" (part of Testimony 5, p. 193 published in 1882) she spoke to this issue, basing her remarks on King Ahaziah's appeal to Baalzebub the god of Ekron for healing (see 2 Kings 1):

> *The heathen oracles have their counterpart in the spiritualistic mediums, the clairvoyants, and fortunetellers of today.* The mystic voices that spoke at Endor are still by their lying words misleading the children of men. *The prince of darkness has but appeared under a new guise....* While they (modern people)

speak with scorn of the magicians of old, the great deceiver laughs in triumph as they yield to his arts under a different form.

His agents still claim to cure disease. They attribute their power to electricity, magnetism, or the so-called "sympathetic remedies." In truth, they are but channels for Satan's electric currents. By this means he casts his spell over the bodies and souls of men.

I have from time to time received letters both from ministers and lay members of the church, inquiring if I think it wrong to consult spiritualist and clairvoyant physicians. I have not answered these letters for want of time. But just now the subject is again urged upon my attention. So numerous are these agents of Satan becoming, and so general is the practice of seeking counsel from them, that it seems needful to utter words of warning....

Not a few in this Christian age and Christian nation resort to evil spirits rather than trust to the power of the living God. The mother, watching by the sickbed of her child, exclaims: "I can do no more. Is there no physician who has power to restore my child?" She is told of the wonderful cures performed by some clairvoyant or magnetic healer, and she trusts her dear one to his charge, placing it as verily in the hands of Satan as if he were standing by her side. In many instances the future life of the child is controlled by a satanic power which it seems impossible to break....

In the name of Christ I would address His professed followers: Abide in the faith which you have received from the beginning. Shun profane and vain babblings. *Instead of putting your trust in witchcraft, have faith in the living God.* Cursed is the path that leads to Endor or to Ekron. The feet will stumble and fall that venture upon the forbidden ground. There is a God in Israel, with whom is deliverance for all that are oppressed. Righteousness is the habitation of His throne....

Angels of God will preserve His people while they walk in the path of duty, but there is no assurance of such protection for those who deliberately venture upon **Satan's ground**. An agent of the great deceiver will say and do anything to gain his object. It matters little whether he calls himself a spiritualist, an "electric physician," or a "magnetic healer." By specious pretenses he wins the confidence of the unwary....

Those who give themselves up to the sorcery of Satan may boast of great benefit t received thereby, but does this prove their course to be wise or sage? What if life should be prolonged? Will it pay in the end to disregard the will of God? All such apparent gain will prove at last an irrecoverable loss. We cannot with impunity break down a single barrier which God has erected to guard

His people from Satan's power. (Testimonies, vol. 5, 193-4, 197-99, emphasis added)

The counsel is clear. In harmony with the Bible, Ellen White recognizes the presence of Satan and evil angels behind the occult systems of healing. To pursue recovery from sickness at such sources simply opens the door to satanic deception and control. The Ellen G. White writings give no support to the holistic health's pantheistic view of reality and emphatically rejects this approach to healing.

Definitions of "**SATAN'S GROUND**" by E.G. White

1. "If we venture on *Satan's ground*, we have no assurance of protection from His power. So far as in us lies, we should close every avenue by which the tempter may find access to us." (Adventist Home 402.4)

2. "We must keep close to the word of God. We need its warnings and encouragement, its threatening and promises. We need the perfect example given only in the life and character of our Savior. Angels of God will preserve his people while they walk in the path of duty; but there is no assurance of such protection for those who deliberately venture upon *Satan's ground*. An agent of the great deceiver will say and do anything to gain his object. It matters little whether he calls himself a spiritualist, an *electric physician*, or a *magnetic healer.* By specious pretenses he wins the confidence of the unwary...."(Christian Temperance and Bible Hygiene p. 116)

3. "I was shown that Satan cannot control minds unless they are yielded to his control. Those who depart from the right are in serious danger now. They separate themselves from God and from the watch-care of the angels of God, and Satan, ever upon the watch to destroy souls, begins to present to such his deceptions, and they are in the utmost peril. And if they see and try to resist the powers of darkness and to free themselves from Satan's snare, it is not an easy matter. They have ventured on *Satan's ground*, and he claims them. He will not hesitate to engage all his energies, and call to his aid all his evil host to wrest a single human being from the hand of Christ." (Messages to Young People 60.1)

4. "Unless you can see that Satan is the mastermind who has devised this science (hypnotism), it will not be as easy a matter as you suppose to separate from it, root and branch. The whole philosophy of this science is a masterpiece of satanic deception. For your soul's sake, cut loose from everything of this order. Every time you put into the mind of other person ideas concerning this science, that you may gain control of his mind, you are on *Satan's ground*, decidedly cooperating with him. For your

soul's sake, break loose from this snare of the enemy."--Letter 20, 1902. (2Selected Messages 349, 350.) (2MCP 715.4)

5. "Cut away from yourselves everything that savors of hypnotism, *the science by which satanic agencies work*."—(Letter 20, 1902 Selected Messages 350)

6. *Spiritualism* is a dangerous phase of infidelity, and we should not go into the assemblies of Spiritualists prompted by motives of curiosity. In so doing we are placing ourselves on *Satan's ground*, and cannot expect help from God unless he has a work for us to do to speak some message to those who are ignorant and deceived, and immediately leave the assembly." (Signs of the Times, Sept. 3 1894)

SATAN'S GROUND:

1. Connecting with unbelievers --- Adventist Home p. 67.2
2. Reading the writings of infidel authors --- Adventist Home p. 413
3. Intemperance --- Christian Education p. 175
4. Yielding to Satan's suggestions --- Counsels on Health p. 166
5. Indulging the appetite --- Counsels on diet p. 22.4
6. Utilizing electric and or magnetic healing--- Counsels on Health p. 459
7. Mind control techniques --- Messages to Young People p. 60
8. Partaking of spurious healings --- 2 Mind, Character, and Personality p. 700
9. Hypnotism --- 2 MCP p. 715.4
10. Making our friends among the ungodly --- Patriarchs and Prophets 204
11. Making excuses for our selfishness --- 2 Special Messages p. 350
12. Mind sciences --- 2 SM p. 350
13. Over confidence in one's knowledge --- 1 Testimonies p. 428
14. Overbearing in personality --- 4 testimonies p. 431
15. Involving one's self in amusements --- The Bible Echo, Oct 15, 1894
16. Impulsive actions in discipline of children puts the children onto Satan's ground as a response to this impulsive action of the parent. Australian Signs of the Times --- March 1903
17. When we tamper with that which we should denounce --- Review and herald Aug. 11, 1903 open letter
18. Attending assemblies of spiritualists unless to warn others of their danger --- Sign of the times Sept. 3, 1894
19. Rebellion --- Sings of the Times De. 13, 1899; Our Besetting Sins
20. Speculating investments --- 4 Testimonies p. 600
21. Discouragement --- Christian Leadership 64.2

22. Disobedience --- D.A. 129
23. Inappropriate expulsion from schools --- Fundamentals of Christian Education 277,8
24. Miracles in our sight --- MYP 61.1
25. Lack of self-effort to overcome --- Testimonies to Ministers 453
26. Allow the mind to come to the superficial and unreal --- MYP 252.3
27. Satan's theories --- Letter 175, 1904
28. Seeking pleasure among those who fear not God --- PP 204
29. Railing accusation --- Reflecting Christ 70.6
30. Criticism --- Sketches from the Life of Paul 233,4
31. Self-rightness, argumentive nature --- 1 testimonies 428
32. Fretting, fault finding --- 4 testimonies 341
33. Careless, unconcerned when one should be --- 4 T. 460
34. Accusing the Brethren --- Misc. Collections Spalding and Magan
35. Fretful, impatient --- 21 Manuscript releases 1501-1598 (1993)
36. Married men placing much attention to married and unmarried girls ---18 Manuscript releases 1301-59
37. Wrong choice in reading material --- 5 Manuscript Releases 347-418

APPENDIX I

Colon Cleansing and Other "Detoxification" Methods

Teaching a need for *colonic cleansing* has become popular, we hear about it on T.V. as well as the radio. The more it is spoken of and advertised the greater people believe what they hear is accurate and true. Unfortunately these teachings and practices are not supported by scientific knowledge and the theory lacks scientific testing to give it support.

Guidelines were formed by the General Conference Department of Health Ministries in the year 2009 for medical institutions within the General Conference of Seventh-day Adventists and are good recommendations for self-supporting institutions. GC Health Institutions Working Policy-2009, Section FH 20--# 3 presents some sound advice concerning practices that have crept into some institutions yet are without Biblical, Spirit of Prophecy or scientific support. Colonic irrigation for cleansing is one such practice.

A copy of section 3 follows:

> 3. The activities of the devil are rampant, both within and without the Church. The Church is warned (Col 2:8) "Beware lest any man spoil you through philosophy and vain deceit, after the tradition of men." Because of the great controversy between good and evil, Health Ministries encourages church members to avoid practices rooted in non-Christian philosophy and belief. The Church and its institutions should promote and provide competent and caring service that respects the dignity and rights of patients.

Adventist health care and ministries are to promote only those practices based upon the Bible or the Spirit of Prophecy, or evidence-based methods of disease prevention, treatment, and health maintenance. *Evidence-based* means there is an accepted body of peer reviewed, statistically significant evidence that raises probability of effectiveness to a scientifically convincing level. Practices without a firm evidence-base and not based on the Bible or the Spirit of Prophecy, including though not limited to aromatherapy, cranial sacral therapy, homeopathy, hypnotherapy, iridology, magnets, methods aligning forces of energy, pendulum diagnostics, untested herbal remedies, reflexology, *repetitive colonic irrigation*, "therapeutic touch," and urine therapy, should be discouraged. (Emphasis added)

Let us consider the *claims* of the discipline of colonic irrigation therapy.

1. We store toxins in our systems and they are not eliminated by the usual methods of metabolism by liver, skin, lungs, and kidneys.
2. Our systems are not competent to clear by products of metabolism along with foreign chemicals that come into our systems.
3. We have waste products in our tissue that our body cannot eliminate and it becomes necessary to use cleansing diets, cleansing herbs, and cleansing colonics.
4. Toxins are surrounded by fats and mucous which cling to the lining of the intestinal track to protect our immune systems, and that we may carry extra weight as a result.
5. Colonics revitalize the systems; rid our body of unwanted bacteria, viruses, and parasites.
6. Cleansing with colonics will prolong life.

When I read or hear the above pronouncements the first thought that comes to mind is, *show me the clear scientific data that substantiates these statements.* In the General Conference *Guidelines for Medical Institutions* we read that practices that are not Biblical, in harmony with Spirit of Prophecy writings, or have not been shown to be true by peer reviewed scientific literature, having undergone randomly selected, double blind, placebo controlled, cross-over testing in large numbers showing statistically significant benefits from several different research institutions showing essentially the same results, the recommendation is not to use. I am unaware of colonic irrigation therapy meeting any of these criteria.

Any health teaching or practice associated with the Seventh-day Adventist name should meet the criteria given in the G.C. guidelines. Colonic irrigation to "cleanse the systems" is not given respect by the medical community as they cannot find any scientific basis for it.

The claim that there forms a lining of the colon of a precipitated mucous, dark and rubber-like which in turn harbors parasites, reduces absorption of nutrients, increases our weight, etc., is especially repugnant to physicians. There have been millions of physicians doing multiple millions of exams by fiber optic instruments so as to view with clarity the lining of the stomach and bowels. Also, surgeries performed on bowel, autopsies, MRI exams, and microscopic histological exams would show an accumulation in the lining of the intestinal track if it were present. There are no reports of such conditions that I am aware of in medical literature.

There are some M.D.'s that are deep into the neo-pagan religions that are recommending cleansing routines, however, it stems from their belief in the Hindu cleansing practices to clear doshas (universal energy), and in the belief that it will raise universal energy up through the chakras to elevate "consciousness" into full godhood. (See chapter 7 on Ayurveda in this book.

DETOXIFICATION—CLEANSING— PURIFICATION FOOT BATHS

A popular *cleansing therapy* is a placing a person's feet in a bath of water that has electrodes from an electrical detox—machine placed within. This is a treatment said to detoxify the system. A pinch of salt is added to the water of the foot bath then for a half hour or more the person keeps his feet in the bath. Black flecks will appear and float on the water, the water turns a brownish color and there may be a bit of foam. Small bubbles of gas rise from the area of the electrodes. It is amazing the debris that may come from clear water and clean feet.

The person receiving the treatment is told that the material seen in the water and clinging to the bath pan are toxins being removed from the body. The patient is very impressed and of course feels immensely improved, even if he or she did not feel bad at the beginning. This *detox* treatment is promoted for all types of ills and even for well people to keep them healthy. It is promoted to supposedly aid people with cancer, arthritis, and most other disorders.

The electrical machines that are made and purchased to do this therapy sell from a few hundred dollars to as much as $4000, or more. However, they are made of simple inexpensive electrical components. Who gives treatments using these machines? Your local medical doctor? Osteopathic doctor? Chiropractor? Naturopath? Nurse practitioner? New Age healer? Self-proclaimed healers?

It is possible that any or all of these various practitioners will be found using the bath but it will be a rare medical doctor, osteopathic doctor, and only occasional chiropractor utilizing the detox bath. Why do not all medical practitioners treat with it so as to remove the toxins from our bodies? Is it that those not using the treatment are just ignorant, have not heard of the method, or do not want to relieve people of their toxins so they will stay ill and so promote more business? Could it be that the medical profession and other scientists do not believe that there is a true benefit from using the detoxification foot bath? Let us ask some more questions concerning toxins.

Do I really have toxins in my body that cannot be eliminated by the liver, lungs, kidneys or skin? How can one know what toxins are present? Yes, the body does receive and contain many chemicals that it needs to discard.

They come from regular metabolism, from outside sources via ingestion, inhalation, and skin absorption. The body eliminates most of these chemicals by the organs designed to eliminate them. Some toxins, such as heavy metals (mercury, lead, etc.) do cling to the tissues and are not eliminated without special chelation treatment. There are minute amounts of some chemicals in various plant sources that have ability to detoxify many chemicals and they may also turn on certain genes that promote their elimination.

It takes special testing procedures to identify toxins and there may be many that are not found by present tests. These tests are not done by the local laboratory in your hospital; they need to be sent to special labs.

A most important question in our minds should be, if I am thinking of receiving *detoxification* therapy either by herbs, colon irrigation, foot baths, or other techniques, does this treatment method do what the therapist claims it does? Have there been quality scientific tests to verify the claims of the therapist? Are highly trained scientists recommending the treatment?

There is a machine used in continuous colonic irrigations that lets one see the material from the colon as it passes through a transparent tube, does this give us proof? When herbs are taken for cleansing there may be passage of black material that the therapists tells you is composed of toxins, how do you know that it is nothing other than the herbs given you? Does the change of color of the water, floating black debris, foamy brown covering of the water from a foot bath convince you that passing toxins from your feet causes those changes seen in the water?

Is there quality medical literature supporting the claims of the *detox therapists* as to the need of and beneficial effects from such *cleansing therapies*? If so, I have not been able to find them.

I wish to share with you more about this electrical detoxification foot bath that many have great confidence in, especially after seeing the *evidence* in the water of toxins coming out of their feet. The electrical machine converts alternating electricity into direct current. The machine has two electrodes, a positive pole and a negative pole. These two poles are fastened close together but not touching, electrical current will pass from one to the other if there are "electrolytes" in water. It will not function if the water is distilled and no electrolytes present. This is why salt is placed in the bath to form electrolytes. The electrical current will move from one pole of electrodes to the other by using the charged (positive or negative) electrolytes of dissolved salt. The electrical poles are made of iron; the action of the electrical current on the iron poles forms iron oxides which are black flakes seen floating on the water, but the patient is told they are toxins from the body. The brown color of the water is from the same change of iron as is rust—iron oxide. Some fats from the feet may float in the water mixing with sodium ion from the salt and form soaps, and hence, the frothy water. Gas in minute bubbles comes up from the water at the site of the electrodes, probably chlorine gas. This comes from the chloride ion of the salt that had been placed in the water.

There is no effect on the body without the body being attached to an electrode (one wire attached to the body). All the chemical action is at the site of the electrodes. The end result, however, is so convincing that this cleansing foot bath has become popular. The physics and chemistry involved are high school level and should not fool anyone with a bit of scientific knowledge. This action of electricity in an electrolyte bath is referred to as "electrolysis." If iron is to be chrome plated it is done by electrolysis. I once visited a gold purifying plant; they were doing the final purification of gold by electrolysis. One of the electrodes attracted the gold that had been dissolved in nitric acid and only gold came to the electrode forming 99.99% pure gold.

The procedure has no effect on a person's body chemistry except for the mental belief in the method. If it were really effective in cleansing the body of toxins what would keep it from removing necessary electrolytes and chemicals from the body? Toxins may not be negatively or positively charged as are electrolytes and then they could not be affected by the electrical current.

I once shared with a therapist the science involved in the foot bath by taking a clean pan with water, placing the electrodes in it as is done with therapy, placing a pinch of salt in the water and turning the machine on for thirty minutes. No feet were placed in the pan. At the end there were black flecks floating on the water, gas had bubbled up, and the water was brown, only difference was the absence of soapy froth.

Usually the people giving the treatments of detox--foot baths believe that the process really does do what has been told to them; unfortunately they are mistaken. However, those who sell the machines are unlikely to be ignorant of the deception being promoted.

E.G. WHITE AND CLEANSING OF IMPURITIES

Searching through the writings of Ellen White for any comments about cleansing or colonic irrigations I found only the following comments about clearing "*impurities*" from our system. In all of her writings on health the word *enema* came up only one time. That was in reference to giving an enema to a sick person to reduce fever, a proper use.

1. "Personal Cleanliness Essential to Health.--Scrupulous cleanliness is essential to both physical and mental health. Impurities are constantly thrown off from the body through the skin. Its millions of pores are quickly clogged unless kept clean by frequent bathing, and the impurities

which should pass off through the skin become an additional burden to the other eliminating organs." (White, E.G., *Child Guidance* 108.2)

2. "Most persons would receive benefit from a cool or tepid bath every day, morning or evening. Instead of increasing the liability to take cold, a bath, properly taken, fortifies against cold because it improves the circulation; the blood is brought to the surface, and an easier and regular flow is obtained. The mind and the body are alike invigorated. The muscles become more flexible; the intellect is made brighter. The bath is a soother of the nerves. Bathing helps the bowels, the stomach, and the liver, giving health and energy to each, and it promotes digestion." (White, E. G., *Child Guidance* 108.3)

3. "It is important also that the clothing be kept clean. The garments worn absorb the waste matter that passes off through the pores if they are not frequently changed and washed, the impurities will be reabsorbed." (White, E.G., Child Guidance 109.1)

4. "More people die for want of exercise than from overwork; very many more rust out than wear out. In idleness the blood does not circulate freely, and the changes in the vital fluid, so necessary to health and life, do not take place. The little mouths in the skin, through which the body breathes, become clogged, thus making it impossible to eliminate impurities through that channel. This throws a double burden upon the other excretory organs, and disease is soon produced. Those who accustom themselves to exercising in the open air, generally have a vigorous circulation. Men and women, young or old, who desire health and who would enjoy life, should remember that they cannot have these without a good circulation. Whatever their business or inclinations, they should feel it a religious duty to make wise efforts to overcome the conditions of disease which have kept them in-doors." (White, E.G., *Christian Temperance & Bible Hygiene* 101.2)

5. "The lungs should be allowed the greatest freedom possible. Their capacity is developed by free action; it diminishes if they are cramped and compressed. Hence the ill effects of the practice so common, especially in sedentary pursuits, of stooping at one's work. In this position it is impossible to breathe deeply. Superficial breathing soon becomes a habit, and the lungs lose their power to expand." (White, E.G., *Counsels for the Church* 218.4)

6. "Thus an insufficient supply of oxygen is received. The blood moves sluggishly. The waste, poisonous matter, which should be thrown off in the exhalations from the lungs, is retained, and the blood becomes impure. Not only the lungs, but the stomach, liver, and brain are affected. The skin becomes sallow, digestion is retarded; the heart is depressed; the brain is clouded; the thoughts are confused; gloom settles upon the spirits; the whole system becomes depressed and inactive, and peculiarly susceptible to disease." (White, E.G., Counsels for the Church 218.5)

7. "The lungs are constantly throwing off impurities, and they need to be constantly supplied with fresh air. Impure air does not afford the necessary supply of oxygen, and the blood passes to the brain and other organs without being vitalized. Hence the necessity of thorough ventilation. To live in close, ill-ventilated rooms, where the air is dead and vitiated weakens the entire system. It becomes peculiarly sensitive to the influence of cold, and a slight exposure induces disease. It is close confinement indoors that makes many women pale and feeble. They breathe the same air over and over until it becomes laden with poisonous matter thrown off through the lungs and pores, and impurities are thus conveyed back to the blood." 371 (White, E.G., *Counsels for the Church* 218.6)

8. "The sufferers in such cases can do for themselves that which others cannot do as well for them. They should commence to relieve nature of the load they have forced upon her. They should remove the cause. *Fast* a short time, and give the stomach a chance for rest. Reduce the feverish state of the system by a careful and understanding application of water. These efforts will help nature in her struggles to free the system of impurities." (White, E.G., *Counsels on Diet and Foods* 190.1) (emphasis authors)

9. "Milk and Sugar.—large quantities of milk and sugar eaten together are injurious. They impart impurities to the system. Animals from which milk is obtained are not always healthy. Could we know that animals were in perfect health, I would recommend that people eat flesh-meats sooner than large quantities of milk and sugar. It would not do the injury that milk and sugar do." (White, E.G., *Christian Temperance & Bible Hygiene* 158.1)

10. "Ministers, teachers, and students do not become as intelligent as they should in regard to the necessity of physical exercise in the open air. They neglect this duty, a duty which is most essential to the preservation of

health. They closely apply their minds to study, and yet eat the allowance of a laboring man. Under such habits, some grow corpulent (fat), because the system is clogged. Others become thin and feeble, because their vital powers are exhausted in throwing off the excess of food. The liver is burdened, being unable to throw off the impurities of the blood, and sickness is the result. If physical exercise were combined with mental exertion, the circulation of the blood would be quickened, the action of the heart would be more perfect, impure matter would be thrown off, and new life and vigor would be felt in every part of the body." (White, E.G., *Christian Temperance & Bible Hygiene* 160.5)

11. "Indulging in eating too frequently and in too large quantities overtaxes the digestive organs and produces a feverish state of the system. The blood becomes impure, and then diseases of various kinds occur. A physician is sent for, who prescribes some drug which gives present relief, but which does not cure the disease. It may change the form of disease, but the real evil is increased tenfold. Nature was doing her best to rid the system of an accumulation of impurities, and could she have been left to herself, aided by the common blessings of Heaven, such as pure air and pure water, a speedy and safe cure would have been effected. (White, E.G., *Counsels on Diet and Foods* 304.2)

12. The sufferers in such cases can do for themselves that which others cannot do as well for them. They should commence to relieve nature of the load they have forced upon her. They should remove the cause. *Fast a short time*, and give the stomach chance for rest. Reduce the feverish state of the system by a careful and understanding application of water. These efforts will help nature in her struggles to free the system of impurities. But generally the persons who suffer pain become impatient. They are not willing to use self-denial, and suffer a little from hunger. . . ." (White, E.G., *Counsels on Diet and Foods* 304.3) (emphasis authors)

13. "The use of water can accomplish but little, if the patient does not feel the necessity of also strictly attending to his diet.'"" (White, E.G., *Counsels on Diet and Foods* 304.4)

All of E.G. White books can be obtained from <u>AdventistBookCenter.com</u>

PART II

Detoxify Your Lymphatics? What is Detoxification? By Ray Foster M.D.

The idea of needing to detoxify your lymphatic system comes from knowledge of how the body works. But perhaps the first questions are what detoxification is and what needs to be detoxified? We all know firsthand about waste. After every meal there are some scrap foods left over called waste or food scraps. If we eat a banana, we do not eat the peel. If we eat an orange, we do not normally eat the peel. The banana peel and the orange peels are left over and we call them waste. The same kind of thing happens in all the body processes. When the body digests our food, there are some indigestible *scraps* left over that we need to get rid of. These indigestible parts of our food never get inside our body and are eliminated with our normal bowel function. These indigestible parts of the food are very important to our health because they absorb harmful waste material that is on or in our food and helps the body gets rid of them in our bowel movements. Another popular name for these very helpful parts of our food is called *fiber*. The function of the colon can correctly be called detoxification as it helps the body get rid of indigestible parts of our foods and other undesirable or harmful aspects of things that we may have eaten.

It is the chemical processes that take place inside our bodies that also generate waste products that is the real "detoxification" process that our body needs to stay healthy. For instance when we exercise strongly our muscles have carbon dioxide waste and if we exercise so vigorously that you can't keep up with the oxygen demand of the muscle activity, then instead of making carbon dioxide and pyruvic acid, your body makes lactic acid. If lactic acid builds up because you do not rest but keep on exercising strongly, then muscle pain can result from the waste build-up of lactic acid. The lactic acid can still be used for energy production, but in excess it presents a problem and needs to be changed back into a useful energy source. This can be called detoxification of lactic acid. The carbon dioxide from the muscles is picked up by the blood and taken to the lungs where it is eliminated in our breathing. These are all normal examples of "detoxification" processes. There are many other examples of waste products that are produced in the body in the course of normal living processes that are many and very complicated. The body has built-in ways to deal with these waste processes that can be considered as "detoxification."

What is the Lymph System? The main organ of elimination of body waste is the skin. That is if you consider the biggest organ (the skin) as the main organ. Sweat is the substance the body makes to get rid of the unwanted substances in the body that can be called "toxins". For instance if you smoke and sweat a lot, nicotine can be smelled and seen as a yellow substance that will come out of your body in your sweat. Now the skin, the lungs, the colon, and the kidneys are the best known organs of elimination of toxins. However there is also a less well known system of elimination called the lymphatic system.

The lymphatic system is like the side-roads compared to the state and national highways. The superhighway of the body is the blood stream. The side roads are the lymphatics. They both take substances like nutrients and hormones and blood cells (the body's army) all over the body. On the return journey from taking nutrients and hormones, they carry wastes and toxins to be eliminated. The differences between the blood and the lymphatic system are many but one of them is that the lymphatics have no heart that pumps the lymph around the body. It depends on muscular action and valves in the lymph vessels to produce a flow of lymph. This is one of the reasons exercise is so vital to good health. *Detoxifying the lymphatic system* simply means increasing the speed of flow in the lymph channels. Once the lymph fluid gets back to the blood – where it is all headed – the body detoxifies any substance that needs to be detoxified. Once toxins are detoxified (rendered less harmful or not at all harmful) – mainly in the liver - then the waste products are eliminated (gotten out of the body) via the skin, lungs, large bowel, and kidneys.

How to Detoxify the Lymphatic System? The lymph system toxins are detoxified by speeding up their passage to the liver for processing and then by the bile to the large bowel for elimination, or to the blood stream where the skin, lungs, and kidneys excrete it. If there is not enough fiber in the large bowel to hold onto the toxic and toxic break down products while they are moving through the colon, then they get reabsorbed and recycled through the blood. One of the best ways to *detoxify the body* is to eat high fiber food so that the toxins the body is getting rid of through the large bowel is moved out in a timely manner and held fast by the fiber in the large bowel while in transit to being eliminated.

So how do I speed up the flow of lymph through my lymphatics? That is the key question in this subject. Two chief ways of speeding the flow of lymph is drinking 8 or more glasses of water a day and exercising 20 to 30 minutes a day. Jumping up and down on a small trampoline, walking, jogging, and weight-lifting are all excellent ways of making your lymphatics move the lymph faster and detoxifying them.

APPENDIX J

COUNTERFEIT MEDICINE

Author: Walter Thompson, M.D. , Chair, Board of 3ABN TV Used by permission

July 31, 2010

Counterfeit Medicine

Definition of a counterfeit: A copy intended to defraud--bogus, fake, fraud, ersatz, false, fraudulent, phony, spurious, deceptive, and imitative.

Intent: to deceive is an important characteristic of a counterfeit object, but the one practicing the counterfeit may simply be deceived with no intent to deceive. Satan is the chief counterfeiter, controlling many unawares. The most effective counterfeit is that which closest resembles the real thing. Therefore one should expect the fake to exhibit many resemblances of truth.

Detection: One cannot determine the nature of an object, teaching, practice, etc., except by comparing it to truth. One can never learn to detect a counterfeit by looking at other counterfeits.

Sources of truth: God is the source of all truth. He has revealed truth in the Holy Scriptures; through prophets; through the "still small voice;" in the natural world as determined by observation and scientific investigation.

Testing for truth: All things must be tested against truth as revealed in the Scriptures and honest scientific investigation—which, when correctly understood, are always in accord.

Dilemma: At times the *ancient healers* recognized healing agents, and, ignorant of the scientific processes responsible for their effects, explained those effects in terms that were familiar to them. Superstitions of all manners thrived, including the use of many, sometimes extreme, practices to *cast out* evil spirits, etc. Sometimes they saw illness as a contest between their gods of gold and wood and stone—some evil and some good. Conscious of the presence of these opposing forces acting among them, but unaware of the true nature of the controversy between God and Satan, many of these ancient peoples understood the contest as being between equals--which were, by some, described as energies—with illness the consequence of in-balance, and healing a matter of balancing these energies (the concept of chi, qi). Thus we have, in certain Eastern cultures, such practices as the use of herbs and combination of herbs, foods, *hot* and *cold* and needles placed in pre-specified points on *meridians* of energy flows (and many others) as a means of restoring balance and improving health.

Many of these concepts and actions remain with us today, though frequently disguised to reveal their true origin. Based upon modern scientific study, we now know that there is a bit of truth in many, and perhaps, most of these. For example, recent studies of acupuncture do suggest improvement of some conditions over placebos—equal to some other recognized treatments for the same condition. We also know from modern research that reflexes in the feet do indeed interface with pathways in the brain and other portions of the body. Many herbs are now found to have definite functions equal or more effective than medications for some conditions.

Acknowledging these apparent benefits, what should be our stance regarding encouraging the practice of them? The dilemma is magnified by the fact that modern, high tech health care also has its limitations and complications.

Should the fact that many of these *alternative* practices have their roots in Eastern concepts of balancing the energies of good and evil, in a sense accepting Satan's claim that evil is a necessary force in the universe for the ultimate benefit of all, eliminate them from applying their demonstrated benefits? How can we know?

Testing! Examine everything and accept only that which passes the test. Does it coincide with the principles of Holy Writ? Does it stand up under careful scientific study? Does it do both?

The Bible takes the position that Jesus is the way, the truth and the life. God is truth. That which is mixed with error is not truth, even though it may contain elements of truth. God is also love. Love always seeks to enhance life. It is not selfish and has no ulterior incentive— wealth, notoriety or power over others. Furthermore, the Bible provides all of the information necessary for optimum life, in this world and for eternity beyond. Tried and tested divine inspiration outside of the Bible may enhance and embellish Biblical truths, but will not in any way diminish or detract from them. Personal messages from the *Spirit* will, like other inspiration, test true when compared with the Holy Scriptures and with honest science. Ultimately, true practices will give all of the glory and praise to God, Creator, Redeemer, Sustainer and true healer.

True science will support all of the above elements of truth. Just as predicted in the Bible, our generation has been blessed with massive volumes of knowledge of how things work. Technology has permitted us to "see" life down to the very atomic level. Never before in history have human beings known so much about the functions of the human body in all of its spheres--physical, mental, social and spiritual. Though knowledge may permit us to do all manner of activities designed to prevent disease and to assist healing of the sick, unless it fulfills the Biblical qualifications, it too may be bogus. It, too, must fulfill the qualities of love to God and to our fellow men, if it is to obtain the endorsement of heaven. Even double blind studies may prove faulty if conducted with even the slightest aspiration for personal or corporate gain. Science, too, must past the Biblical test. Does our modern, high tech, health care pass the test of love for God and for our fellow men? Does God receive the glory of our apparent successful treatment programs?

In order to pass the scientific test, "alternative" practices and procedures must pass the same tests as generally applied to modern high tech medicine— blinded and double blinded tests; and reproducible, statistically demonstrated benefits that measurably exceed the potential risks. (Emphasis added)

Modern medicine, when practiced by God-fearing practitioners meets the Biblical standard. It provides the knowledge and opportunity to apply all Biblical principles of love and truth. Though it possesses the potential to pass the Biblical and scientific tests, it can be abused if God is ignored.

Many forms of *alternative* medicine contain elements of truth, but also contain detectable fallacies, and are thereby unable to fulfill the requirements of the test. Some may meet the Biblical standard, but miss the scientific standard. Others may meet the scientific standard while missing the Biblical mark.

Those utilizing these alternative approaches to health care and those seeking care from them would do well to place the practice under consideration to the scrutiny of the tests. Do they satisfy the standards of the Bible? Can they be defended by scientific methodology? If they fail on either account, they must be considered counterfeit and inspired by the conspiracy deceits of Satan. They are dangerous.

Just one example: Mary's only son (let us call him Mathew) was admitted to the local hospital intensive care unit in extremis. In spite of extensive lab tests, imaging studies with MRI's, PET scanners, and all the rest high tech has to offer, it appeared that Mathew was going to die without even having a diagnosis. Mary was frantic. Is there not anyone that can figure out what is wrong and give her son the right treatment, she wondered, and sometimes expressed to sympathizing friends. Just when it appeared the battle would be lost, Mary was told of an old "holy man" who was skilled in balancing the forces of energy that are believed by some to be the cause for illness. Mary figured she had nothing to lose by hiring his services for Mathew. He was already dying. What could be worse, she thought. The "holy man" came and performed his rituals. Not long afterward Mathew began to improve, and little by little recovered completely.

There is an ancient truism; *all that glitters is not gold!* The fact that Mathew's recovery appeared to coincide with the service of the holy man does not prove cause and effect. Neither does it prove the old man's god was more concerned for Mary or more powerful than Mary's God. But on this day, Mary's faith was shaken, and Mary will never forget the act of the "holy man" or his god on Mathew's behalf.

Frequently I encounter patients and/or their families who have sought help from caregivers, either by modern high tech, or by those using "alternative" means, who have recovered health after long sessions of intercessory prayer in combination with the physical measures. Not uncommonly credit is given to the healer who has applied the technology or practice, rather than to God, the true healer—just as illustrated by the foregoing account. Are we truly ministering to a patient if we succeed in relieving pain, or even prolonging life, if we fail to offer them, or more un-lovingly, lead them astray by our witness of word or example?

I noted above that the Bible provides all that is necessary for optimal health and long life, both for the here and now, and for eternity. For many reasons most people are unwilling and/or unable to abide by these principles— both for preventing disease, and for treating it when it appears. While no God-inspired care giver would refuse to minister to such a patient, neither would he/she offer such a one less than Bible consideration to the scrutiny of the tests. Do they satisfy them as God loves them!

Knowing this, how does one living today make wise decisions in choosing his/her health care? There can be only one answer to this question. Principles of truth have been well described in the Bible, and we are admonished to test all things by these principles. Health care is no exception. Whether we are speaking about modern, high-tech medical care, or some type of alternative health care the principles are the same. The Bible is a fit standard by which to judge the validity of scientific "facts" as well as claims that have no real scientific confirmation. The bottom line is this. Life comes from God. He is the only source of life. He created us, redeemed us and sustains us. He is our only true source of health and healing. Anything that leads us away from Him and causes us to put our trust in some other person, concept or procedure has its roots in the underworld and should be avoided at all costs.

Relief of symptoms – or even miraculous healing of malignant disease, is not a safe determinant of truth and validity. In fact, all through the centuries, hurting people have been led away from the only true source of life by miraculous relief of symptoms and/or cure, apparent or real, from some terrible disease. On the other hand, the healing power of God administered by dedicated lay persons and professionals often softens hard hearts and opens doors for the reception of the gospel whether or not a miracle of healing occurs.

The fact that much of what we call alternative care has its roots in deception does not necessarily indicate that all alternative care is either evil or ineffective any more than modern medicine is either evil or ineffective. All of the devil's *tricks* begin with a kernel of truth that he then distorts and reshapes to direct one's attention away from God, our Creator, to himself. Let us look at one example. The Bible tells us that God placed the rainbow in the sky after the flood as a covenantal promise that such a flood would never again destroy the earth. Yet, Satan has taken that symbol of a rainbow and linked it with *New Age* philosophies and healing and with homosexuality. This fact does not in any way detract from the promise God made to His followers so long as they remember the truth, recognize the lie, and shun it.

Moses, author of the first five books of the Bible, wrote by inspiration that if the people were faithful to the words of God they would not suffer any of the ills of the Egyptians among whom they lived. (Exodus 15:26) And even though Moses had been raised and educated by the Egyptians and trained in health care practices by them, he did not include those practices in the inspired writings of the Bible.

The following critical criteria are proposed as guides to help one determine the safety and validity of all forms of health care, including alternative care. These principles alone will lead to true healing of body, mind and spirit and fit one for optimizing life here and now and in preparing one for eternal life with God when life on earth is over.

Alternative care that meets the following criteria may be considered true and valid:

> It acknowledges that God is the source of all healing – in word and in practice.

> It follows the principles outlined in the Bible and inspired writings when planning and administering health care.

> It passes careful scientific investigation.

> Physical healing is frequently followed by spiritual healing.

> The health care provider recognizes his/her role as servant of God and gives Him the glory for the good results rather than taking the glory for him/herself.

The following alternative care practices should raise red flags when encountered:

> They may appear to give healing, or may indeed heal a given illness, but come short of offering one a faith relationship with God that alone is able to heal the whole person-- body, mind, and spirit--and to take away the alienation that sin has caused between man and God.

The health care giver depends upon his/her own powers, i.e., education, intellect, special training, etc., as the primary agent of healing.

Products designed or created for market value rather than for the benefit of the client's health.

Marketing schemes that discredit tested and tried truths, procedures, techniques, products, etc.

Marketing designed to make a profit rather than to make the product available to as wide a cliental as possible at the most economical price.

The caregiver claims special qualities to his/her therapeutic technique, medication, procedure, etc.

Healing is credited to manipulation of universal energy – example: yin and yang.

It utilizes mind "emptying" meditation and/or communications with the universal mind.

It uses all forms of magic, paranormal phenomenon, communication with the dead, etc.

The caregiver stands to profit from "hidden" benefits!

Nature, rather than nature's God often gets the credit for the healing that occurs.

It may appear to be scientifically defensible, but fails to conform to the Word of God in the Bible – a valid test for true science.

APPENDIX K
CHARACTERISTICS OF MODERN SPIRITUALISM

Characteristics of Modern Spiritualism listed in this appendix are direct quotations from the book, *The Great Controversy* by Ellen G. White.

1. Power to heal: "He doeth great wonders, so that he maketh fire come down from heaven on the earth in the sight of men, and deceiveth them that dwell on the earth by the means of those miracles which he had power to do." Revelation 13:13. *"No mere impostures are here foretold. Men are deceived by the miracles which Satan's agents have power to do, not which they pretend to do."* p. 553. (emphasis added)

2. "Ye shall be as Gods," he declares, "knowing good and evil." Genesis 3:5. p. 554.

3. Spiritualism teaches "that man is the creature of progression; that it is his destiny from his birth to progress, even to eternity, toward the God head." "Each mind will judge itself and not another." "The judgment will be right, because it is the judgment of self." p. 554.

4. "The throne is within you." Said a spiritualistic teacher, as the "spiritual consciousness" awoke within him: "My fellow men, all were unfallen demigods." p. 554.

5. And another declares: "Any just and perfect being is Christ." p. 554

6. And to complete his work, he declares (Satan), through the spirits that "true knowledge places man above all law;" that "whatever is right is right;" that "all sins which are committed are innocent." that "God doth not condemn;" and "that all sins that are committed are innocent." p. 555.

7. When the people are thus led to believe that desire is the highest law, that liberty is license, and that man is accountable only to himself, who can wonder that corruption and depravity teem on every hand. p. 555.

8. The reins of self-control are laid upon the neck of lust; the powers of mind and soul are made subject to the animal propensities. p.556

9. If there were no other evidence of the real character of spiritualism, it should be enough for the Christian that the spirits make no difference between righteousness and sin, between the noblest and purest of the apostles of Christ and the most corrupt of the servants of Satan. pp. 556-7

10. The spiritualists teachers virtually declare: "Everyone that doeth evil is good in the sight of the Lord, and He delighteth in them; or, where is the God of judgment?" Malachi 2:17, p. 557.

11. They deny the divine origin of the Bible, and thus tear away the foundation of the Christian's hope and put out the light that reveals the way to heaven." p. 557.

12. Satan is making the world believe that the Bible is a mere fiction, to be lightly regarded, obsolete." p. 557.

13. It is true that spiritualism is now changing its form and, veiling some of its more objectionable features, is assuming a Christian guise. pp. 557-558.

14. While it formerly denounced Christ and the Bible, it now professes to accept both. p. 558.

15. Love is dwelt upon as the chief attribute of God, but it is degraded to a weak sentimentalism, making little distinction between good and evil right and wrong. p. 558.

16. The people are taught to regard the Decalogue as a dead letter. p. 558.

17. God's justice, His denunciations of sin, the requirement of His holy law, are all kept out of sight. p. 558.

18. In the class here described are included those who in their stubborn impenitence comfort themselves with the assurance that there is to be no punishment for the sinner; that all mankind, it matters not how corrupt, are to be exalted to heaven. p. 560.

19. Satan has substituted the sinful, erring nature of man himself as the only

object of adoration, the only rule of judgment, or standard of character. p. 554.

20. All whose faith is not firmly established upon the word of God will be deceived and overcome....But he can gain his object only as men voluntarily yield to his temptations. p. 560.

Addendum on Yoga:

A most dangerous concept is that we can separate yoga and yoga exercises from their roots, practice them, and be free of their spiritual influence. Connie J. Fait is a former Tibetan nun, yogi, and head of a Tibetan Buddhist Temple who practiced, studied, and taught yoga and it traditions for forty years prior converting to Christianity. She warns of the spiritual association of the practice of yoga exercises and postures even devoid of meditation. She makes the following comment: (see gtto://winebifgrace,cin/blog/?p=29077) posted April 7, 2014 "The knowledge of the Yogic Tradition is deeply hidden in mystery, and only understood by accomplished yogis who have passed on those secrets orally to one another for 5000 years. Yoga asanas (postures) are recognized as the main tool to realize these secrets and is accomplished only through a process of experience. Anyone who is doing yoga asanas is in that same process – whether or not they are aware of it or intend it."

She further explains that yoga asanas are the basis for the theology of Hinduism. From the start of Hinduism, recluse yogis sat yearning for union with their believed creator "Brahman." As they sat in mystical mind altered states, spontaneous physical movements occurred, referred to as "kriyas" now called "asanas." In the practice of these postures they would experience high meditative states and experience contact with deities who appeared to them. Specific poses were named for those gods. Frequently various types of unexplained physical distress occur to those doing these postures.

APPENDIX L
HOW CAN I TELL GOOD FROM BAD? QUESTIONS TO ASK

Set 1. What is the origin of the method? By whom, where, when, why?
Was it tested by other independent scientists and were the results positive?
Does it have a history of occult or mystical associations?
Does its originator have a history of psychic and or Eastern mysticism beliefs?
What is the long term history of the originator?

Set 2. What other treatment methods does it utilize or associate with?
Who uses it? Is it similar to other alternative treatment methods yet with a slight variation and with a name change?

Set 3. Is it said to balance, unclog, infuse, or correct energy? Does it promote concepts of "frequency," "vibrations," "electromagnetic forces?" Does it find the power of correction or healing from inside our bodies, from self? Where does it lead to? Do the proponents of it claim that it raises level of consciousness? Do you receive electric like shock sensations, feeling of great warmth, deep love, tingling of your body or extremities, etc.?

Set 4. Does the treatment harmonize with known laws of science?
Does it promote known laws of health and point to God's laws of health?
Is there solid data from science testing that supports it value?
Does it have a track record of observation by qualified appraisers?
What are the critics saying about it and what are their credentials?

Set 5. What or who receives the credit for healing?
What qualifications does the promoter or practitioner have?

Set 6. **DOES IT MAKE COMMON SENSE?**

Origin of Martial arts:

In the mid-fifth century, an Indian Buddhist Monk, Bodhidharma came from India to the Shaolin Temple (Hall of Three Buddha's) in the Hunan province of China. He had revised Hinduism (referred to as Chan Buddhism), and he brought yoga to the Shaolin Temple monastery. "Legend tells that it was he who taught the monks the methods of physical movement combined with their meditation to enhance spiritual (occult) abilities. Through certain breathing, visualization techniques, and acts of worship, the monks were said to develop almost supra-natural psychic and physical powers." Bodhidharma had written a small book *The Muscle/Tendon Change Classics* which was found at the temple following his death. The book outlined spiritual and physical exercises which would enable the Buddhist to reach *enlightenment*. Thus, from Indian yoga developed the martial arts of the Buddhist. The practice spread to Japan, Okinawa, and Korea. Each country brought forth additional styles and names for the practice.

This book by Bodhidharma is given great respect by martial artists worldwide. It outlines the foundation of all martial art forms including qi gong. The book presents meditation, attention to breathing, and visualization practices which have great similarity to a book written in 1522-1524, *The Spiritual Exercises of Ignatius Loyola.* The philosophy of Ignatius's book has very close similarity to those of Hinduism, Buddhism, and Taoism.

GLOSSARY

A

A.A.—abbreviation for Alcoholics Anonymous, at times "AA"

Abrams' black box—box that was used in divining

Abram's box—electrical—mechanical box used for divination

absent healing—healing a patient from a long distance

aconite—very poisonous plant used as a remedy in homeopathy

Acupuncture according to Voll—a special method of doing acupuncture by using electrical contacts on supposed acupuncture points. Also known as "EVA"

acupuncture points—localized places on skin said to give access to movement of chi in meridians, supposedly channels for carrying chi

Acupuncture Watch—an Internet web site that reports on and critiques or exposes acupuncture (www.acuwatch.org)

acupuncture—placing needles in skin on acupuncture points for therapy

Adonay—term used in Free—Masonry to apply to Jesus Christ and considered to be the God of darkness and evil

Agni—fire in the body, actually normal metabolism, also a Hindu deity

Ahaziah—son of Ahab, King of Israel following death of Ahab

aikido—one form of martial art

Akron, Ohio—city where beginning of Alcoholics Anonymous began and Dr. Bob & Anne Smith lived

alchemical—refers to a pre-chemistry discipline of medieval times, attempt by chemical changes to bring transformation of one thing into another. Example—base metal into Gold; mortality into immortality

alchemist—person practicing alchemy, looking for secret of life

alchemy—forerunner of chemistry, however an alchemist was attempting to change one substance into another by physical means, but also to change the soul from mortal to immortal (spiritual alchemy)

Alcoholic Foundation—foundation established by Rockefeller organization to help AA in its start

Alcoholics Anonymous Comes of Age—book written after 20 years functioning of AA, written by a cofounder (Bill Wilson) , official book published by Alcoholics Anonymous World Services Inc.

Alcoholics Anonymous World Services, Inc.—business organization which is controller of the program of Alcoholics Anonymous worldwide and holds copyrights to their books

Aldous Huxley—a well know author in his day, New Age promoter, participated in use of LSD with Bill W.

Alexander, Jack—writer for the *Saturday Evening Post* who wrote in an article 1941 about AA which initiated the growth of AA

Alice Bailey—author of books directing the growth of New Age movement, all were messages channeled from a spirit guide, "The Tibetan Master" or "Djwhal Khul"

allergen—substance that stimulates our immune system to produce antibodies

Allison, Nancy—author of *The Illustrated Encyclopedia of Body/Mind Disciplines*

alpha—first

omega—last, end

altered state of consciousness— referring to a change of mental state from the active mind

alternative—non-evidence-based, non-conventional therapy, refers to acupuncture, reflexology, etc., any treatment not shown to be scientifically evidence-based

aluminum—mineral of the earth, found in some gems

Alzheimer's Disease—mental disorder, memory fades causing senility

ama—imaginary white sticky substance in colon said to be spread through the cells of the body, called a toxin, term from Hinduism's Ayurveda concepts. Has never been seen or isolated

amber—petrified pitch, usually from pine tree

American Medical Society—society of American physicians organized to promote their interest, does not have any legal control over individual physicians

amulets—objects, artifacts, symbols, etc., worn to ward off bad luck or harm and illness, believed to possess supernatural powers

anatomist—person who is instructor or has special knowledge of anatomy

Ancient Wisdom—pagan religion of ancient Babylon and mystery schools secret doctrine, man is God.

anesthesiologist—medical doctor, specialist in giving anesthesia

animal magnetism—same as universal energy, vital force, etc.

animate—living substance

animism—attribution of conscious life to nature as a whole or to inanimate objects, same as paganism and basic same beliefs but more specific to Africa and some Far Eastern peoples. Belief in a universal energy, nature worship

Ankerberg, John—Minister and co-author of *Can You Trust Your Doctor?*

anthroposophy— definition— knowledge concerning man: similar to theosophy but stresses the spiritual path as outlined by Rudolf Steiner, who had been member of Theosophy Society, but left it to establish his own following.

antibodies—usually a protein made by an animal to fight foreign invaders, germs, viruses, etc.

antidote—solution for a problem, often referred to a potion to cure some ailment

aphrodisiac—a substance felt to stimulate sexual powers

Apollo—Greek God, in Mythology

apothecary—pharmacy

applied kinesiology—mystical testing of muscles to determine weak internal organ, allergies, etc.

Aries—ram of the zodiac

aromatherapy—using fragrances and aromas from plants in medical treatment

asanas—postures of yoga

ascended masters—deceased individuals who supposedly have become immortal spirits and communicate with the living. Actually fallen angels of Satan

Asclepios—Greek God of healing

assessment—a process of running the palms of the hands above a body to feel the energy pattern said to be present

astral body—one of several imaginary energy bodies or levels of universal energy above the material body. From this energy body astral travel is said to occur i.e., out of body experiences, etc. At death, this body is said to leave the material body and exist in an astral plane.

astrologer—one practicing astrology

astrologic medicine—medical therapy practiced by using information obtained from the zodiac

astrological concepts—beliefs in sun, moon, and stars having strong influence and association with man and the earth

astrology—belief that the gods live in the planets and that the sun, moon, and stars guide the destiny of man

atheistic—denies existence of God

atonement—at-one-ment with God achieved through Jesus Christ **attuned**— initiated into being a Reiki practitioner. occultic/ spiritistic

aura—presumed body of energy arising out the chakras and radiating ten to twelve inches from the body, supposedly in colors of the rainbow. Cannot be scientifically demonstrated. A Hindu concept

auricular therapy—using the external ear for acupuncture/acupressure instead of the body. Supposedly represents the whole body

Ayurvedic system—Ancient Indian Healing Tradition, involves believing in universal energy called prana, energy which is believed to travel through the body via chakras

Aztecs—civilization in Mexico prior to the Spaniards arrival

B

Baalzebub—idol god of city of Ekron in Bible days

Babylon—city in ancient times and now in ruins, in country of Iraq

Babylonian mysteries—religious secret initiatory rites and ceremonies originating from the ancient city of Babylon. Consisted of the principles of pagan religions and promoting the "Deity of Man."

Bach Flower Remedies—38 flower essences originated by Dr. Bach an English physician. Flowers are placed in water and the sun allowed to shine on them which is believed to impart vital energy. Water then used as medicinal

Bach, Edward, M.D.—originator of flower essences, English physician

Baiame—name of supreme spirit god of Australian Aborigines

Baker, Douglas—author of *Esoteric Healing,* and occultist

Bavarian Academy of Science—organization of scientists of Bavaria

Beatles—British musical group

belladonna treatment—the mixture of two hallucinatory medicines taken from plants and given to patients in detoxification treatment for alcoholism

Benson, C. Irving—minister who was an Oxford Group member

Benson, Herbert, M.D.— Professor at Harvard School of Medicine and author of book, *The Relaxation Response, Your Maximum Mind,* on the faculty of Harvard Medical School and who has had influence in the field of mental health treatment. He advocates the "Relaxation Response" which is similar to autogenic training and/ or Eastern meditation. Teachings similar to Buddhism

Bergson, Anika—co-author of *Zone Therapy*

Bernard, Theos— an American author and practitioner of yoga and Buddhism

Besant, Annie (Aka Bessant)—directed the Theosophy Society afterdeath of Blavatsky, also vice pres. of the French Co-Masonry

Bewitched— attracted with pleasure to something

Biblical World View—belief in the origin of life as described by the Bible, the purpose of life, the future and after life, as presented by the Bible.

Bill Wilson (Bill W.) —cofounder of Alcoholics Anonymous

biochemical—chemicals involved with cellular chemistry, activity of chemicals in bio-systems

bioelectric energy—electricity formed within a biological system

biofeedback—autogenic training (self-hypnosis) using an electrical measuring device to observe temperature, blood pressure, brain wave patterns, etc., while placing oneself into theta brain wave status and self-hypnosis

bioplasma—universal energy, the name that Russians use

biopsy—to take tissue from the body for microscopic exam for analysis

bio-resonance—referring to sound resonance as ascertained by voice analysis

Bird, Christopher—author of *The Divining Hand*

black magic—sorcery, to cause to happen something bad or destructive

Blavatsky, Helena—one of the originators of the Theosophy Society, 1875, spiritualist and by channeling wrote foundational books for the Theosophy Society and New Age

blue book—refers to the official book, *Alcoholics Anonymous* used in fellowship meetings

Bob, Smith, M.D. —an alcoholic and cofounder of A.A. who lived in Akron, OH

bobbing—a form of water divining by use of a straight wire extending from the knee when in the sitting position. A reaction is when the end of the wire that has been curled and a light bulb placed in it rises and falls indicating the distance by increments to water. Each rise and fall indicates a certain distance as pre-chosen by the diviner.

body therapy—various types of body treatments such as massage, Rolfing, etc.

body/mind/spirit—a whole person with equal influence of each part

breastplate—rectangular heavy cloth with three rows of four gemstones worn on chest of high priests of Israel

Breath of Life—power involved in craniosacral therapy, same as chi, prana, vital force etc.; power that Dr. Upledger attributes to healing in craniosacral therapy

Brint, Armand—astrologer and iridologist

Buchwald, Dedra, M.D. —faculty member of University of Washington, Seattle, WA. Wrote article appearing in the *Annals in Internal Medicine* reporting study on acupuncture for fibromyalgia

Buckman, Frank—founder of Oxford Group

Buddhism—religion of Buddha's philosophy, a religion split off from Hinduism

Burns, Dick—An alcoholic who had gained sobriety through AA and then wrote thirty or more books promoting AA as a Christian organization

C

Cabbala (Cabala, Kabalah, Kabbalah, Kabbala)—Jewish secret society

Cachora—an Indian Shaman of the Yaqui tribe

caduceus—a symbol of a rod with wings at the top and with two snakes ascending it; ancient symbol of medicine

calcium—mineral of earth and found in some stone formations

calomel—mercury chloride preparation used as medicine

cantharides—an extremely irritative substance made from Spanish fly

Carl Jung—a Swiss psychiatrist, founder of analytic psychology, had profound influence on theories of psychology in 20th century

Carl Rogers—prominent psychologist known for humanistic teachings

Caro, Edgar—third year medical student in 1893 wrote a question to E.G. White on def. of "drug"

Carruthers, Malcolm, M.D.—author of *Meditation of the Heart,* in *Yoga Today*

Carruthers—husband and wife team of physicians performing biofeedback sessions

causal body—body of mystical energy at higher plane or frequency than etheric or astral, and is involved with reincarnation concepts. Is supposed to be able to remember past life experiences and future life experiences

cell com system—a machine that is supposed to increase cell intercommunications and so bring health and healing from all types of disease

Celts—ethnic group of people found in the British Isles

centering—meditation

chi, qi, ki—universal energy, Chinese and Japanese names for such

chakra balancing—using any method that is believed to affect the chakras and so balance the proclaimed energy within

chakra—a supposed focal area of concentrated universal energy in the body. The body is said to have seven chakras which are claimed to be in color. Each chakra will be one of seven colors of rainbow

channeled—refers to receiving messages from spirits

channeler—a person who is able to contact spirits and communicate with them

charmer—a person who can affect by a magic spell

chelation—chelation therapy is wherein chemicals are placed within the body that will remove substances that the body can not remove on its own. Lead in the body can only be removed by using a chelating agent. Usually intravenous administration

ching—conduit

ching-mo—conduit vessel

chiromancy—palm reading, palmistry

chiropractor— type of medical practitioner trained in the philosophy of "chiropractic," that is belief in an innate energy traversing the body via spinal nerves and that by manipulation movement of the back this vital energy may be unclogged or moved to clear congestion

Cho, Paul—author *Solving Life's Problems*

choleric—angry, easily irritated, irate

Christ Consciousness—term used in New Age jargon to refer to Divinity within

Christian Science—a religious body with pantheistic concepts. Believes that all healing can be done with prayer

Church of the New Jerusalem—Swedenborgian church also known as The New Church, followed teaching and interpretation of scriptures as interpreted by Emanuel Swedenborg

Circe—personality in Greek Mythology

Cirlot—author of *Dictionary of Symbols*

clairvoyance—discerning or seeing objects or thoughts not observed by others

clairvoyant—one having power of discerning objects not present to the senses. Occultic power

coccyx—anatomical spot on the body, often referred to a "tail bone"

colonic cleansing—repeated enemas or use of machine that gives continuous cycling of water through large bowel, also use of herbs to cleanse bowel

color therapy—use of color to affect the chakra's energy balance

co-masonry—Masonic order for females in France

complementary—usually referring to non-conventional style of medical therapy

concepts—beliefs

Confucius—a Chinese who was a renowned ancient philosopher

Constance Cumby—a lawyer who also authored the book, *The Hidden Dangers of The Rainbow*

contemplation—concentration in thought or study

controls—a term used to describe a spirit talking through someone, it may materialize at times

correspondence—synonym of association and/or sympathy

cosmic energy—universal energy of the cosmos

cosmological correspondence—refers to the belief in close association & relationship between cosmos, earth, and man

cosmology—science or subject of the cosmos, or suns and planets of the universe and their relationship to one another and to earth

cosmos—the sun, moon, stars, and the heavens

counterfeit—fake, false, fraud, phony, deceptive, imitative (see Appendix J)

Cousens, Gabriel, M.D. —a popular physician who promotes integrative medicine

Craig, Winston, Ph.D., R.D. —author of book *Nutrition and Wellness*, *A Vegetarian Way to Better Health,* Chair Department of Nutrition, Andrews University

cranio-sacral (cranial—sacral, craniosacral)—one style of body therapy wherein very light massage or touch is applied to the base of the neck and back side of the skull, and at times over the sacrum. This particular discipline claims that the bones of the skull are not in proper position and the massage is to re-position them. However, these bones are fused solid and cannot be manipulated. The fluid of the brain and spinal canal are supposed to be manipulated as well by the placing of hands about the head region

Creative energy— often referred to as prana, chi, life force etc.

Creative Principle—synonym of universal energy, supreme Self, One, god, etc., referring to highest level of mystical energy

Creative visualization—an act wherein a person attempts to create by the power of his mind a happening, attitude, change, circumstance etc.

crystal healers—healing by use of crystals that are supposed to influence universal energy of the body

crystal—stone with formation of internal structure of repetitive molecular formations

Cummings, Stephen—co-author of *Science of Homeopathy*

Cush—son of Ham but also had mythological names of Mercury, Thoth, Hermes

D

Dark Ages—period of history in Europe from between 500 A.D. to 1600 A.D.

decubiti ulcer—an ulcer of the skin that forms usually from continuous pressure on the skin which causes loss of circulation and death to the cells in that location.

deification—making something god, such as a person made god

Deists—belief that God created the earth and then went off and left it with out divine influence to control and manage the earth

Deleuez, Phillippe Jean—author of several books and coined the term "animal magnetism"

Delores Krieger—instructor in nursing profession and promoter of Therapeutic Touch therapy

deluge—flood

detoxification—the breakdown of a toxin or toxins and removal by various methods

Di Mina, Alfonso—biophysicist of United States

diuretic—substance that causes increased flow of urine and loss of water from the body

divination—act of divining to obtain information by occult method

Divine Mind—a term used by Christian Science; also it is a synonym of universal mind, universal intelligence, energy, etc.

diviner—one who divines

divine—the act to obtain information by an occult method, The word may be referring to the Divinity of God

divining rod—stick or physical object used to divine

Djwal Kul—spirit being that channeled messages to Alice Bailey the New Age doctrine and to Elizabeth Prophet the information in *Intermediate Studies of the Human Aura*

dogma—a doctrine or body of doctrines or beliefs

doshas—refers to three divisions of prana energy in Ayurveda medicine, similar to the two divisions in Chinese medicine, yin and yang

Dowling, Fr. Ed—Jesuit Priest who became friend to Bill W.

dowse—to divine, usually by pendulum

dowsing—using a pendulum of any type to divine

Dr. Silkworth—physician at the Towns Hospital who first called alcoholism a "disease"

dualism—concept of opposing forces within universe expressed as positive—negative, or negative— positive, dark—light, cold—hot, yin—yang, etc.

E

Eastern religions—religions based on pantheism, Hindu, Taoism, Buddhism, Shintoism, Shikh, etc.

East—West—combination of Eastern mysticism with Western occultism

Ebby Thatcher—friend of Bill Wilson who introduced him to the Oxford method of treatment for alcoholism

eclectic—eclectic physician is one that uses many medicinals but in small doses, something for every symptom

ego—psychology term referring to the mental status of pride or self worth

Egyptian Mysteries—Egyptian religion came originally from Babylon and was formed out of the same basics, sun worship, nature worship, life after death, man having divine spark

Ekron—Philistine city on Mediterranean coast in country of Israel

electrocardiogram—a tracing on paper of the electrical activity of the heart

electroencephalogram—a tracing on paper of the electrical activity of the brain revealing the frequency of electrical brain waves

electrolysis—movement of ions through a solution powered by electrical force to cause precipitation of the ion onto an electrode or some metal object

electromagnetic bodies—Hindu concept that there are additional bodies to our physical bodies and are composed of electrical forces. Not recognized by modern science.

electromagnetism—electrically induced magnetism

Elijah—prophet of God in Israel

Elixir of Life—Life Force, substance that sustains life

Emily Rose—nine-year-old girl who exposed therapeutic touch by her school project

empathy—the capacity to experience another's feeling as if it were one's own; emphasis is on spirit power for healing, known to use spirit power of animals in therapy

Emperor Fu Hsi—developed the circle of harmony, pa kua, in 2900 B.C.

Emperor Hwang Ti—wrote the Nei Ching medical text near 2600 B.C.

Emperor Shen Nung—2800 B.C. compiled a text "pen-tsao" on herbs

enchanter—one who influences by charms

enchantment—to be in a state of charm

enchant—to influence by charm

encyclopedists—refers to the movement and people of at the time of the "enlightenment" late 1780's-90's. At that time the encyclopedia was written and printed.

Endor—a village location near Mt. Tabor in a large plain east of Nazareth and west of Sea of Galilee.

energy cyst—hypothesis of energy bound up in muscle, ligament, etc. where it has continued over years. Not connected with science or reality.

energy medicine—medical therapy by balancing universal energy

enlightenment—A period of late 18th century where reason was worshiped and religion put down; also refers to having reached the state of godhood, one with the universe etc.

Ephesians—people living in Ephesus in Asia Minor, now Western Turkey

Ephod—a special chest cloak worn by Jewish high priests in Bible

Epler, Jr., D.C.—author of *Bloodletting in Early Chinese Medicine and its Relation to the Origin of Acupuncture*

Ernie T.—alcoholic who established early in the history of A.A. a fellowship group in Cleveland Ohio

esoteric Christianity—refers to Christianity that practices mysticism

esoteric—occult or hidden

essence—having the qualities of the original, when referring to God it refers to His very person or presence being in something. It may refer to a substance taken or extracted from something for application to something else. Universal energy is sometimes called essence. A fundamental nature or quality

essential oils—aromatic oils taken from plants that are supposed to contain universal energy

etheric body—this refers to an imaginary body said to be made of energy, and some authors describe it as having frequencies of a faster speed than light. It is said to act like a template for our bodies. Energy disturbance at that level is said to later show up in man as disease.

Ethiopia—country in Africa

ethnopharmacology—science of the study of plants for medicinal values relative to various ethnic groups

etiology—source or cause of illness or disorder

evidence-based—"evidence-based" means there is an accepted body of peer reviewed, statistically significant evidence that raises probability of effectiveness to a scientifically convincing level.

Ezekiel— a prophet in Israel of Old Testament times and a name of a book written by him which is in the Bible

F

familiar spirit—demon spirit

fascia—connective tissue in animal and man: ligaments, tendons, etc.

Faulun gong—Chinese martial art

fibromyalgia—medical disorder consisting of painful muscles, joints,and points of insertion of tendons on bones. Cause unknown.

Finke, Ronald A.—author of *Creative Imagery*

fire walk—pertains to walking or running through hot bed of coals

Fitzgerald, Robert, S.J.—Jesuit priest, author of book, *The Soul of Sponsorship,* member of same Order of Jesuits as Ed Dowling, the close friend of Bill W.

Fitzgerald, William, M.D. —originator of zone therapy later called reflexology

Flower essences—mystical energy removed from blossoms of flowers and placed in water to be used for therapy

forbidden ground—a term used by E.G. White to refer to locations, instances or influences, subjects, etc. where the power of Satan will be manifest. Has reference to area of the Tree of Knowledge of Good and Evil in Garden of Eden. Adam and Eve advised to not go near it.

Foster, Ray, M.D. —physician at Black Hills Health Center, author of *lymphatic detoxification* article in Appendix I

Founders Watch—a group of the members of A.A. who would stay close to Bill W. when he was at A.A. functions to prevent him from "hustling" young women

Fox, Emmet— New Thought minister who authored *The Sermon on The Mount* used by Oxford Group in their working with alcoholics to gain sobriety

Free Masonry (Freemasonry or Freemason)—secret fraternal society, often called masonry

G

Galen—(129-200 AD)—a physician who lived in Pergamum (Western Turkey) and was instructor of medicine. He was a brilliant writer of medicine and his opinions were the basis of medicine for more than 1500 years.

Gall, Franz Joseph, M.D. —first to recognize that different locations on the brain controlled specific areas of body motion and other functions, developed phrenology as a result.

Galyean, Beverly—(now deceased)author of article on psychology and consultant for the Los Angeles school system in psychology, promoted New Age doctrine.

games of chance—gambling games

Garrison, Fielding, M.D.—author of *History of Medicine*

Gasner—Catholic priest who healed by use of hands only, lived at the time of Mesmer, an exorcist

gemstone—stones of beauty and of value

geomancy—divination by figures formed when a handful of dirt is thrown on ground, or by lines randomly drawn. Gems used as divination by throwing out many gems on a cloth with locations marked signifying certain pre-assigned meanings.

geometry—science of measuring angular areas; areas not always rectangular or square

Gerber, Richard, M.D.—medical doctor, believer in energy medicine and author of *Vibrational Medicine*

Gerome, Stan—wrote article about synchronicity and cranio-sacral subject. Instructor at Upledger clinic

Gnosticism—secret society in early Christianity time, "a *thorn*" to Christianity. A mixture of Cabala, Judaism, and Zoroastrianism from Persia. Believing in hidden spiritual knowledge. Emphasis on knowledge instead of faith

God Calling—name of book written by two ladies that called themselves "Two Listeners"

Gods of the New Age **Video**—a two hour video illustrating the movement into the west the Hindu teachings of the East. Produced by Jeremiah Films.

Grand Orient Lodge of France—Masonic lodges in and aroundFrance in mid 1700's and later. Approximately 150 such lodges.

Grand Orient Lodge—Masonic lodges of Paris, France in mid to later 1700;s

Great Reality—term referring to universal energy, higher self, chi, prana, higher consciousness, etc.

Green, Elmer and Alyce—co-authors of the book *Beyond Biofeedback,* researchers in biofeedback

guided imagery (mental imagery, visualization)—using imagination to conjure an image in the mind, such as an animal or bird, which in turn becomes one's guide. actually a demon in disguise.

Gumpert, Martin—author of *Hahnemann: The Adventurous Career of an Adventurous Rebel*

Gurudas— Aka Ronald Lee Garman author of *Flower Essences and Vibrational Healing*

H

Hahnemann, Samuel, M.D. —originator of homeopathy discipline 1755-1843

hallucinogen—substance that will cause hallucinations

Hank P.—business partner of Bill W.

Hardinge, Mervyne, M.D. —author of book, *A Physician Explains Drugs, Herbs and Natural Remedies,* Professor of Pharmacology, founder of School of Health, Loma Linda University

Harner, Michael—a shaman, teacher of shamans and author of *The Way of the Shaman*

Hartigan, Francis—author of biography of Bill W. and a member of AA, secretary to Bill W.'s wife

hatha yoga—type of yoga wherein the sun's energy is breathed in through the right nostril and the moon energy through the left. Ha = sun, tha = moon; joining of sun and moon energies by use of yoga

Henry Mason—author of text *The Seven Secrets of Crystal Talisman*

herbal medicine—using herbs for medicinal use, often for their occult energies

herbalism—using herbs for health and healing

herbalist—one who practices the art of healing by use of herbs

herbs—plants used as special sources of nutritional substances and in the field of Eastern mysticism, yin—yang, hot—cold, status

Hermes—Thoth to the Egyptians, Hermes to the Greeks. Mythical god figure; originator of alchemy. Originally referred to Cush son of Ham, son of Noah.

Hermetic tradition—following after the lore of Hermes Trismegistus, magical, alchemical, esoteric etc.

Hester, Ben—author of *Dowsing—an Exposé of Hidden Occult Forces*

hieroglyph—a drawing or carving depicting a message or information

higher consciousness—refers to higher planes of the seven levels of universal energy, up to state of godhood

higher power—in Eastern thought refers to the subconscious that is at a higher level than your conscious thought process and near to god-hood level. In Alcoholics Anonymous it can refer to any entity that one may choose to be his "higher power" or "god"

Higher Self—mystical concept of being a god, having godhood

Hill, Ann—author of *A Visual Encyclopedia of Unconventional Medicine*

Hippocrates—famous physician around 400, B.C. and was a great medical writer. Recognized that lifestyle was connected to disease, a new concept at his time.

Hitching, J. Francis—author of *Earth Magic*

Hoizey, Dominique and Marie-Joseph—authors of *A History of Chinese Medicine*

holistic health—health, of body/mind/spirit as a result of a proper balance with nature

holistic—term used by New Age (neo-pagan) worldview relevant to subject of health emphasizing the interconnection of body, mind and spirit.

hologram—a small localized area or substance which is a template of a greater area, such as the cell of the body as a template of the universe. Often refers to a small localized area on the body which is considered to represent the entire body. Not accepted in science.

homeopathy—alternative medical style of practice with therapy consisting of using minute (at times no original molecules of the substance left in the solution) doses of substances as medicinals.

Homer—ancient Greek poet who wrote about mythology

Homo-Vibra Ray—machine, that it is claimed, will detect electromagnetic disturbances in an individual and then send back into the body electromagnetic frequencies to correct the supposed imbalance and thus effect healing.

Hopp, H.J. —author of *Homeopathy*

Houck, James—only surviving non drinking member of Oxford Group who knew Bill W.

house party—a gathering of members of the Oxford Group for two or more days of fellowship

Howard, Michael—author of the book, *The Occult Conspiracy: Secret Societies—Their Influence and Power in World History*

Huang-ti-nei-ching text—most important Chinese text at end of first century

Hubard, Reuben—author of *Historical Perspectives of Health*

human potential—generally used in reference to a belief that man has divinity within and it can be raised to a higher level. A Pantheistic concept

humanism—doctrine coming forth at time of enlightenment (mid and late 1700's), Man is center of all and Self reigns supreme, Divine within etc. self sufficiency of man, does not derive assistance from a God.

humanistic—life centered on man himself as the ultimate, God is left out.

humors—fluids, referring to the supposed four humors of the body; concept for the last 2500 years until scientific medicine revealed its fallacy

Hunt, Dave—author and Evangelical minster; Co-author of *America—The Sorcerer's New Apprentice, The Rise of New Age Shamanism.*

hydrotherapy—treatment using water in many different ways

hypnosis—being in a state of mind alteration so that another person can control you. Can be to a point of full trance or unconscious state

hypnotism—mind therapy wherein one submits his mind to the control of another

I

I Ching sticks—stick of wood used in divination acts, Chinese in origin

Ignatius Loyola—established the Jesuit Order in early 1500's

illuminist—one belonging to Illuminati secret society. The Illuminati led by Adam Weishaupt infiltrated the Masonic lodges of France starting around 1776 and was an influence leading to the French revolution of 1789.

immortality—life never ending

inanimate—nonliving substance, such as metal, rock, mineral, etc.

incantation—chanting some phrase or word

Ingham, Eunice—advanced the therapy of reflexology after Dr. Fitzgerald passed on

innate—name given to universal energy by chiropractors, the flow of which is said to be facilitated by manipulation of "subluxations" of vertebrae in the spine

inner self—similar to higher self, the subconscious that functions at higher level than conscious thought and has access to wisdom of universe

integrative—blending or mixing of conventional and non-conventional medical practices

intuition—an ability to receive extrasensory intelligence and/or directions from a source not of the conscious mind but from the unconscious and/or possible spirit source

iridology chart—chart of the iris with ninety different divisions to it; each section is believed to relate to some specific part or organ of man

iridology—alternative medicine discipline used to divine from iris of the eye, past, present, and future disease and its location in the body

iron—mineral of the earth, common substance used in hundreds of manufactured products, made into steel by adding carbon

Ironside, H.A.—A prominent Pastor who wrote a small book exposing Oxford Group as not Christian and promoting Eastern style meditation

irrational—no cause and effect consideration. In medical treatment often referring to mystical considerations

Isis—mythical Egyptian goddess

J

Jaggi, O.P., Ph D., M.D.—surgeon and author of the book, *Yogic and Tantra Medicine*

James, William, M.D. —professor of psychology at Harvard, author of *Varieties of Religious Experience*, a spiritualist

Jensen, Bernard, D.C.—author of *The Science and Practice of Iridology*, New Age healer

John—John an Apostle of Christ and wrote the Bible books of John and Revelation

Johnston, Dale P.T.—physical therapist in LA Grande, OR, author of Underground Oasis

judo— form of martial art

K

Kabbala, Kabalah, Caballa, Cabala—secret society of Israel; considered "grandfather" of secret societies

Kah, Gary—author of *En Route to Global Occupation*

Kamiya, Joe, M.D.—San Francisco physician who coined the word "biofeedback" in his research on "autogenic training"

kapha—third division made up of a combination of the other two divisions (doshas) of prana energy

Karagulia, S.—author of *Energy Fields and Medical Diagnosis, The Human Aura*

karate—form of martial art

Keating, Thomas—Catholic priest promoting Emergent Church movement

Kellogg, John, M.D.—physician from the mid 1800's until late 1940's. Director of Battle Creek Sanitarium, and authored many books. Known as a great leader in healthful living, also originator of breakfast cereals and other health food products

kenpo—form of martial art

Kent, James Tyler—author of *Lectures on Homeopathic Philosophy*, 1979, reprint from original published in 1900.

Khalsa, Dharma Singh, M.D.—author of *Meditation as Medicine*

Kinesiology—true science of the action of muscles

ki—synonym for universal energy

Knights Templar—Catholic organization that went to the Holy Land to protect crusaders but became involved in secret organizations of the Arabs and came back to Europe where eventually the King of France subdued them. Evolved into many other secret orders over time

Koch, Kurt—a German Lutheran Pastor who is known for his wisdom in counseling people and authoring articles connected with the occult.

Krieger, Delores, R.N.—nurse that promoted and made popular Therapeutic Touch therapy.

kundalini—"serpent power" supposed to be latent energy laying in the bottom chakra

Kunz, Dora—author of Therapeutic Touch discipline and past president of Theosophical Society and a spiritualist

Kurtz, Ron—Buddhist psychologist

L

Laban—nephew of Abraham of Bible history

lactic acid—a chemical produced by muscles when exercised. When builds up to high concentrations pain occurs in the muscle and at very high levels action of muscle may cease

Lanagan, John—author of Worldview Times web site <http://www.worldviewweekend.com/worldview-times>

laparoscope—instrument used to view inside of abdomen and often surgical procedures done through the instrument called laparoscopy

laser puncture—use of laser light on skin instead of using a needle as in acupuncture

latent forces—mystical forces supposedly stored in human mind or elsewhere in the body until liberated by various occult methods

lattice—formation of molecules arranging themselves in a repetitive physical position creating a crystal

leukemia—form of cancer of white blood cells

levitation—raising objects by power of occult

Leviton, Richard—author of article in *East-West Journal of Natural Health and Living*

Levy, Robert—co-author of *Shamanic Reiki*

ley lines—power lines of energy said to travel through the ground; and is said to emanate increased power at points where the lines cross; universal energy power is believed to be accessed by humans where lines intersect each other; example, stone circles

Li Xiao Ming, —Qi Gong master from Beijing College of Traditional Chinese Medicine

life force energy—synonym for universal energy and all other synonyms

life force—synonym to universal energy, vital force, prana, chi, etc

Linder, Rosa—Author of article in *JAMA, Lancet, and British Medical Journal* exposing Therapeutic Touch

Living Temple, The—book written by John Kellogg containing pantheistic sentiments

Llyn, Roberts—co author of *Shamanic Reiki*

Lockie, Andrew—Author of *Natural Health, An Encyclopedia of Homeopathy*

lodestone—naturally—magnetized piece of mineral magnetite, which draws iron particles to it

Logos—Greek term for universal energy

Lois Wilson—wife of Bill Wilson

Lotus—term referring to having reached godhood

LSD—"lysergic acid"—diethylamide, a chemical used to bring mind changing experiences to the person taking the substance. Often induced a hallucinating mind change. At one time it was legal to use

Luciferian Occultism—hidden knowledge and/or activities directed by Lucifer or Satan and used to promote worship of Satan

Lucifer—Satan, when he was an unfallen angel. Means *light-bearer*

Luthe, Wolfgang, M.D.—German doctor and student of Johannes Schultz M.D. , and a leading exponent of autogenic training following Shultz's death.

lymphatic—non blood vascular system in animal and man which drain fluids from the body into the blood system

M

M.R.A. (Moral Rearmament Association)—Oxford Group changed name to this name

MacArthur, John—author of *The Truth War*

macrocosm—refers to sun, moon, stars and the 626

magenta—an added color to the seven colors of the rainbow, deep purplish-red

magic arts—sorcery, various paranormal acts or practices usually for healing, synonym with sorcery

magician—one skilled in magic, one involved in occult practices

magnesium—a mineral

magnetic energy—energy produced by magnets, such as electricity when magnets are moved against each other. Also used in holistic health to refer to universal energy, etc.

magnetic field therapy—giving therapy by altering an magnetic field about someone

magnetic fluid—synonym for universal energy

magnetic healer—one who claims to heal by using magnets or electromagnetic energy frequencies

magnetic therapy—therapy given by use of magnet or magnets, may be by pulsating magnets or use of static magnet

magnetism—a true physical force found in the earth and seen in iron and some other substances having positive and negative poles

magnetoelectric energy—a synonym for universal energy. The term is coined by William Tiller retired physics instructor of /Stanford University.

magnets—iron that has been magnetized

Magus, Simon—a Biblical character (Acts 8) who was a magical healer in the day of the Apostles, he asked of Peter to buy the power of laying on of hands to pass on the power of performing miracles. The originator of the Gnostic movement in early Christianity which opposed Christianity

mana—synonym for universal energy; name used in Polynesia for universal energy

mandala—in Sanskrit it means circle. Artwork of various designs placed in a circle to depict the theology of paganism. Depicts the universe and the power of the gods

Manichaeism—secret order and movement that followed Gnosticism in the second and third centuries A.D. Had its doctrine out of Cabala, Gnosticism, and Zoroastrianism of Persia

Manley Hall—author of many books for the Masonic Lodge. *The Secret Teaching of All Ages*

mantra—word, phrase, sentence or even Bible verse, repeated over and over

Marcy, E. E.— author of *The Homeopathic Theory and Practice of Medicine*

marma points—localized position on the body where universal energy is said to flow through the connective tissue and where channel junctions of flow occur. Points on body where pressure is said to unblock congested flow of universal energy, similar to acupuncture points in traditional Chinese medicine. Originates from Ayurvedic medicine

martial arts—physical type of exercise or movements used as a form of meditation and for defense through balance. Qi gong is the name first assigned to this art, then many variations developed, such as judo, tai chi, etc.

massage, Swedish—massage given to facilitate blood and lymph circulation of the body

massage, trigger points—[marma points]—massage given to particular points believed by Ayurvedic medicine to move universal energy when blocked

Ma-wang-tui graves—Chinese graves discovered in 1970's and contained writings of all medical treatment types in third and second century B.C.

Ma-wang-tui— text from ancient Chinese graves (168 B.C.)

Maxwell, Jessica—author of *What Your Eyes Tell You About Your Health,* iridology article (in Esquire magazine)

McCarty, Michael—author of article in *The Lancet* exposing Therapeutic Touch

McMahon, T.A.—co-author of *The Seduction of Christianity*

McNamara, Sheila—author of text *Traditional Chinese Medicine*

meditation—placing the mind in a neutral state (detached awareness), or concentrating on only one thing so as to turn the thoughts inward

medium—a person who connects between earth and the spirit world

mediumistic trances—altered state of consciousness facilitated by a medium

mediumistic—being a spiritualistic medium

melancholic—depressed, sad

Menninger Foundation—psychiatric research institution in Topeka, Kansas

mental imagery (guided imagery)—forming in the mind a picture of what one may desire to have or create, to change things. Does not refer to regular thought and planning or creative ideas

Mercandante, Linda—author of *Victims and Sinners*

mercury—fluid-like metal, silver in color (quick-silver), comes from cinnabar ore, very toxic to living creatures. Used for millennia as a medicinal

Mercury—mythology figure in Greek, same as Hermes in Egyptian mythology, synonym for Cush

meridian—an imaginary channel in the body claimed to transport energy

Mermet, Alexis—priest who felt he was first to use pendulum to diagnosis medical abnormalities

Mesmer, Franz, M.D.—known for his making popular hypnotism, and the use of hypnotism was called mesmerism (late 1700's into 1800's)

mesmerism—hypnotism

Mesopotamian civilization— past civilization that existed in present-day Iraq

meta-analysis—combining the data of many different similar studies and analyzing them as one study

metabolism—normal internal chemical process of living creatures

metaphysics—physical phenomena unexplained by conventional science of physics. Has to do with paranormal—occult.

Meyers, Frederic—past president of the American Society of Psychical Research (early 1900's) and friend of William James, M.D.

microcosm—refers to man as the microcosm of the universe

Miller, Edith—author of *Occult Theocracy*

mind sciences—pertaining to various disciplines relating to explaining workings of the mind and related therapies.

mind set—belief system of an individual, example: creationist mindset or understanding of origin in contrast to evolutionists' beliefs

modality—method

monism—belief that all substances of the universe are parts of one basic energy. One is all and all is one. Pagan concept of association of all substance of the universe

Moonies—individuals following cult leader, Rev. Moon, from Korea

Morgana— feminine for sun god of Celts

mother tincture—base substance from which dilutions of homeopathy remedies have their origin

moxibustion—burning of small cones of plants on the skin to effect localized heat. Ancient Chinese custom; same effect as acupuncture

MRI—magnetic resonance imaging machine uses magnets and computers to image the interior of individuals. Works by laws of physical science

mumio—mixture of medicinals popular in Russia. Contains around fifty different substances

myography or electromyography —tracing graphs made of electrical activity of muscle action

mystical medicine—medical therapies which are actually using spiritualistic power in an attempt to promote health and healing

mysticism—the act of seeking union with the godhead. Noah Webster dictionary of 1828—The doctrine of the Mystics, who profess a pure, sublime and perfect devotion, wholly disinterested, and maintain that they hold immediate intercourse with the divine Spirit

mystic—one who through meditation or self-surrender seeks union with the godhead and one who believes in universal wisdom, cosmic consciousness. May believe that he holds direct communication with God

Mystics—Noah Webster Dictionary 1828: A religious sect who professes to have direct intercourse with the Spirit of God

N

nature worship—worship of the *creation* rather than the *Creator*

naturopathy—medical discipline, promotes the concept of existence of toxins in the system and that must be removed by colon irrigation or special herbs to cleanse the colon. There is no scientific information to back up these claims

Navaho—native Americans found in Southwest USA

Nebuchadnezzar—King of Babylon 600 B.C.

necromancer—one who practices the art of conferring with the spirits of the dead (a channeler)

Nei Ching—most celebrated text of Chinese medicine, written in 2600 B.C.

Nell Wing—secretary to Bill Wilson

neo-paganism—a return in beliefs to old nature worship, doctrine of pagans brought into modern day setting packaged in new terms and made to appear as a new and great improvement in philosophy and religion.

Neutral— this word is used in reference to whether a method of therapy that had a long history of use in the occult could be taken out of that context for use in Christian setting and be spiritually safe

New Age Movement—name given to a large number of groups and organizations and many people not in organizations who have a common philosophy. Trend is toward nature worship in philosophy

New Thought Movement—supposedly Christian renewal movement arising in 1800's and attempting to infiltrate other religious organizations with their teachings, pantheistic in nature but hidden

Newhouse, Sandy—co-author of *Native American Healing*

ninjutsu—form of martial art

nirvana—land of paradise for the pagan, Buddhist. Similar concept as heaven to the Christian

nitrosamine—chemical that has carcinogenic properties

noetic sciences—paranormal, mystical

Norse—early people of Norway

Nuga Best—a massage table mimicking chiropractic treatment for the spine

numerics—determining meanings from a word or object by use of numbers; mystical application of numbers

O

oasis—a place in the desert with water and vegetation that gave refuge and rest to the traveler of the harsh desert environment. Underground Oasis used in this text refers to a place of refuge for the weary soul in addiction.

observer of times—astrologer, horoscope user, etc.

Occident—Western civilization

occult—hidden, obscure, secret, connected with spirit world

occultist—one using occult theory or practice

odic force—synonym for universal energy

Odyssey—Homer's Greek mythological epic chronicling Odysseus

Olcott, Henry—co-originator of the Theosophy Society in New York 1875

omega—last, at the end

omen—a sign or warning of a future event, situation or condition

One—term used in pagan theology to refer to the highest level of the universal energy, godhood, Supreme Self, etc.

Ophiel—author of a book on creative visualization (aka Edward C. Peach)

optometrist—Doctor of Optometry, non-medical doctor of vision care

orenda—universal energy name used by a certain Indian tribe. Each tribe had its own name for such

organon energy—synonym for universal energy, associated with homeopathy

origins—explanation of origin of cosmos, earth and man

Oschman, James—scientist and author of *Energy Medicine*: *the Scientific Basis*

oscilloscope—instrument that is used in physics to demonstrate electromagnetic waves of energy invisible form. Television screen for example.

osteopathy—discipline of medicine, originally practiced by manipulation of joints as treatment for disease but now same as main stream scientific medicine practice.

Ouija board—instrument of divination with alphabet and numbers and "yes" and "no" words. Questions asked of the board are answered by a pointer going to the different numbers, letters, or words on the board.

Oxford Group—refers to a quasi-Christian movement in the early 1900's.

oxygen—gas of the atmosphere, may combine with certain minerals and form various stones

P

pa kua—Chinese circle of harmony

pagan—one who is not a Christian, Jew or Moslem; is a nature worshiper, lunar goddess worshiper, dedicated to establishing "Old Religion"

palmistry—using the palm of the hand to divine the future

pantheism—a doctrine that equates God with the forces and laws of the universe, universal energy. God in everything and everything god

Pantheistic World View—belief in the origin of life as described by

pagan religions (created out of a two sided energy by the perfect balancing of the two parts), the future is "Nirvana" in the spirit world but only after many lives by reincarnation.

Paracelsus—very famous16[th] century physician who believed in universal energy, also an astrologer and believed in vital energy and dualism

Pass it On—another official book published by AA World Services Inc. for use in AA fellowship

passive mind—a mind that has been brought to the state of non-thinking

Paul Yonggi Cho—author of *Solving Life's Problems*

peer review—scientific articles reviewed by other scientists before publishing to make certain that the study has followed proper methods of investigation thereby giving the study greater probability of accuracy in its results.

Pegasus—producers of flower essences

Pelletier, Kenneth, M.D.—author quoted in article written by Biblical Research Committee of SDA, General Conference of SDA's. (1987) Pelletier is a believer in New Age concepts

pendulum—divining instrument, usually an object hanging from a string swinging independently so as to give answers to questions by predetermined parameters

Pen-ts'ao—text on 365 herbs, earliest text on herbs written

Pergamos—city in Western Turkey or Asia Minor in Biblical days

Pergamum—city in Asia Minor or now days country of Turkey (same as Pergamos)

peyote—cactus that has hallucinatory properties when ingested

Pfeiffer, Samuel, M.D.—author of *Healing at Any Price*

phallic symbol—symbol of male sex organ

Philistines—people or small nation next to Old Testament Israel and occupied territory on south part of coast

phlegmatic—showing steady temperament

phrenology—pseudoscience with belief that the shape of the head determined personality and character. These were believed to be changed by applying pressure on the head in specific locations

physiology—normal function of living creatures

piezoelectric effect—electrical charge generated from a crystal when crystal is compressed

Pike, Albert—in mid 1800,s he was the Grand Master of the Masonic Order and authored the book, *Morals and Dogma of the Ancient and Accepted Scottish Rite of Freemasonry*

Piper, Mrs. L.E.—spiritualist with whom William James joined in séances for over 25 years

pisces—zodiac symbol of the fish

pitta—second division of prana energy

Pittman, Bill—author of *AA The Way It Began*

polarity—term applied to a "non recognized" condition of one side of the body being of positive polarity and the other side the negative

potassium—a mineral

potentizing—making more potent or adding strength by thumping the mixture

potion—a substance to be taken internally that would have some magic effect on the creature that took it

power object—a object used by a shaman in his treatment of the ill or injured, often a quartz crystal

power of the will—power of choice

prana—air, breath, and said to carry universal energy into body with the breath

pranayama—mystical meeting of the sun and moon energies via breath at the level of the nasopharynx (back part of nose and throat) and providing exceptional influence on wellbeing of the individual. Belief is from Ayurveda teachings.

pre Christian mystery tradition—Babylonian mysteries and/or pagan religion

precepts—doctrine, teaching, law of, etc.

Priessnitz, Vincent—initiated hydrotherapy clinic in Austria.

primordial—original, first created or developed state

prognosticator—one who foretells from signs or symptoms

Prophet, Elizabeth Clare—authored the book, *Intermediate Studies of the Human Aura,* as received dictation by the spirit Djwal Kul

psora—Samuel Hahnemann, M.D. , determined to his satisfaction that all disease, apart from surgical maladies and syphilis, originated from a basic infectious disease he called "psora." All acute and chronic disorders he believed originated from this. He states in his book, *Organon,* p. 78, that it took him 12 years to discover this fact. Such a basic infectious disorder—the source of all other disease is not recognized by science.

psychedelic—referring to a chemical, when ingested, causes mind-altering changes

psychic healing—healing another by the power of one's mind

psychic therapy—directing by mind; supernatural forces to effect therapy

psychic—effect or status of mental state. Refers to sensitivity of a person to supernatural forces or one that uses such

psychology—science of the mind and behavior, or science of the soul in the word's early meaning

psychometry—diagnostic technique of determining the characteristics of people who are not present by means of objects that have been in their possession. The practitioner might use a personal object such as a watch, a ring, or other jewelry, and hold the object with the eyes closed, in order to receive psychic impressions of its owner.

psychoneuroimmunology—science or study of the influence on the immune system by mental activity and the thoughts

psychophysiology—study of function of the brain processes

psychotronic radionics—use of electronics and machines combined with mental activity to divine and/or treat

pulse diagnosis—using the nature of the pulse to diagnose disorders in the human body. Has its origin in Chinese traditional medicine.

purer consciousness—synonym for One, Supreme Self, god etc.

pyruvic acid—one of the chemical metabolites of body

Q

qi gong (ki gong)—most fundamental of Chinese martial arts. Meditation in action or without motion to effect balance of chi

quartz—crystalline form of silica

Queen's Work—Catholic magazine published by Jesuit Society in St. Louis, MO

R

Radiaesthesia—is the ability of a person to perform as medium in divining information by use of pendulums or machine pendulums. Ability depends upon degree of connection with occult powers

radionics—use of electrical machines for divination for diagnosis and at times treatment

Ragon—Masonic author of *Maconnerie Occulte*

Ramacharaka—Yogi, pseudonym for William Atkisnson

Raman, R.V.—Sage of astrology in India

Rand, William Lee—author of *The Nature of Reiki Energy*

Raphael, Matthew J.—author of *Bill W. and Mr. Wilson*

Raso, Jack—author of *Expanded Dictionary of Metaphysical Health Care...*

Raso, M.D., R.D.—author of *Mystical Diets*

rational therapies—therapies given that are based on cause and effect relationship

Ray, Barbara, Ph.D.—author of *Reiki Factor*

Raynaud's disease—disorder of spasms of arterioles of hands and feet causing reduction of blood flow to the anatomical part and may result in pain, sometimes death to tissue.

reflexology—alternative treatment method, rubbing the palms of the hands or the bottom of the feet to affect healing of various areas of the body

Rei—ghost, spirit, soul, etc

Reiki guide—a spirit that assists in Reiki healing. Often embodied. occultic, spiritistic

Reiki Master—one who has reached the third level in training and practice of Reiki healing.

reiki—a form of body therapy from Japan and is closer to psychic therapy than to soma therapy. Uses, if any, very light touch for therapy

reincarnation—the doctrine of re-birth and many lives

Reisser, Paul C., M.D.—medical practitioner and co-author of *New Age Medicine*

Relaxation response—title to program of yoga-like actions which is taught by Dr. Herbert Benson. This technique made yoga acceptable to medical profession.

religion of nature—paganism, Wicca

re-pattern—to reform a pattern of action or appearance

Reuter's Health Information—Internet web site which gives daily review of new science reporting's on medicine

Rife machine—machine that is supposed to measure the frequencies of electromagnetic waves said to be coming from infectious agents (fungus, bacteria, viruses) within our bodies. The machine is said to send corrective waves of proper frequencies back into our bodies to rid the body of these agents. This is said to cure infectious disease and sometimes cancer, since its founder believed that all cancer is a result of virus infection.

Ritter, Johann Wilhelm—German scientist member of Bavarian Academy of Science in early 1800's

Rodriquez, Cardinal Caro—Bishop of Santiago, Chile, who recognized that the Theosophy society was supported by the Masonic Lodge in that city

Roeckelein, Jon E.—author of *Imagery in Psychology*

Rogers, Carl—leader in secular humanistic psychology

Rohr, Richard—Catholic priest promoting Emergent Church movement

Rolf, Pauline—originator of Rolfing massage, correcting the flow of universal energy

rolfng—heavy, painful massage therapy, to point of bruising the tissues

Rosicrucian—one of the prominent secret societies existing for past several centuries

Rudolph Bauman—wrote summary of effectiveness of acupuncture for Academy of Sciences of the German Democratic Republic 1981

rune dice—special dice used in divination

Russian parapsychology—psychology involved with the use of supernatural forces

S

Sage—Hindu holy man

Sampson, Wallace, M.D.—wrote a critique on the report on acupuncture put out by the National Institute of Health.

sanguine—cheerful, hopeful

sanitarium—treatment facility usually involving the use of more "natural" treatment methods. Use of exercise, rest, sunshine, diet, physical therapy, etc. as main treatment methods. This word first used by John H. Kellogg M.D. at Battle Creek, Michigan.

Sanskrit—ancient Indian language that the Vedas were written in

Satan's Ground—At the Garden of Eden the immediate area around the Tree of Knowledge of Good and Evil would be considered Satan's ground. God had directed Adam and Eve to not go near it. If they placed themselves in an area where the devil had influence they would be more susceptible to his wiles. E.G. White uses the expression "Satan's ground" to refer to not only locations, but to associations, reading material and author's works, therapies, attitudes, etc., that when utilized or we become exposed to we are on Satan's ground and our protecting angel is hindered in his work for us.

Satanism—Satan worship or following of

Saturday Evening Post—a very popular weekly magazine which had very wide circulation

Schultz, Johannes, M.D.—neurologist in Berlin who continued Oskar Vogt's work on auto hypnosis

sciences—a term referring to physics, chemistry, engineering, medicine, dentistry, nursing, etc.

scientific medicine—medical care based on known laws of physics, chemistry, and physiology as learned by demonstration and testing through scientific methods

scrying—crystal ball gazing, divination act

SDA—Seventh-day Adventist

Seal of Solomon—same as star of David

Seiberling, Henrietta—lady who connected Dr. Bob Smith with Bill Wilson in Akron

sensitive—one who has special psychic powers or special senses in the occult

Seventh-day Adventist—religious denomination

shaman—name given to native "medicine man," a witch doctor

Shiatsu—body therapy of specific type from Japan. Very gentle

Shi-Chi text—acupuncture first found in these Chinese writings of 90 B.C.

Shing Moon—Oriental name for female sun god

Shiva—Hindu god

Siberia—North Eastern part of Russia with natives similar to American Indian.

signature—refers to association "like cures like" where a substance may influence another due to its similar appearance;

silicon—a mineral of the earth. One seventh of the earth's surface, sand is silicon dioxide.

Simon Lilly—Crystal Healer and author of *The Complete Illustrated Guide to Crystal Healing*

Smith, Anne —wife of Dr. Bob Smith/co-founder of A.A.

sodium—a mineral

solidified light—claim made by shaman of Australia that light can turn into a quartz crystal

Sol—sun and name used referring to the sun a god

soma body work (somatic)—physical treatment to the body by various massage-type methods

SomatoEmotional Release—act of the "inner physician" bringing healing by releasing bound up energy in "energy cyst"

sonopuncture—use of ultra sound to affect acupuncture points instead of using needles

soothsayer—one that foretells events

sorcerer—one who uses witchcraft or occult forces, one who by enchantments or charms persuades another to make decisions that are detrimental to his eternal wellbeing.

sorceries—all forms of witchcraft and their acts; all actions that persuade or influence an individual so as to cause a decision to be made that ill effects his eternal destiny

sound therapy—application of sound or music to affect the chakras to effect electromagnetic balance

spirit guides—Satan's angels, demons acting as if a beneficial guide to a human

Spirit of Prophecy—often the term is used to refer to writings of E.G. White

spirit—intelligent entity of the unseen world, Satan's angels

Spiritual Counterfeits Journal—a journal exposing spiritualism in New Age, Holistic healings

Spiritual Exercises of Ignatius Loyola—principles applied in the training of a Jesuit Priest to bring the person to total surrender and loyalty to the Jesuit Order.

spiritualism—belief that spirits of the dead communicate with the living. Any act or belief that connects us to the power of Satan

spiritualist—one who uses spirit powers

spook sessions—sessions of contacting the spirits or doing paranormal acts such as automatic writing, Ouija board use, telepathy, etc. Bill Wilson of Alcoholics Anonymous referred to "spook sessions" in regards to his occult activities.

spurious healings—false or counterfeit

Sri Aurobindo—a Yogi

Stalker, Douglas—author of *Examining Holistic Medicine*

Stan Gerome—Instructor in craniosacral therapy at Upledger Institute

Star of David—a symbol of one triangle placed over another so as to form six points in the star

Star Wars—Hollywood movie that featured "universal energy" under the name "The Force"

stargazer—astrologer

statistically significant—results of a test reach a level that is likely to indicate significant relationship.

Stein, Diane—author of *Essential Reiki*

Stewart, David Ph.D.—author of *Essential Oils of the Bible*

subluxation—supposed congestion or obstructive focus of *innate energy* (universal energy) flow along the spinal column and outward to the periphery of the body. This does not refer to "out of place" vertebrae as many believe. Spinal manipulation is believed to unclog the energy congestion. This teaching is the basis upon which chiropractic medicine was founded. Subluxations have not been demonstrated by science.

subtle energy medicine—using universal energy to effect healing, producing an effect upon etheric body

subtle energy—same as universal energy

subtle teachings—doctrine of universal energy or pantheism

successed— homeopathic remedy that in its preparation has been shaken hard or "thumped" in the mixing

Sufis—secret society of the Islamic peoples

Sumerian—ancient civilization of Babylon or from the land of Mesopotamia (Iraq), same as Mesopotamian

sun worship—to worship the sun as a deity

Sunna—feminine name for sun god

super soul—synonym for reaching godhood

Supreme Self—synonym for godhood.

Supreme Self—the divine within raised to its zenith of development so that it connects with the cosmic intelligence and power of the universe

supreme ultimate—synonym for One, Supreme Self, god, highest level of theoretical universal energy

Sutherland, William, D.O.—Osteopathic physician considered originator of craniosacral therapy

Swain, Bruce—author of article in *East—West Journal*

sway test—method of divination where in an object is held near the chest and questions asked will be answered by one's body being pushed forward by a yes answer and pushed backwards with a negative answer. (Described as a stand up Ouija board.)

Swedenborg, Emanuel—Very influential writer and spiritualist of late 18th century and early 19th.

sympathetic remedy—remedy which is founded upon the doctrine of association, sympathy, and/or correspondence

sympathetic—showing relationship such as correspondence

synchronicity—a hypothesis of Carl Jung wherein release of a physical distress relieves a mental condition

Szurko—ex-mystic

T

tae kwando—form of martial art

tai chi chuan—Chinese exercise, form of qi gong, meditation in motion

Takata, Hawayo—Japanese woman that came to US and popularized Reiki

talisman—an object thought to act as a charm, may be of letters, numbers or sentences, may be a gemstone worn on the body as a charm or for protection, then called an amulet

Taoism—Chinese religion meaning "the way" based in astrological beliefs, man is a microcosm of the cosmos (macrocosm)

Taoist— Believer in Chinese religion based out of mystic philosophy and Buddhist religion

tarter emetic—an old-style medicine used to cause vomiting (contains antimony)

template—a mold or pattern used to form some other object

The Force—universal energy .

The Voice Divine—article written by one of the "Two Listeners" authors of the book *God calling* tells of the meditation sessions of those two ladies. One made contact with a spirit every time and the other never did.

theology—study of God, doctrines of

Theosophical Research Center—an organization and center within Theosophical Society dedicated to experimentation with mystical methods

theosophy—divine wisdom, term used to describe esoteric and mystical beliefs that describe the relationship of human beings to the universe and the Godhead. These belief systems may describe emanations from the "Supreme God" who reveals different aspects of transcendent reality through various intermediary deities, spirits, or intelligences.

Therapeutic Imagery and Dialogue—name given additional acts in craniosacral therapy. Patient uses imagination to visualize "inner physician." Therapist dialogues with inner physician as a part of healing therapy. Occultic, spiritistic in nature

Therapeutic Release and Dialogue—a contribution of Dr. Upledger to therapy of craniosacral, spiritistic in nature

therapeutic touch—healing therapy by using the hands to balance energy. No real touching is done. Hands are held a few inches from the body

therapeutic—a remedy for disease

Theriac—prime medicinal of Galen, formed of more than 70 substances grew to 230 substances through the centuries. Considered the universal antidote

theta—a specific frequency of brain wave that correlates with neutral state of thought process. Same frequency of brain wave that biofeedback takes place in and at times the same wave frequency that occurs with yoga meditation. Alpha wave may also occur with yoga.

theurgic—magical, miracle, supernatural intervention, white magic

Thomsen, Robert—author of biography, *Bill W.*

Thoth—same as Mercury, Hermes or Cush

Three ABN—television network, Christian—SDA

times—used in the Bible referring to prognostication to times of events determined by astrology

Tisserand, Robert—author of *The Art of Aromatherapy*

Tom P.—friend and neighbor of Bill Wilson who at times attended "spooking sessions" and wrote about them

Towns Hospital—alcoholic rehab hospital in New York operated by William Silkworth, M.D.

Trachetenberg, Dr. Alan—arranged for summit on acupuncture for National Institute for Drug Abuse of the National Institute of Health.

transcendental meditation—basis is same as Eastern meditation (relaxation and use of mantra to obtain passivity of mind) with minor changes to make it acceptable in the West. The mantra consists of a secret word or phrase, popular form of meditation in the US, England, Australia, New Zealand. Popularized in West by Maharishi Mahesh Yogi.

Trojan horse—refers to ancient story of city of Troy where a large wooden horse filled with soldiers was left out side the city as the surrounding army left and the horse was pulled into the city and the gates were opened in the night by these soldiers and the besieging army returned and entered the city to conquer.

Tuchak, Vladimir—co-author of *Zone Therapy*

Tunks—a minister connected with the Oxford Group in Akron, Ohio

Twelve Steps and Twelve Traditions—a book written by Bill Wilson to amplify the Twelve Steps of Alcoholics Anonymous and to present the Twelve Traditions that are the governing principles of conducting the program and which helps keep it the same around the world.

Twelve Steps—the principles followed in reaching for sobriety in the fellowship of AA

Two Listeners—pen name for two ladies who wrote the book, *God Calling*

U

Ullman, Dana—co-author of *Science of Homeopathy*

unified energy field—synonym for universal energy

universal energy—one of one hundred terms to describe an unmeasured, unproven, mystical force said to permeate the universe and from which all things are made. Popular terms are vital force, vitalism, universal intelligence, etc.

universal intelligence—refers to universal energy, ch'i, prana, etc. All the knowledge of the universe is supposed to be in the composition of universal energy, prana, ch'i, etc.

universal magnetic fluid—synonym for universal energy

unrufling—a movement of the hands sweeping across a body supposedly to smooth out the energy pattern of the body

Unschuld, P.U. —author of *Medicine in China: A History of Ideas*, and *Nan-ching: The classic of Diffi cult Issues*

Upledger, John, D.O.—osteopathic doctor who has continued the craniosacral therapy technique and popularized it, developing the Upledger Institute to promote the technique

Usui, Mikao— (1865-1926) known as the originator of Reiki, Japanese

usurp—to take possession of something from someone or power

V

V.C. Kitchen—author of *I Was A Pagan*

Varieties of Religious Experience—book written by William James, M.D. , and used by Oxford Group and A.A. for text in their programs

Vata—one division of prana

Vedas—writings or books in Sanskrit language of ancient Indian times

Vibrational Medicine—synonym of energy medicine, focus is on electromagnetic wave frequency concept

vibrational therapies—reference to special attention to treatmentmethods claiming to alter or correct electromagnetic vibrations

viscera—internal organs

visualization—making a picture in one's mind with the belief that the picture that is formed will come about, more relevant to situations and attitudes than to material substance.

Vita Florum—flower essences brand

vital energy—synonym for universal energy, a non entity but believed to permeate the cosmos, the Creative Principle, etc. E.G. White spoke of "vital force" etc. She was speaking of our system of metabolism, immunology, etc., as guided by our genes, kept in strength by right habits of life and nutrition. She does not refer to the universal energy we have been exposing in the occult and Neopaganism of today.

vital essence—synonym for vital force or universal energy

Vitz, Paul—professor of Psychology at New York University

Voegeli, Dr. Adolph—famous homeopathic doctor

Vogel, Marcel—author of *The Science of the Mind, The Healing Magic of Crystals*

Vogt, Oscar, M.D.—brain physiologist in Berlin used hypnotism and his patients developed auto-hypnotism

volition—the will of a person, the power of choice

von Peczely, Ignatz—founder of iridology concepts

von Reichenbach, Baron—student of Mesmer's and is credited with forming the Ouija board.

von Schelling, Friedrich Wilhelm Joseph—German philosopher

W

Walker, Richmond—author of *Twenty-Four Hours a Day*

Walters, Dale, Ph.D. —co-researcher on biofeedback with Drs. Greens in Menninger Clinic, Topeka, Kansas.

wand—a rod, often referring to staff or stick of a diviner, it may be a precious stone ground to a length and diameter to simulate a pencil or small stick

Warrier, Gopi—co-author of *The Complete Illustrated Guide to Ayurveda*

water witching—searching for water with various divining techniques

Weil, Andrew, M.D.—medical doctor with Hindu-type beliefs that has become somewhat of a guru in influencing people in alternative medical beliefs and practices

Weldon, John—co-author of *Can You Trust Your Doctor?*

Western occultism—same doctrine as paganism but coming from the West

White, E.G.—Author of more than 100,000 pages and the most translated woman writer in history. Wrote on theology, family life, and health. Most accurate health writer in history. Heavily involved in development of Seventh-day Adventist Church. She had a deep understanding of the spiritualistic doctrines and basis upon which they were formed.

wholistic health—proper balance of body/mind/spirit as taught by the **Bible**

Wicca—organization of witches

Wikipedia—encyclopedia on internet

Willis, Richard, M.D.—author of *Holistic Health Holistic Hoax?*

Winemiller, Mark, M.D.—author and researcher on magnet use for Achilles tendonitis

witch—a person believed to have magic power

witchcraft—the practices of a witch (sorcery); an irresistible impulse or attraction

witchdoctor—medicine man, shaman, native healer usually connected with the spirit world

witness—some object having been worn, touched or from a person and supposed to conduct vibrational patterns said to be specific to the person it came from. Used in Radionics the person it came from. Used in Radionics and not found to be science-based.

Witt, Claudia, M.D.—author of article on acupuncture, faculty of Charité University Medical Centre in Berlin

wizard—diviner

Woodstock—name of the location of a festival held for young people in 1969. 500,000 people were estimated in attendance. The name is commonly used to refer to that particular festival.

world view—a person's understanding and orientation to the question of one's origin, purpose and future

Worwood, Valerie Ann—author of *Aromatherapy for the Soul,* and other aromatherapy books.

Y

yang—positive energy force, Chinese **yin**—negative energy force, Chinese

yoga exercises—various types of snake-like physical movements and/ or postures with the purpose of moving kundalini—serpent energy up through the chakras to reach the crown chakra and become "one with the universe"

yoga—meditation— means to yoke, involves practice of maintaining different postures (asanas) for extended time, object is to move out of the re-incarnation cycle and enter the bliss of the spirit world with the ascended masters. Purpose is to yoke up with the spirit world.

Yogi—practitioner of yoga, teacher

Youngen, Ray—minister, author of *A Time of Departing*

Yuman—tribe of American Indians in southern California

Z

zapping machine—a small hand-held battery operated electrical instrument that is supposed to kill a specific type of parasite which is said to live in the intestines which, when it moves to organs, causes all types of disease and especially cancer. The person making and selling the machine is the only one who makes such claims

zodiac—pathway of the planets in the cosmos, represented by a round circle illustrating the pathway, twelve houses, thirty-six rooms to the zodiac

zone therapy—reflexology of hand and foot massage to correct energy imbalance

Zoroastrianism—pagan religion of ancient Persia prior conversion to Islam.

RECOMMENDED READING: CHRISTIAN AUTHORS

1. *New Age Movement and Seventh-day Adventists*: Biblical Research Institute of General Conference of Seventh-day Adventists,12501 Old Columbia Pike, Silver Spring, MD 20904, (301-680-6000) (see appendix E)
2. John Ankerberg, John Weldon; *Can You Trust Your Doctor?* , Wolgemugh & Hyatt, Pub. Inc., Brentwood, TN (available at public library)
3. John Ankerberg & John Weldon, *The Facts on Holistic Health and the New Age Medicine,* Harvest House Pub., Eugene, OR 97402
4. Richard J.B. Willis; *Holistic Health Holistic Hoax*? Pensive Publications, 10 Holland Gardens, Watford, Hertfordshire, WD2 6JW, England [available at Adventist book stores]
5. Manuel Vasquez; *The Mainstreaming of New Age,* Pacific Press Pub. Assn., Nampa, Idaho. (available at Adventist book stores)
6. Mervyn G. Hardinge; *A Physician Explains Ellen White's Counsel on Drugs, Herbs, & Natural Remedies,* Review and Herald Pub. Assn., Hagerstown, MD 21740 (available at Adventist book stores or call 1-800-765-6955)
7. Ben G. Hester; *Dowsing: an Exposé of Hidden Occult Forces,* Leaves of Autumn Books, Payson, AZ, 1982
8. Will Barron; *Deceived by New Age*, Pacific Press Pub. Assn. Boise, ID (available at Adventist book stores)
9. Constance Cumby; *The Hidden Dangers of the Rainbow*; Huntington House, Inc. 1200 N. Market Street, Suite G, Shreveport, LA 71107 (318-222-1350)
10. Gary Kah; *En Route to Global Occupation*, Huntington House Pub. Lafayette, LA, 1992.
11. Gwen and Richard Shorter; *JEWELRY, Adornments, Personal decoration and More–SPIRITUALISM CONNECTION,* Homeward Publishing Ministries,
12. Dave Hunt, T.A. McMahon; *America The Sorcerer's New Apprentice The Rise of New Age Shamanism,* Harvest House Publishers, Eugene, Oregon 97402 Available at Amazon used Books
13. Daniel L. Gabbert, *Biblical Response Therapy, Healing God's Way*, Aardvark Global Publishing C. LLC, Black Hills Health and Education Center, PO Box 19, Hermosa, SD 57744, ph. 605-255-4101, website—www.bhhec.org
14. Magna Parks, Ph.D., *Christians, Beware! The Dangers of Secular Psychology,* Teach Services, Inc. Brushton, New York, email info@bingoodhealth.com

INDEX

Ingram Content Group UK Ltd.
Milton Keynes UK
UKHW010815260623
424053UK00004B/418